Microvascular Surgery in Head and Neck Reconstruction

Microvascular Surgery in Head and Neck Reconstruction

Edited by

Leandros Vassilios F. Vassiliou

Consultant Oral Maxillofacial and Head and Neck Reconstructive Surgeon, Manchester University NHS Foundation Trust, Manchester, UK; and

Visiting Professor, University of Greater Manchester, UK

Panayiotis Kyzas

Consultant Oral Maxillofacial and Head and Neck Surgeon, East Lancashire Hospitals NHS Trust, Blackburn, UK; and

Visiting Professor, Edge Hill University, UK

Nicholas Kalavrezos

Head and Neck Reconstructive Surgeon, University College London Hospital, London, UK; and President of the European Association of Craniomaxillofacial Surgery (EACMFS)

OXFORD
UNIVERSITY PRESS

OXFORD
UNIVERSITY PRESS

Great Clarendon Street, Oxford, OX2 6DP,
United Kingdom

Oxford University Press is a department of the University of Oxford. It furthers the University's objective of excellence in research, scholarship, and education by publishing worldwide. Oxford is a registered trade mark of Oxford University Press in the UK and in certain other countries.

Published in the United States of America by Oxford University Press
198 Madison Avenue, New York, NY 10016, United States of America.

British Library Cataloguing in Publication Data
Data available

Library of Congress Control Number: 2025949645

ISBN 978–0–19–284982–3

DOI: 10.1093/med/9780192849823.001.0001

Printed and bound by
CPI Group (UK) Ltd., Croydon, CR0 4YY

I wish to thank my children Christina, Lucian, Aurelia, and Maximilian for the inspiration they gave to me. This book would have never become reality without the love and encouragement from my parents Francis and Uka who made me believe in myself. I wish to dedicate the book to my teacher Anna Patrikiou who made me the surgeon I am today. I apologise to her for not finishing it earlier so she could see it.

Leandros Vassilios F. Vassiliou

I want to dedicate this book (and an apology) to my wife, Despoina, and my daughter Rafaela. Without their love and tolerance, I wouldn't be able to deliver what was needed from my end for this book.

Panayiotis Kyzas

To the memory of my father Dimitri who inspired my love for the Patient and Surgery.

To my teachers Klaus Grätz and Iain Hutchison who taught me the knowhow of head & neck surgery.

I am grateful.

Nicholas Kalavrezos

Foreword

Historically surgery has been the mainstay of definitive treatment for most head and neck cancers over two centuries. Advances in *radical* ablative surgery, introduced in the mid-20th century, took centre stage and remained the standard of care until the second half of the past century. The ultimate goal at that time was to eradicate the cancer, but not much attention was paid to restoration of form, function, and quality of life. Attempts at reconstruction of major pharyngolaryngeal defect required multistage operations with tube pedicles. Introduction of the deltopectoral flap in the 1960s and the pectoralis myocutaneous flap in the late 1970s ushered in an era of immediate reconstruction. However, it was not until the mid-seventies and eighties that a major revolution took place in the surgical armamentarium with the introduction of microvascular free tissue transfer, which enabled reconstruction of *any* surgical defect in one stage with an increasing focus on restoring form, function, and improving quality of life. From a technical standpoint, the crux of the viability of a free flap is the long-term patency of the vascular anastomosis.

The editors are to be complimented for putting together a textbook compiling the "nitty gritty" of selecting the right patient, the right flaps, the right donor sites, and the right vessels, as well as the technical details to assure a successful anastomosis and the eventual reconstructive outcome, from a variety of global leaders in the specialty sharing their experience and pearls of wisdom. Microvascular surgery for head neck reconstruction is amongst the most technically demanding procedures in contemporary surgery. The ultimate determinant of reconstructive success is flap viability, and that viability rests squarely on the quality and reliability of the microvascular anastomosis. The editors and contributors have painstakingly put together a detailed treatise on the essentials for safe and successful reconstructive microsurgery, from the operating room environment, instrumentation, selection of appropriate flaps to match the goals of reconstructing the defect, anaesthetic considerations, algorithms of selection of vessels, minute details of anastomotic techniques, monitoring and troubleshooting, as well as what to do in a patient with a vessel depleted neck.

This is truly an encyclopaedia of microvascular surgery, of immense value to the beginner who wants to learn microsurgery "the right way", to perfection, and equally of value to the practising microsurgeon to hone his or her skills. Input from the doyens of microsurgery from around the globe adds the concrete of experience and wisdom to this highly technical book. This treasure trove of pearls and prisms of microvascular surgery is a unique publication, and is a must-have book for the one who wants to learn microsurgery, the one who wants to perfect microsurgery, and the one who desires to continue to refine the art and science of microsurgical reconstruction. Needless to say, this book should have a place on the shelves of all medical libraries around the world. The editors have done a remarkable job, and deserve a big thank you from the readership.

Jatin P. Shah
Professor of Surgery, E.W. Strong Chair in Head and Neck Oncology
Memorial Sloan Kettering Cancer Center
New York, NY, USA

Preface

We are delighted to see this textbook being published. Head and neck oncologic surgery frequently demands extensive resection followed by complex reconstruction, with free tissue transfer. Microvascular surgery for head and neck reconstruction is amongst the most technically demanding procedures in contemporary surgery. The ultimate determinant of reconstructive success is flap viability, and that viability rests squarely on the quality and reliability of the microvascular anastomosis.

For many, microsurgery has long been regarded as an elusive 'art'—a skill passed down by apprenticeship, guarded by experience and the myth of 'magic hands'. This textbook dispels that myth. It aims to translate the principles and techniques of microvascular anastomosis into a clear, stepwise, and reproducible framework that trainees can learn, and experienced surgeons can refine.

This book seeks to fill a gap in the literature by assembling contemporary techniques, practical tips, and importantly, a methodical, algorithmic approach to troubleshooting and salvaging compromised flaps.

The chapters are the product of a collaborative effort by internationally respected microvascular surgeons who bring decades of collective experience to the reader. Without the help, dedication, and support of our co-authors and colleagues, this textbook would never have materialized.

The photos and videos of microvascular surgical operations demonstrated in this book correspond to successful cases of free tissue transfer. The graphic illustrations that complete the content of this book are the result of the hard work and talent of Francis Vassiliou.

Readers will find not only detailed instructions for constructing reliable arterial and venous anastomoses, but also structured pathways for diagnosing problems, prioritizing interventions, and executing effective solutions when complications arise.

A universally accepted surgical quote suggests that one learns way more dealing with surgical complications rather than smooth successful cases; we wanted to share this knowledge and help current and future H&N colleagues to develop and improve their own practice.

Whether you are a resident beginning to learn microsurgical principles, a surgeon consolidating your technique, or an expert seeking to broaden your repertoire, this book offers clear, evidence- and experience-informed guidance designed to improve patient outcomes and advance the practice of head and neck reconstruction.

Leandros Vassilios F. Vassiliou
Panayiotis Kyzas
Nicholas Kalavrezos

Contents

Videos

Some chapters in this book are accompanied by online videos.
You can watch these by searching for this book's title or ISBN at https://academic.oup.com/
A list of the videos is provided at the end of the book.

Abbreviations

AF	Atrial fibrillation
AJV	Anterior jugular vein
ALT	Anterolateral thigh
ASA	American Society of Anesthesiologists
ASIS	Anterior superior iliac spine
AT	Anaerobic threshold
BMI	Body mass index
CBS	Carotid blowout syndrome
CO	Cardiac output
COPD	Chronic obstructive pulmonary disorder
CPET	Cardio-pulmonary exercise testing
CSA	Circumflex scapular artery
DBE	Deep breathing exercises
DCIA	Deep circumflex iliac artery
DSA	Dorsal scapular artery
DVS	Deep venous system
EBSLN	External branch of the superior laryngeal nerve
ECA	External carotid artery
ECMO	Extracorporeal membrane oxygenation
EJV	External jugular vein
ERAS	Enhanced Recovery After Surgery
ESRD	End-stage renal disease
ETE	End-to-end
ETS	End-to-side
FCR	Flexor carpi radialis
FFF	Fibula free flap
FHL	Flexor hallucis longus
FONA	Front of neck access
GA	General anaesthetic
HELLP	Haemolysis, elevated liver enzymes, and low platelets
HNC	Head and neck cancers
HR	Heart rate
IADL	Instrumental activities of daily living
IJV	Internal jugular vein
IM	Interosseous membrane
IPPB	Intermittent positive pressure breathing
IS	Incentive spirometry
LCD	Liquid crystal display
LCFA	Lateral circumflex femoral artery
LD	Latissimus dorsi
LFCA	Lateral femoral circumflex artery
LFCN	Lateral femoral cutaneous nerve
LMWH	Low-molecular-weight heparin

LRTI	Lower respiratory tract infection
MACD	Microvascular anastomotic coupler devices
MAD	Microvascular anastomotic device
MAP	Mean arterial pressure
MDT	Multidisciplinary team
MH	Malignant hyperthermia
MI	Myocardial infarction
MRA	Magnetic resonance angiography
OCT	Optical coherence tomography
OSA	Obstructive sleep apnoea
PAC	Pulmonary artery catheter
PAP	Profunda artery perforator
PCA	Patient-controlled analgesia
PL	Palmaris longus
PONV	Postoperative nausea and vomiting
PRN	Pro re nata
PVA	Poly-vinyl alcohol
PVR	Pulmonary vascular resistance
QoL	Quality of life
RFFF	Radial forearm free flap
ROS	Radical oxygen species
SCAIF	Supra clavicular island flap
SCIA	Superficial circumflex iliac artery
SCIV	Superficial circumflex iliac vein
SMA	Superior mesenteric artery
SSD	Sterile services department
SV	Stroke volume
SVR	Systemic vascular resistance
SVS	Superficial venous system
TCA	Transverse cervical artery
TDAP	Thoracodorsal artery perforator
TIS	Transverse intermuscular septum
TIVA	Total intravenous anaesthesia
VC	Vena comitans
VDN	Vessel-depleted neck
VG	Vein grafts
VL	Vastus lateralis

Contributors

Julio Acero, Professor of Oral and Maxillofacial Surgery, Ramon y Cajal University Hospital, Madrid, Spain; and Past President of the European Association of Craniomaxillofacial Surgery (EACMFS)

Danny Adam, Consultant Oral Maxillofacial and Head and Neck Surgeon, East Lancashire Hospitals NHS Trust, Blackburn, UK

Nidal Al Deek, Associate Professor of Surgery, Division of Plastic and Reconstructive Surgery, Department of Surgery, University Hospitals, Cleveland Medical Center, Case Western Reserve University, Cleveland, USA

Fernando Almeida, Clinical Professor, Department of Surgery, Alcalá University (UAH), Alcalá de Henares, Spain; and Oral and Maxillofacial Surgeon, Department of Oral and Maxillofacial Surgery, Ramon y Cajal University Hospital, Madrid, Spain

Basim E.S. Dawoud, Consultant Oral Maxillofacial Surgeon, Manchester University NHS Foundation Trust, Manchester, UK

Eleonora O.F. Dimovska, Consultant Plastic and Reconstructive Surgeon, Uppsala University Hospital, Uppsala, Sweden

Andrew Goodall, Consultant Oral Maxillofacial and Head and Neck Surgeon, East Lancashire Hospitals NHS Trust, Blackburn, UK

Nicholas Kalavrezos, Head and Neck Reconstructive Surgeon, University College London Hospital, London, UK; and President of the European Association of Craniomaxillofacial Surgery (EACMFS)

Panayiotis Kyzas, Consultant Oral Maxillofacial and Head and Neck Surgeon, East Lancashire Hospitals NHS Trust, Blackburn, UK; and Visiting Professor, Edge Hill University, UK

Gonzalo Mallarino, Surgeon in Head and Neck Oncologic and Reconstructive Surgery, University Hospital Mederi, Bogota, Colombia

El Muiz Mustafa, Maxillofacial Surgeon, Head and Neck Oncology, Microvascular Reconstruction, Nottingham University Hospitals NHS Trust, Nottingham, UK

Danielle Ormandy, Consultant Anaesthetist, East Lancashire Hospitals NHS Trust, Blackburn, UK

Phil Pirgousis, Associate Professor of Otolaryngology—Head and Neck Surgery, Reconstructive Surgery, Neurological Surgery; Co-Director of Head and Neck Oncology/Reconstructive Surgery and Skull Base Surgery, Mayo Clinic Florida, Jacksonville, Florida, USA

Leandros Vassilios F. Vassiliou, Consultant Oral Maxillofacial and Head and Neck Reconstructive Surgeon, Manchester University NHS Foundation Trust, Manchester, UK; and Visiting Professor, University of Greater Manchester, UK

Fu-Chan Wei, Professor of Plastic Surgery, Department of Plastic and Reconstructive Surgery, Chang Gung Memorial Hospital and Chang Gung University, Taipei, Taiwan

1
Theatre set-up and essentials for microvascular surgery

Leandros Vassilios F. Vassiliou, Panayiotis Kyzas, and Nicholas Kalavrezos

1.1 Theatre set-up

Introduction

Major head and neck operations constitute a multitude of shorter, separate independent procedures, and therefore ideally require large theatres with ample space. It is important to allow enough space not only for the multitude of equipment but also the number of trolleys with the necessary surgical instruments, including saws and drills and the separate trays dedicated to the microvascular part of the procedure.

Ambient temperature

The temperature of the room, although it is controlled within a specific range, should be comfortable for the surgeon. Too low or too high temperatures would lead to distraction, irritation, and loss of focus. The optimum ambient temperature range is between 20–22°C.

Space and set-up

See Figure 1.1.1 and Figure 1.1.2. The theatres must be well-lit with good IT/computer support with wide screens in visible locations for the surgical teams.

It is important to consider that the majority of major head and neck operations when microvascular free flap reconstruction is involved will require—for a significant part of the surgery—a two-surgical (and nursing) team approach, hence provision should be made to accommodate two teams working around the patient.

The space should not only be designed to accommodate two surgical teams, composed of two or three surgeons and a scrub nurse on each side, but also the runners that need to supply the team with additional materials and equipment.

The most optimum set-up has the patient's head facing away from the anaesthetic machine or anaesthetic station. In other words, the anaesthetic station being placed next to the

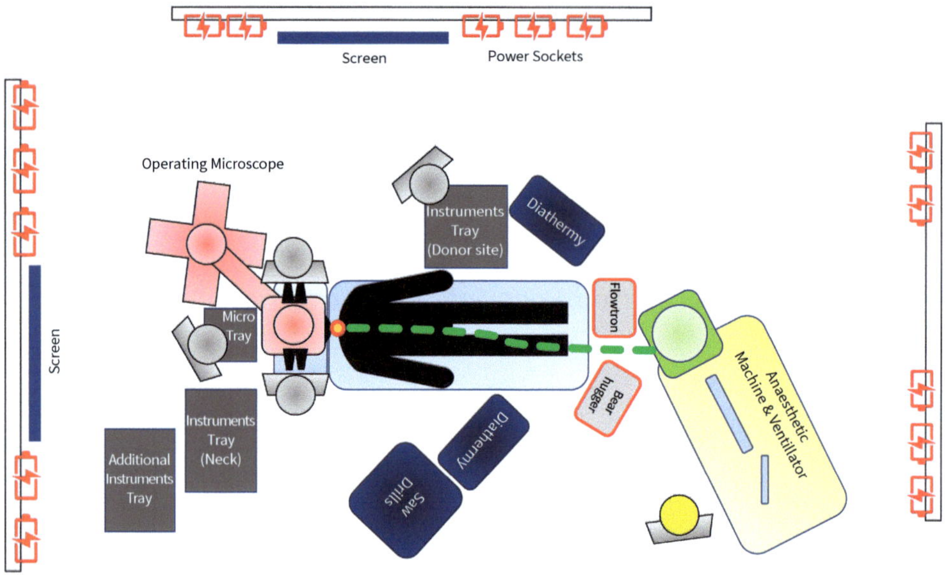

Figure 1.1.1 Indicative schematic operating theatre floor plan, demonstrating the position of the operating table, microscope, equipment, instrument trays, for a head and neck major operation involving cancer ablation and reconstruction. The example refers to a hypothetical case of an oral reconstruction with a harvested free flap from the left radial forearm.

patient's feet. Of course, that will require long tubes and cables for the anaesthetic gases and monitors.

Importantly, there should be adequate space around the head of the table, not only to accommodate multiple trolleys with the variety of instruments required for the head and neck operation and tumour ablation but also enough space for the microscope including the scrub nurse sitting on top and in between the microvascular surgeons.

The presence of external medical and nursing observers must be also considered, as well as the comfort of the multiple teams involved in the operation for several hours.

Lighting

The theatre should be equipped with new technology LED main lights. In many units, lights can also be supplied with cameras in order to stream live or record the operations for teaching purposes. This is effectively of value for head and neck operations as the operating field is quite narrow, not allowing many theatre observers to have a meaningful direct visual exposure to the actual procedure.

Theatre lights could be supplemented with mobile satellites to provide adequate lighting for free flap harvesting, such as radial forearm, fibula, deep circumflex iliac artery (DCIA) flaps, or anterolateral thigh flap (ALT). In modern days, headlights are becoming more and more essential as they can provide quite strong light focused on the operating field and following the surgeon's head movements. Headlights ideally should be battery-powered rather than cable-powered in order to seamlessly allow free movement without restriction.

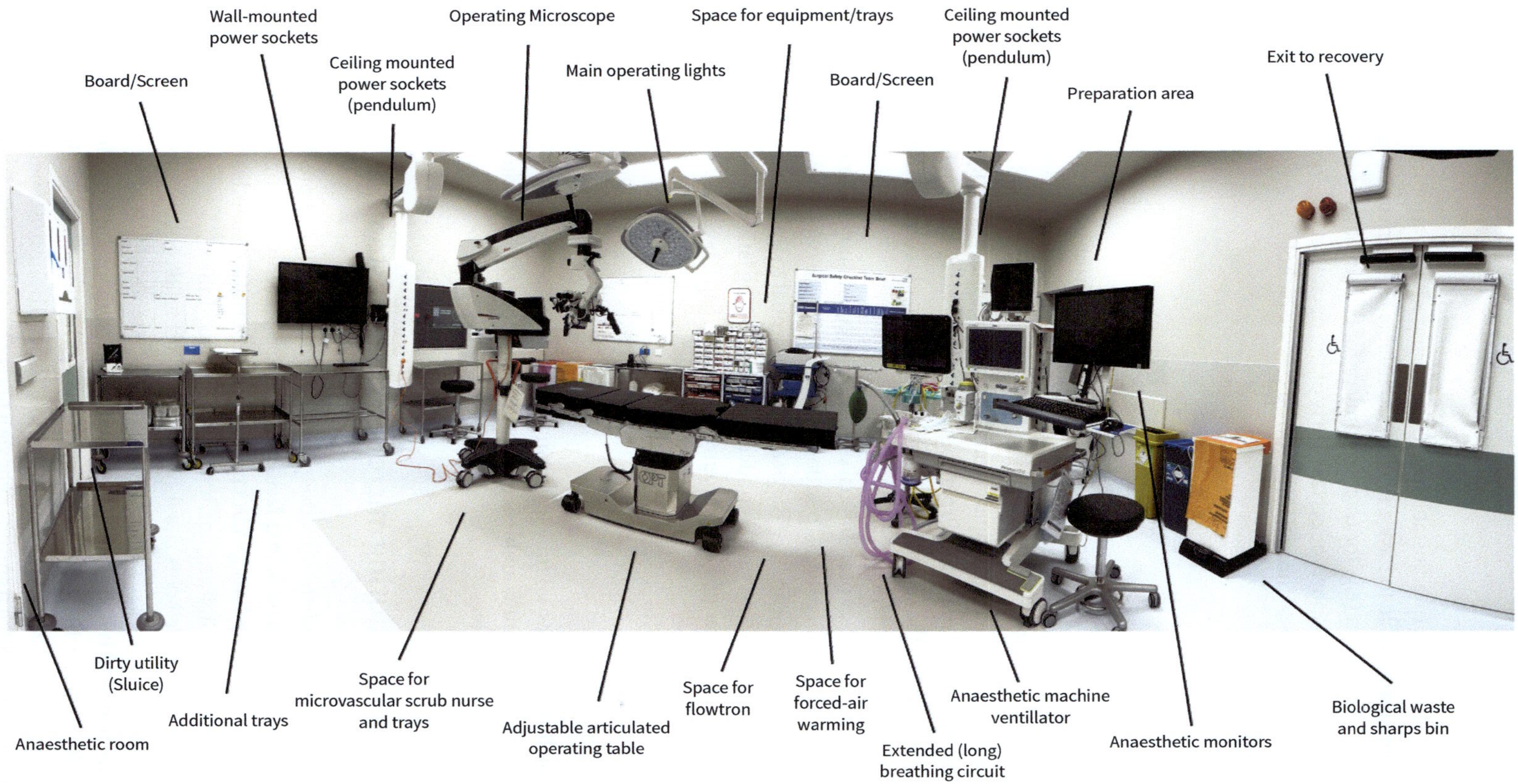

Figure 1.1.2 Photograph demonstrating an indicative theatre arrangement for a head and neck major operation involving cancer resection and reconstruction with the microscope in position.

Operating table

The operating table should be of adjustable position, ideally with electronic controls. It is important for the operating table to have a separate adjustable component for head support that allows neck hyperextension (e.g. for tracheostomy or for certain parts of the operation), as well as flexion to provide support for certain parts of the operation (e.g. resection, post-anastomosis), or to accommodate the patient's cervical c-spine pathology (e.g. osteoarthritis or ankylosing spondylitis).

Equipment

The vast majority of equipment will be monitoring devices requiring electric supply, hence the side wall of the theatre next to the anaesthetic machine has to be supplied with an adequate number of power sockets and extensions. Provision should be made to cover the cables to avoid accidents and hazards, apart from the essential surgical equipment such as diathermy and the anaesthetic machine. Provision should be made for adequate space to accommodate the Bair Hugger, the Flowtron (intermittent pneumatic compression) boots and of course the respective cabling and power supply.

The theatre should have a variety of additional support such as arm support for radial forearm free flaps, gel supports for certain patients' positioning, and avoidance of pressure ulcers.

A separate mention is of the bean bag. The bean bag is essential to immobilize the patient, especially when in lateral decubitus position, such as for harvesting latissimus dorsi, scapula, and even fibula flaps. Equally, sandbags are required for DCIA flap harvest.

Music

Finally, some 'easy listening', low-volume music in the background is advisable contributing to the necessary calm and seamless ambience necessary for such long procedures, which are resource and manpower intensive.

Theatre environment during microvascular anastomosis

Microvascular anastomosis is the task that requires the utmost focus and precision. To this end, the environmental and surrounding factors/parameters have to be optimized to allow the surgeon to concentrate fully. Background noises and conversation sounds should be kept to an absolute minimum while lighting and temperature are optimized.

The overhead operating table lights should be switched off to allow concentration, focus, avoid light reflection and shadows. The main operating theatre should be lit as normal. The surgeon's microvascular field is lit by the microscope light. It is important to avoid the microscope light intensity to get to 100% as this can produce overheating of the surgical field and tissue or vascular dryness and damage to the delicate soft tissues. The microscope light is usually an integrated halogen bulb, which transmits light via a fibreoptic cable into the operating field.

1.2 Microsurgical instruments

Introduction

This chapter analyses the most commonly used microvascular surgery instruments and materials in order to help the microsurgeon to become familiar with the essential toolkit and principles in preparation for the chapters of actual microsurgery.

Vessel preparation instruments

Micro-suction

See Figure 1.2.1. A bloodless field under the microscope helps the surgeon to visualize the microsutures and see inside the vessel's lumen. Clamp removal for checking vessel flow and the functional status of the anastomosis often leads to a blood-filled field in the working area. Irrigation with heparin saline is an important step during the vessel anastomosis, which will also flood the field. The normal suction cannulas are not suitable to use during microsurgery, because they may endanger the anastomosis through their powerful suction.

We advocate utilizing the 'Single-Use Zoellner Suction Tubes', which are used to remove fluids from the operating area during ear, nose, throat (ENT) otology procedures. These suction tubes are manufactured from medical-grade surgical stainless steel and are supplied in individual, easy-to-open sterile packs. Contents are wrapped in a sterile field.

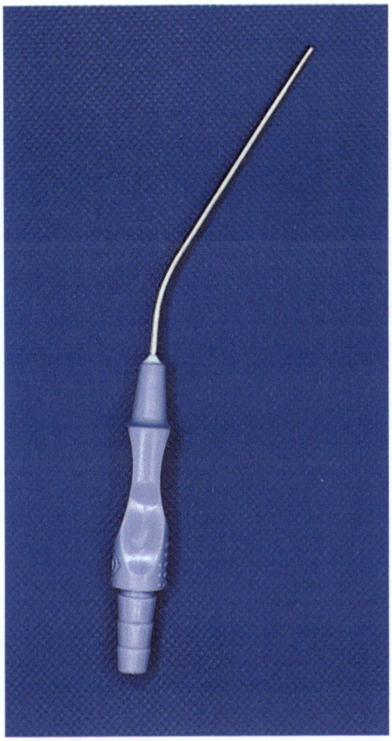

Figure 1.2.1 Photograph of a microsuction tip.

Non-ratchet forceps

See Figure 1.2.2. These are modified 'mosquito' type artery forceps without the jaw-lock ratchet component. The smooth, rounded tips allow atraumatic vessel preparation as they can be gently introduced in the plane between the adventitia and the perivascular tissue. By gentle opening of the tips the plane is bluntly dissected allowing quick and atraumatic denuding of the vessel.

Micro-ligaclips

See Figure 1.2.3. Micro-ligaclips are essential for ligating small side branches during the pedicle vessels' separation and preparation under the microscope. They are usually made of titanium (non-ferrous, MRI safe). The clip is chevron-shaped to allow optimum adaptation for complete vessel occlusion while the clip is closing. The tips are specially designed with diamond grooving and striated 'jaws' to provide secure interlocking non-slipping grasping of the vessel in atraumatic fashion.

Iris scissors (straight)

See Figure 1.2.4. Iris scissors are even finer than metzenbaum and are used for cutting fine structures. They are short, straight, and sharp. Iris scissors are great surgical instruments that make incisions in the iris (coloured part) of the eye. They have a small, sharp blade and come in straight or curved. Iris scissors are also called portioning scissors or lid margin scissors.

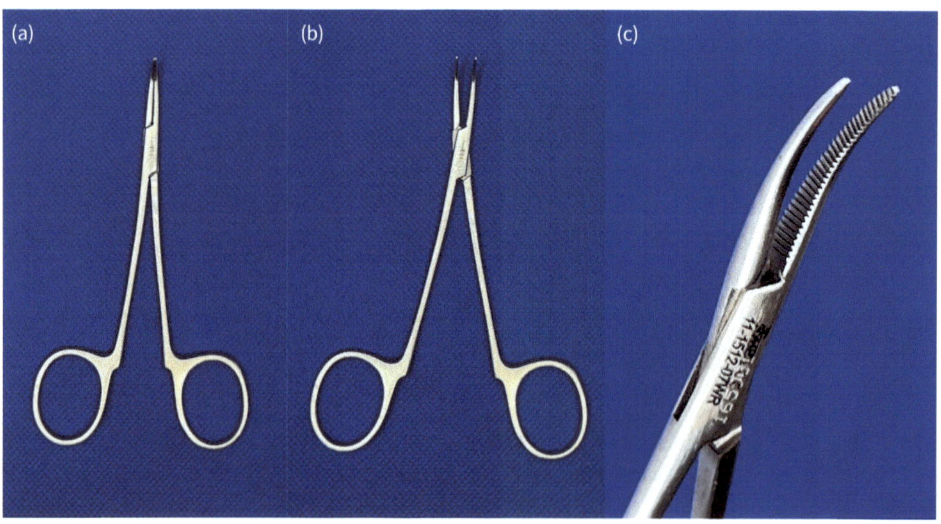

Figure 1.2.2 Photograph of the non-ratchet forceps.
a. Closed.
b. Open.
c. Close-up demonstrating the striated atraumatic jaws of the tips with rounded tip edges for blunt and atraumatic vessel dissection.

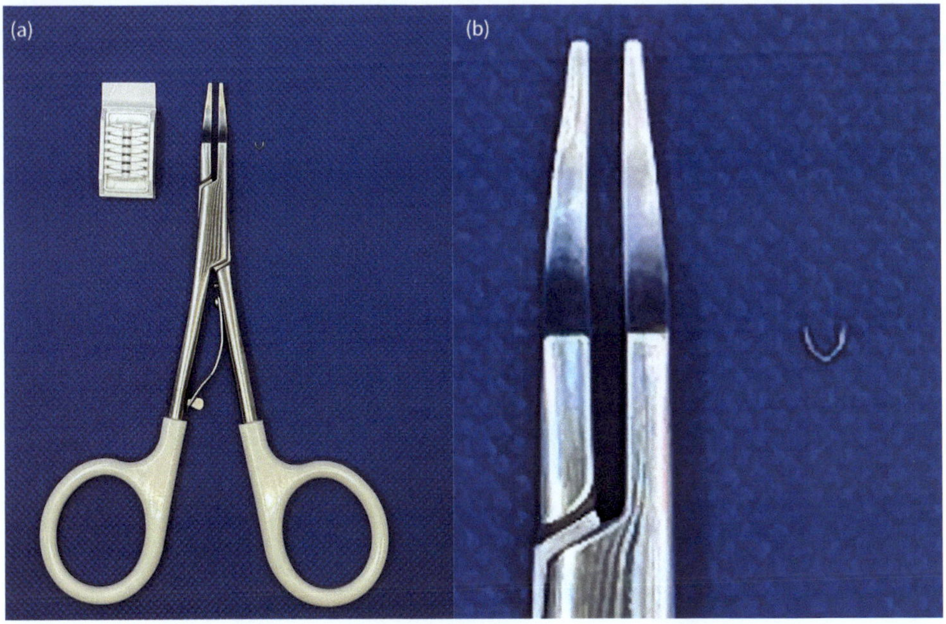

Figure 1.2.3 a. Micro ligaclips cassette with handle and a single clip demonstrated.
b. Tip of microvascular ligaclip applicator and 'chevron' shaped ligaclip.

Microvascular surgery instruments

Vascular clamps

Micro-clamps

See Figure 1.2.5. Vessel clamps come in different sizes, shapes, and clamping forces. The main division is the 'A' or 'V' prefix, which refers to a different tip design; the 'A' type clamps have a slightly incurved tip allowing a firmer stable grip of thick-walled vessels. Clamps with 'V'

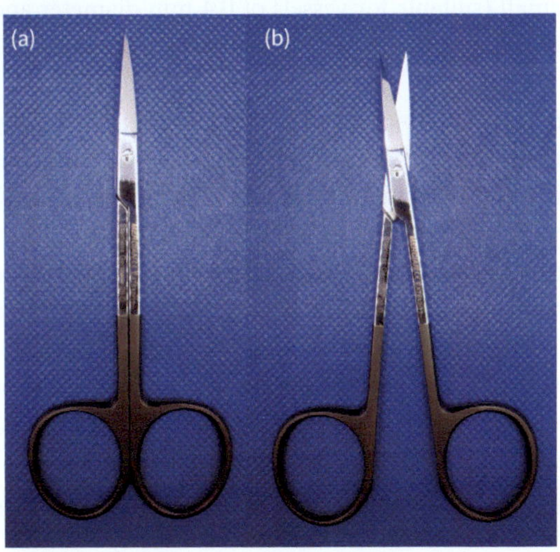

Figure 1.2.4 Iris scissors.
a. Closed.
b. Open.

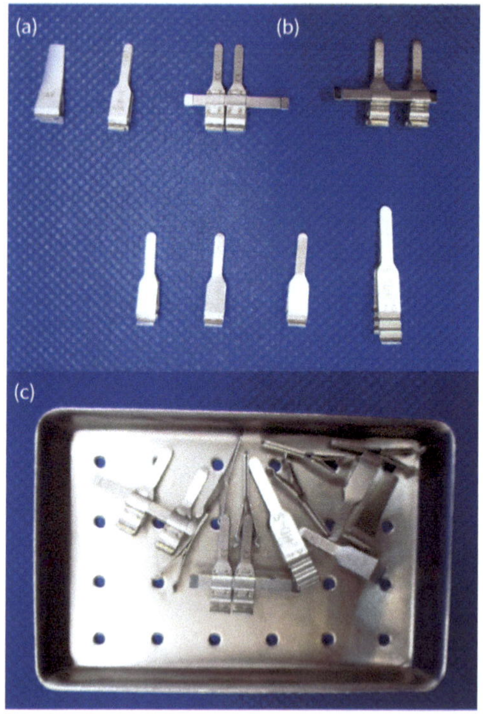

Figure 1.2.5 Microvascular clamps.
a. Single microvascular clamps with a different-width tip.
b. Double microvascular clamps with sliding bar.
c. Tray containing the microvascular clamps for sterilization.

pattern can be used as all-purpose in any vessel, although traditionally V-clamps are used for veins and A-clamps for arteries.

They range from small (suitable for vessels of 0.4 mm diameter and above) to large (for vessels up to 5 mm diameter) and with variable spring tension, exerting clamping forces from 10 g to 140 g.

The pressure exerted by the clamps on an artery is approximately 30 g. The compression is calibrated to be atraumatic for vessels even as small as 0.4 mm in diameter.

It is important to use A-clamps for arteries and V-clamps in veins. V-clamps have weaker spring strength. They are gentler for thin-walled vessels; however, the closure grip may not be adequate to obstruct the arterial flow should they be used for arteries. Conversely, arterial clamps may have too strong a spring force, which could crush delicate venous walls. Vessel clamps should always be applied with the appropriate clamp applicator.

A very useful type of vessel clamp is the double clamp (approximator clamp). This system comprises of two clamps mounted on a bar or frame. These clamps can slide along the bar in order to bring two vessel ends closer together or move them away.

These small vascular clamps require a 'clamp applicator' (Figure 1.2.6), which has single-toothed ended tips that fit onto the groove of the micro-clamp handle.

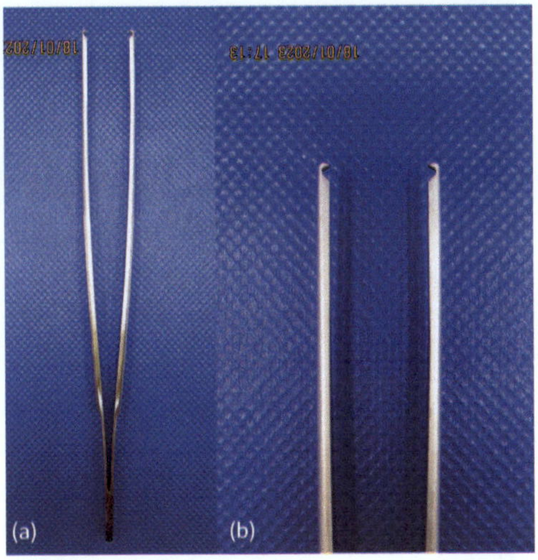

Figure 1.2.6 a. Microvascular clamp applicator.
b. Microvascular clamp applicator tips under magnification (close-up).

Bulldog vascular clamps

See Figure 1.2.7. These come in various sizes and widths of tips and are used for clamping larger vessels. They come in variable designs and closure pressures ranging from 30 g to 180 g. These are especially useful for clamping the internal jugular vein (IJV) for an 'end-to-side' anastomosis or anastomosis with the external jugular vein (EJV) in an 'end-to-end' fashion.

Satinsky clamp

See Figure 1.2.8. These are specially designed vascular clamps that can isolate only a segment of a vessel (if placed longitudinally to the axis of the target vessel), allowing blood flow outside the clamped segment, hence only partially obstructing the flow.

They are particularly useful for anastomosis into the IJV, either end-to-side or end-to-end with a short recipient stump of a tributary, when a V-clamp cannot be applied.

Jeweller's forceps (also known as watchmaker's forceps)

See Figure 1.2.9. Jeweller's forceps are essential for microvascular anastomosis. Jeweller's forceps should be checked, and tips should meet evenly for a length of at least 2 mm. These are the workhorse instruments for microvascular anastomosis as they provide fine vessel handling and a good, stable grip for vessel preparation and manipulation during the anastomosis.

Jeweller's forceps come in different handle shapes and lengths. The main surgeon should hold the shorter forceps so that any tremor is eliminated, and the grip is closer to the manipulated vessel. The assistant is sitting on the opposite side and should use a pair of long jeweller's forceps (Figure 1.2.10).

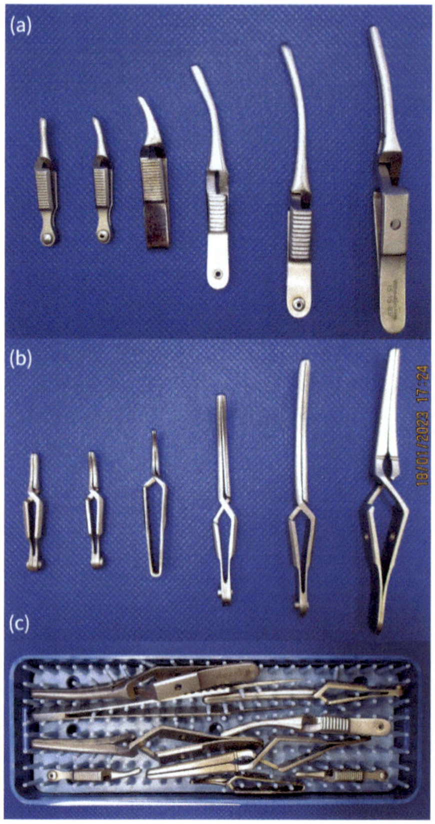

Figure 1.2.7 a. Set of different-sized and shaped bulldog clamps (lateral view).
b. Set of same microvascular bulldog clamps (vertical view).
c. Tray containing all microvascular clamps securely placed for sterilization.

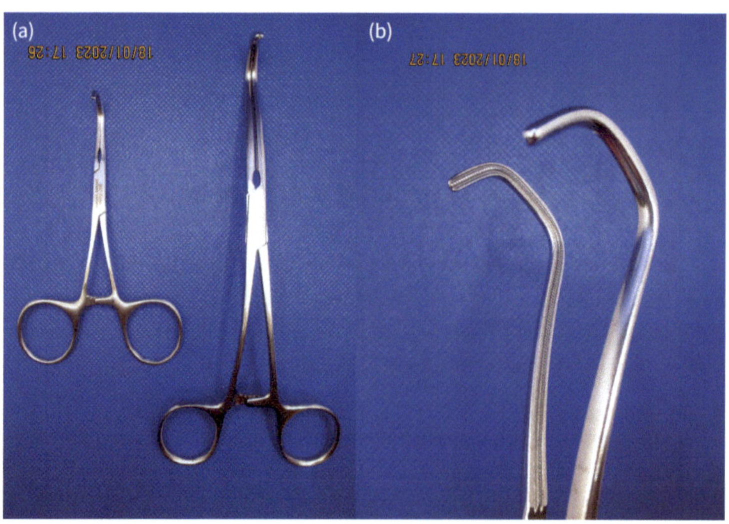

Figure 1.2.8 Satinsky clamp.
a. Small left (large size right).
b. Close view demonstrating the striated jaws that secure and immobilize the vessel in an atraumatic way.

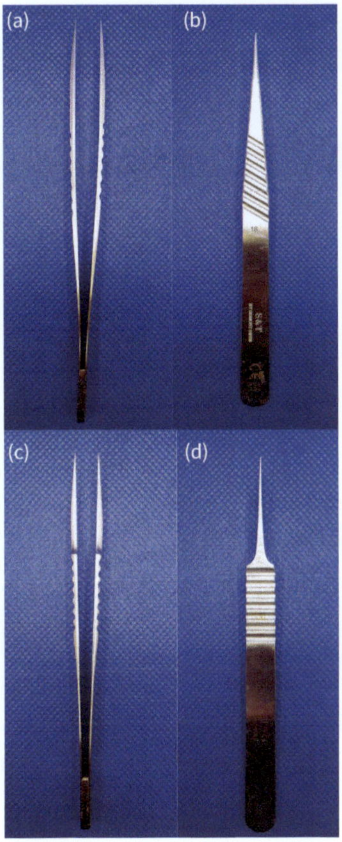

Figure 1.2.9 a. Microvascular jeweller's forceps (vertical view).
b. Microvascular jeweller's forceps (lateral view).
c. Different type of microvascular jeweller's forceps (vertical view).
d. Different type of microvascular jeweller's forceps (lateral view).

The forceps are held by the non-dominant hand of the main microsurgeon who performs the anastomosis. The tips of jeweller's forceps must align with a 1/1,000 inch precision, as this is the thickness of a 10/0 suture and a minimum of 3 mm length to allow grip of the suture thread or the needle.

Dissecting scissors

See Figure 1.2.11. Microvascular dissecting scissors are spring handled and curved, which could be short or long. Microvascular sutures are used for vessel preparation and adventitia trimming. There is a variation of straight blades (adventitia scissors), although these are rarely used and on most occasions are used to trim off protruding 'tongues' after imperfect cutting of the vessel, especially intima projections.

An important element of the microvascular dissecting scissors is the rounding of the tips that renders the instrument safe for dissecting closely along the vessel adventitia without the risk of puncturing it.

Vessel dilators

See Figure 1.2.12. These modified jeweller's forceps have a rounded, polished tip, so that insertion into the vessel lumen does not damage the delicate intima.

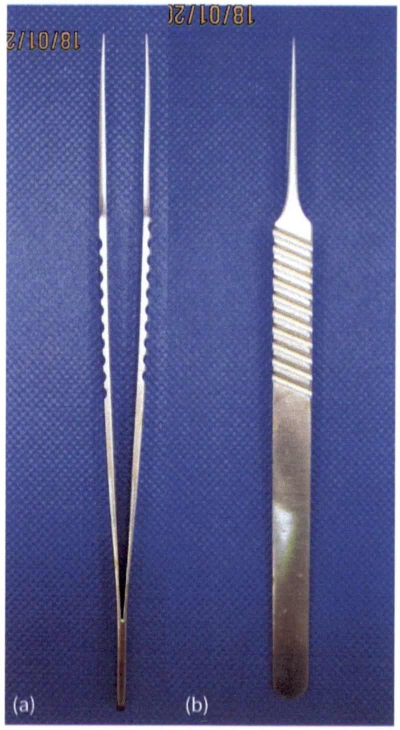

Figure 1.2.10 Long jeweller's forceps for the assistant working on the contralateral side of the anastomosis.

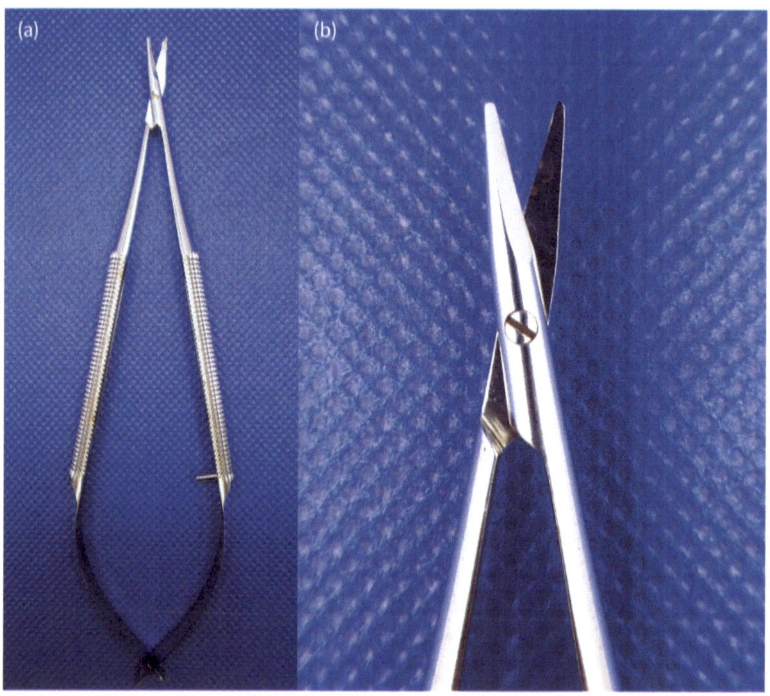

Figure 1.2.11 a. Microvascular dissecting scissors.
b. Close view of microvascular dissecting scissor tips.

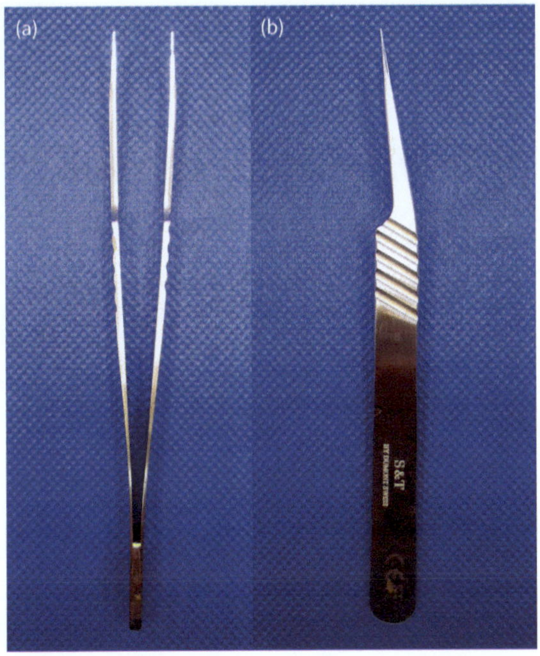

Figure 1.2.12 a. Vessel dilators (vertical view).
b. Vessel dilators (lateral view).

The vessel dilator tips stem from the edge of the handle in an angulated direction. This allows gentle insertion into the vessel lumen with the tips closed. Relaxed release of the handle allows the dilatators to open and gently dilate the blood vessel intima and media. This movement also allows stretching and alignment of the intima on the underlying median layer. It also allows detailed inspection of the vessel lumen and recognition/identification of any intraluminal defects such as atheromatous plaques, intima dissection, or loose projections due to imperfect cutting of the vessel end.

The vascular lumen should be dilated in all its quarters. This is achieved by dilation in one direction, then removal and reinsertion of the dilator with a 90-degree rotation to allow differential dilation.

Microvascular needle holders

See Figure 1.2.13. Microvascular needle holders can be straight or curved and of different grip (round or flat), depending on the surgeon's preference. We recommend round-handled curved needle holders. Microvascular needle holders are of paramount importance, and they should be checked regularly for any bent ends.

Microvascular instruments case

See Figure 1.2.14. It is important that all instruments are contained in an instrument case which is metal-lined and with rubber spigots that provide protection against any instrument damage. The microvascular instruments should be carefully cleaned after use and placed in the case prior to autoclaving.

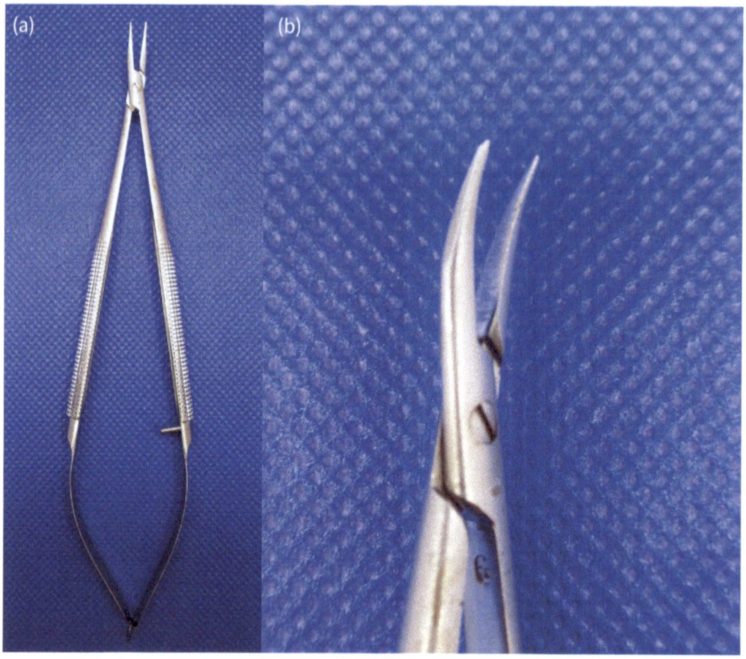

Figure 1.2.13 a. Microvascular needle holder.
b. Close view of microvascular needle holder tips.

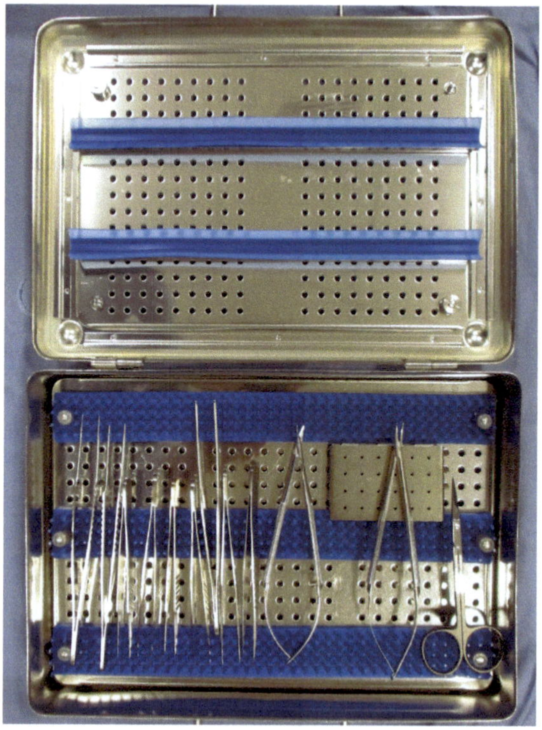

Figure 1.2.14 Microvascular instruments case with rubber rests for secure placement.

Background (contrast) material

See Figure 1.2.15. Background is a sheet of coloured smooth material that is placed under the vessel stumps prior to and during the anastomosis to set the plane of the microvascular surgery and improve visualization. Materials must be sterile and include silicone, plastic, rubber, polyethylene, and polypropylene in various shapes that include square (tetragonal), octagonal, and hemispherical shapes. The colours of the background sheets used are mainly green, blue, and yellow. Relevant studies have concluded that high-luminance green or blue coloured background sheets can enhance the visibility of nylon thread and vessels, as well as relieve the visual discomfort for microsurgeons.

Irrigation syringes with soft (intravenous cannula) tip

See Figure 1.2.16. Syringes with soft tips from intravenous catheters (cannulas) are used to irrigate the blood vessels with heparinized saline (1,000 units of heparin in 50 cc or 100 cc of normal saline, sodium chloride 0.9%, Figure 1.2.17). Usually, 20 cc syringes are the standard, fitted with different coloured cannulas (pink 20 gauge, or blue 22 gauge) to match the vessel calibre attached to them.

Neurosurgical patties (neuro-patties)

See Figure 1.2.18. Neurosurgical patties, originally used in neurosurgery, are sterile pads made of textile material (usually 100% cotton) that are extremely useful in microvascular surgery. They can be placed under the anastomosis plane, alternatively with a background silicon material, in order to manage the fluid environment.

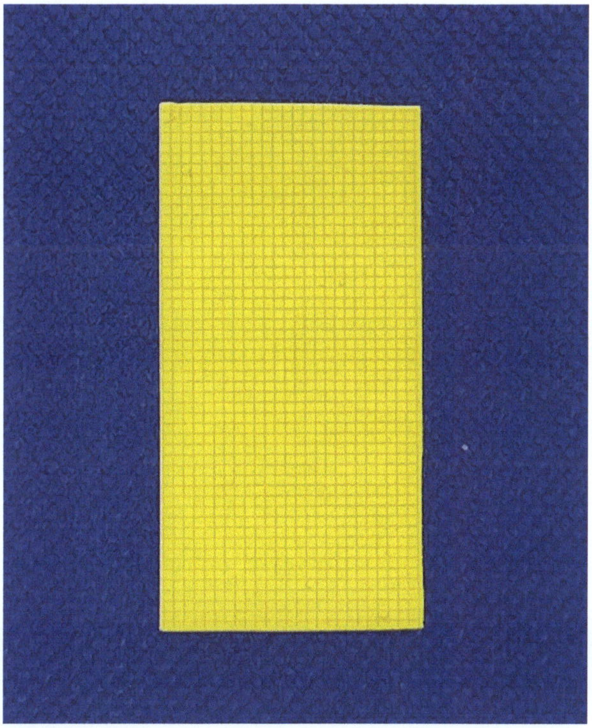

Figure 1.2.15 Background material in fluorescent yellow colour.

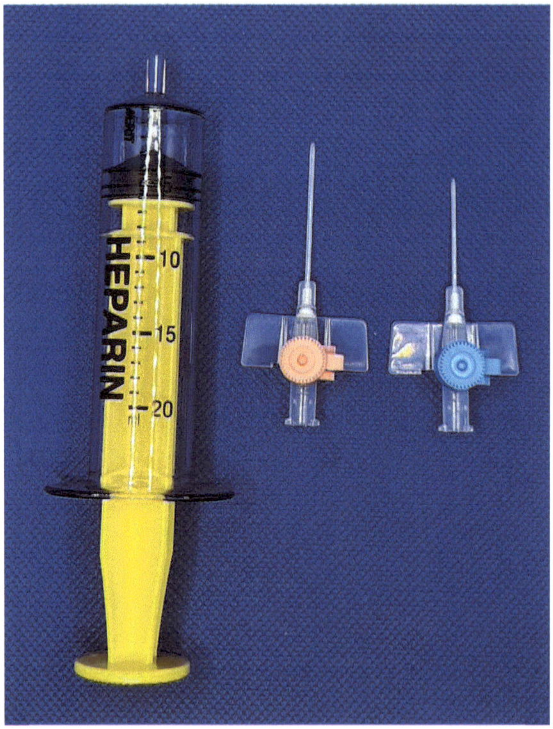

Figure 1.2.16 Irrigation kit for heparinized saline and most commonly size intravenous catheter tips for vessel irrigation.

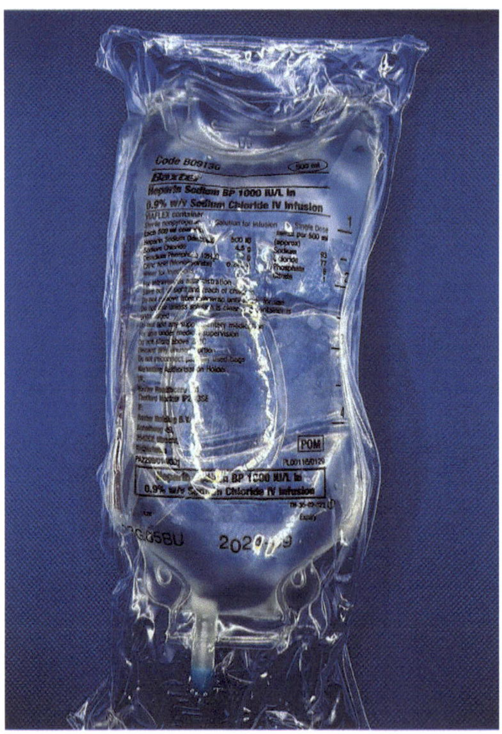

Figure 1.2.17 Photograph of ready-to-use sterilized heparinized saline (1 litre).

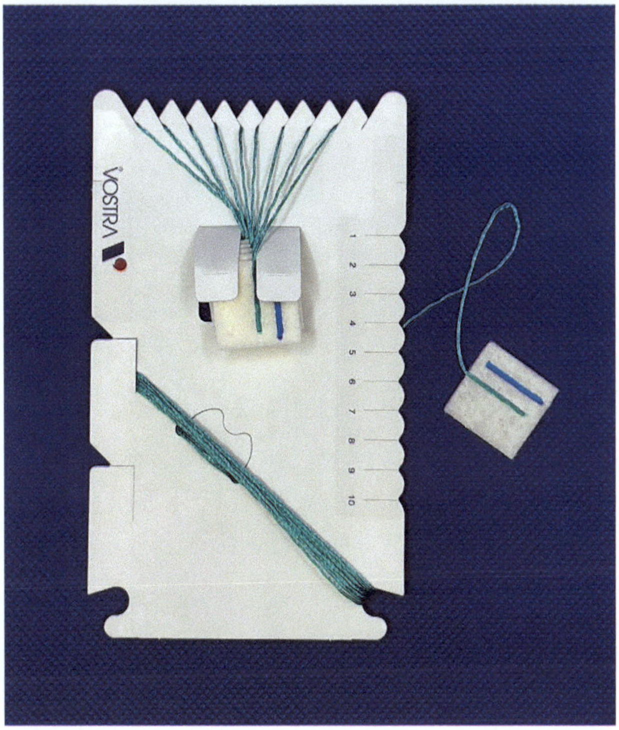

Figure 1.2.18 Photograph of neuro patties.

Neuro-patties are easy to handle as they are very pliable when wet. From a safety point of view, as they are part of the countable items, they are attached to a locator string that increases visibility and assists in identification and carry an X-ray detectable element secured on one side of the pad.

Post-anastomosis, they are useful in assisting in haemostasis while handling the delicate vessel tissue, as they are highly absorbable and gentle with the vessel tissue. Application of two patties—one below and one above—the anastomosis with mild gentle pressure usually helps control minor bleeding from the stitch holes.

Arrows (K-sponge spears)

See Figure 1.2.19. K-sponges, originally used in ophthalmic surgery, are made of highly absorbent compressed hydrocellulose or ultra-smooth micropore PVA (poly-vinyl alcohol) sponge. They come in an arrowhead shape in a stick for pinpoint-accurate application. They can absorb fluid volume even 20 times their weight and are extremely efficient in clearing the vascular lumen from fluid. They can be used by the assistant to gently manipulate or retract the vessel's lumen edge, or at the end of the anastomosis for haemostasis of small leaks between stiches or bleeding points from stitch holes.

Tonsil swabs

See Figure 1.2.20. Tonsil swabs have excellent absorbing ability. They can be placed under the anastomosing vessels to provide cushioning and a resting plane for vertical anastomoses.

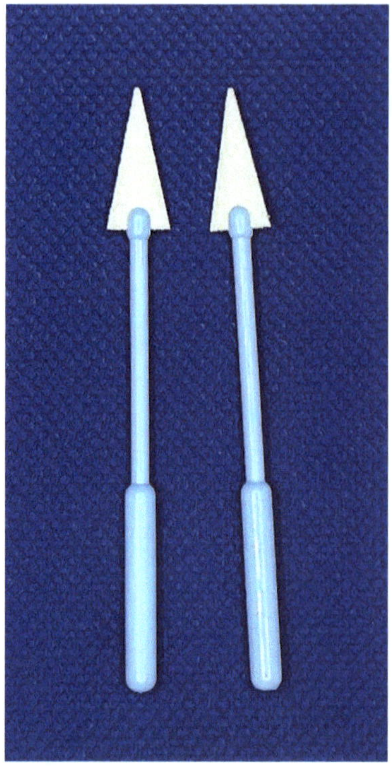

Figure 1.2.19 Photograph of cotton spears (arrows).

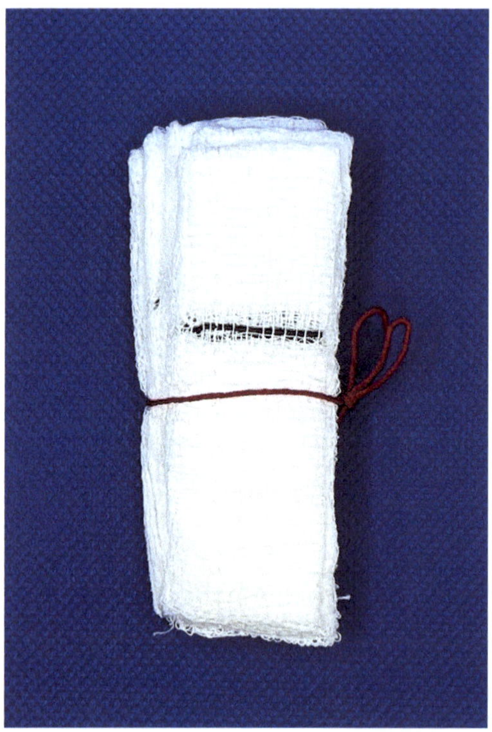

Figure 1.2.20 Tonsil swabs.

Also, during preparation of the recipient vein, they can be placed in a way where one end lies under an open running vein, following completion and release of the arterial anastomosis, and the other outside the neck, absorbing and diverting the blood flow outside the neck, preventing flooding of the operating field.

1.3 Microvascular sutures and suturing technique

Introduction

This chapter discusses the most commonly used microvascular surgery sutures and the basic suturing techniques and manoeuvres in order to help the microsurgeon familiarize with the basic microvascular surgery principles as they will be further applied in the next chapters.

The microscope due to its central role in microvascular surgery is separately described in Chapter 4.

Microvascular sutures

The most commonly used suture material for microvascular anastomosis is a monofilament nylon (ethilon) stitch. Suture sizes from 8-0 to 10-0 can be used. In our experience 8-0 size is suitable for the majority of the anastomoses. The ideal needle is a flat bodied (spatulated) microvascular needle (micropoint); round-body needles are more difficult to control and shouldn't be considered as the first needle of choice -unless extremely atraumatic conditions are required with imminent risk of intima layer dissection. The needle is 3/8 of circle with 6.5 mm length. Indicatively the diameter of an 8-0 suture is 4:1/000th of an inch and a 10-0 suture is 1:1,000th of an inch. The length of an 8-0 is 13-30 cm and of a 10-0 is 13 cm long.

An 8-0 suture (Figure 1.3.1) provides accuracy and adequate tensile strength, especially for arterial anastomoses, enough to withstand the changes of the blood pressure flow in the carotid artery system.

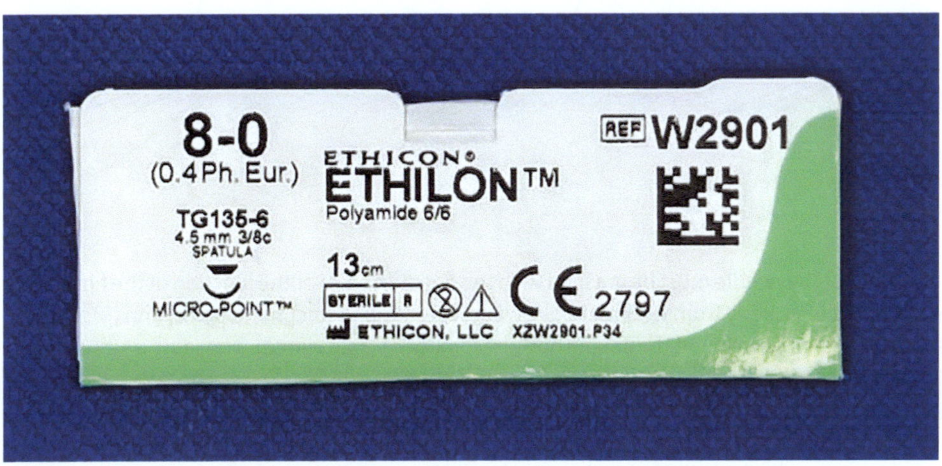

Figure 1.3.1 Pack of Ethilon 8.0 suture for microvascular anastomosis.

For smaller-calibre vessels and anastomosis of venae-comitantes (VCs), or small vessels of perforator flaps, 9-0 or 10-0 sutures can be used. The choice should take into account the fine balance between possible anastomotic leaks, the strength of the anastomosis against the flow pressures and the number of sutures required in total. In our experience, even for small, thin-walled VCs, an 8-0 is usually adequate and the number of six sutures is sufficient for almost every venous anastomosis.

Technique—basic microvascular suturing skills

Holding the needle

It is important to mount the needle correctly on the microneedle holder. The needle can be initially grasped with the jeweller's forceps and is then mounted at approximately one-third of its body in the needle holder (Figure 1.3.2).

For a right-handed surgeon, the needle should always point from right to left, so that it can be advanced through the tissue following its curvature via a gentle wrist rotation.

If the needle is in a stable position, it should be set at 90 degrees to the axis of the tips of the needle holder (Figure 1.3.2b). The flat surface of the needle body should be grasped by the flat tips of the needle holder for stability. It is important to note that if the needle is held too near to the tip, it will point downwards (Figure 1.3.2a) and if it is held too near to the thread end it will point upwards (Figure 1.3.2c).

The needle tip should point horizontally and at 90 degrees, as mentioned, to allow tangent penetration through the vessel wall (Figure 1.3.3). Attention should be given to avoid at any cost a downward-pointing needle, as this is high risk for suturing through the back wall (through stitch), which will lead to one of the fundamental failures of the anastomosis.

Advancing the needle through the vessel wall

The needle should be inserted through the vessel wall in a completely perpendicular to the plane of entry orientation, and to achieve this the vessel wall edge must be everted (Figure 1.3.4). Gentle

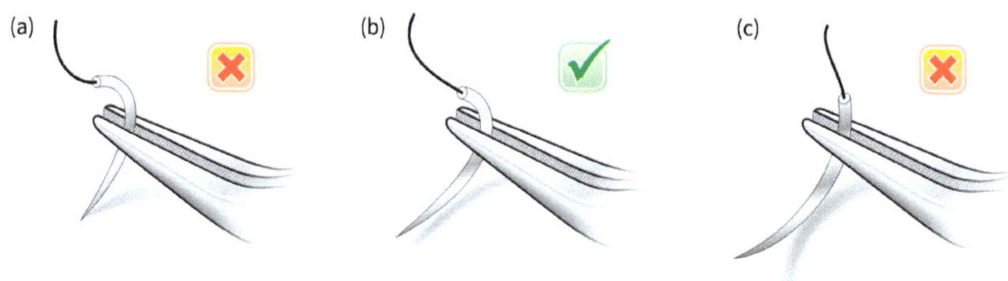

Figure 1.3.2 The needle must be grasped with the needle holder at the junction of the first and second third of its body from the proximal (swage, eye, suture attachment point) end (B). This is where the cross-section of the needle body becomes flat (spatulated), providing a safe and stable grip. The shape of the needle in the proximal third is cylindrical and hence unstable to hold (C) as it can rotate between the tips of the needle holder. Also, importantly, holding the needle at the junction of first with second third provides 90 degree angle with the needle point, ensuring perpendicular insertion to the vessel wall. If the needle is held too close to the tip, then it points downwards and endangers hitting the back wall (A).

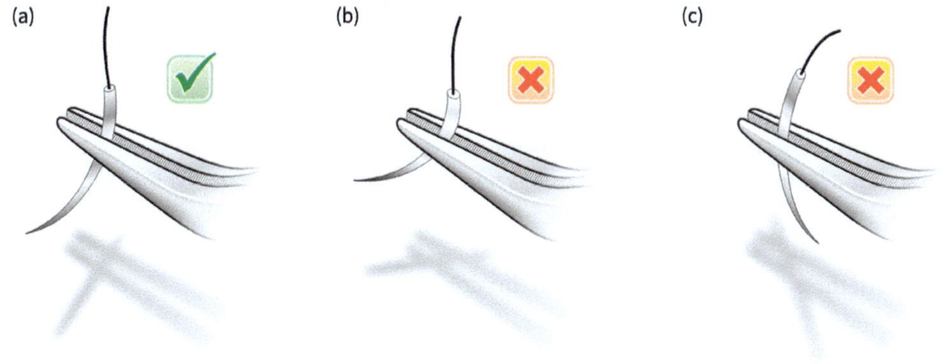

Figure 1.3.3 a. Correct way to mount the needle on the needle holder allowing 90-degree angle (perpendicular insertion) through the vessel wall via gentle wrist rotation. For the right-handed surgeon this configuration renders the tip of the needle the extension of the wrist and fingers and with gentle rotation the needle effortlessly passes through the vessel wall. Figures b and c demonstrate the wrong mounting of the needle resulting in poor control and unfavourable motion pattern when advancing the needle.

insertion of microvascular forceps (preferably vessel dilator, jeweller's, or arrow) everts and also provides counterpressure, for the needle to pass effortlessly through the vessel wall. This tangent course of the needle through the vessel wall is important to minimize vessel wall injury and subsequent bleeding. This is further assisted by the appropriate rotation of the surgeon's wrist.

The width of the 'bite', otherwise the distance between the vessel wall edge and the penetration point should be a minimum of three times (3×) the thickness of the needle itself. It is usually bigger for arteries and much thinner for veins and should roughly equal one to two times (1–2) the thickness of the vessel wall at its edge.

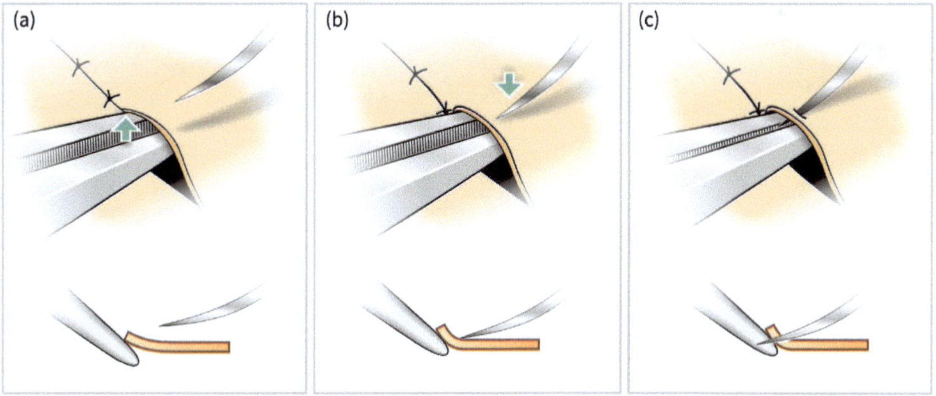

Figure 1.3.4 a. Prior to the insertion of the needle in the vessel adventitia layer, the vessel wall is gently everted by inserting a vessel dilator or a jeweller's forceps (caution with this instruments' tips to avoid traumatizing the inner intima layer). b. The needle is inserted at 90-degree angle (perpendicular) to the vessel wall. The pressure of the needle insertion is counteracted by the eversion from the other side (insertion of the forceps inside the vessel lumen with concomitant eversion and counterpressure). c. The forceps inside the lumen lift the vessel wall, protecting the back wall and also receive the needle point once it passes through the full thickness of the vessel, in order to pull the whole needle through.

Grasping the whole thickness of the tissue between the jaws of the forceps must be avoided at all costs as this as this will jeopardize the atraumatic suturing technique and result in damage of the intima and thrombosis.

Receiving the needle from the other end

Once an adequate length of the needle is visualized through the inner wall of the vessel it should be grasped with the needle holder and with a gentle rotation, following the curvature of its shape, the needle should pass through the vessel wall in its entirety. The needle and the attached thread are subsequently pulled through.

Passing the needle through the opposite vessel

This step is crucial. It is important to be able to visualize the inner aspect of the lumen and bring the tip of the needle with precision to the exact point that it needs to be inserted. The lumen is carefully inspected for imperfections (atheromas, intima tears). The vessel wall must be stabilized and again everted. This requires accurate coordination between the surgeon and the assistant:

- The surgeon can grasp gently the adventitia, pulling the vessel wall outwards while inserting the needle from inside out. At the same time, the assistant can apply gentle pressure at a point further behind the vessel edge in order to evert the vessel edge and offer counterpressure to assist with the passage of the needle through the thickness of the wall.
- The assistant can gently hold the adventitia, lifting it up either with forceps or an arrow, simultaneously everting the vessel edge, while the main surgeon passes the needle through and with a forceps held with the left hand applying counterpressure onto the vessel wall (Figure 1.3.5). Pressing down with the forceps and upwards with the needle as it passes through the wall everts the vessel edge.

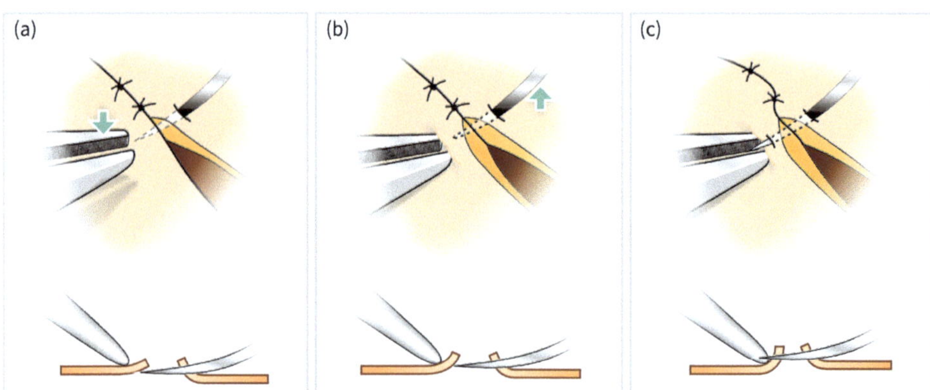

Figure 1.3.5 a. The figure shows how the needle is navigated under the vessel's edge. At this point it is important the edge of the wall is everted and the exit point carefully inspected and aimed with the tip of the needle. b. One the needle starts penetrating the inner wall (intima layer) the counterpressure with the forceps by gently pushing the wall down provides eversion and guides the needle to pass through the thickness of the wall in perpendicular manner. c. The image shows how the mildly open tips of the forceps are ready to receive the needle as it continues to advance through the vessel wall, continuing to apply constant counterpressure allowing atraumatic pass of the needle.

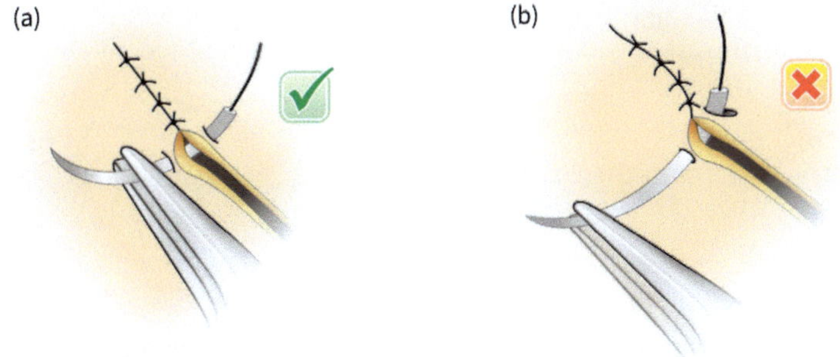

Figure 1.3.6 a. The figure shows the correct way to hold the needle as it passes through the vessel. Holding the needle from its body allows rotation consistent with the curvature of the needle. This ensures perpendicular and hence atraumatic pass through the vessel wall. b. Holding the needle from its tip prevents natural rotation and results in 'pulling' motion, which can damage the vessel wall or create stitch holes that later bleed.

Once the needle is through, it needs to be grasped with the needle holder (Figure 1.3.6) and, again, with a wrist's rotational movement, following the curvature of the needle, it passes in its entirety through the wall.

For the first few stitches, decrease the magnification in order to allow better visualization of the field and thread length. The thread is kept parallel to the direction of the needle entry/exit course and at 90 degrees to the line of the anastomosis and is pulled until only a few centimetres are left free at the short end, for the creation of the loop prior to tying the knot.

Tying the knots

It is important to tie square surgical knots. For an anastomosis under tension or when correcting leaks (with the anastomosis running), a double surgical knot is recommended; otherwise, a single knot is adequate as long as it is flat, square, and locked.

Prior to tying the knot, grasp the thread with the jeweller's forceps in the left hand (right-handed surgeons) (Figure 1.3.7) and with the needle holder the end of the thread. It is

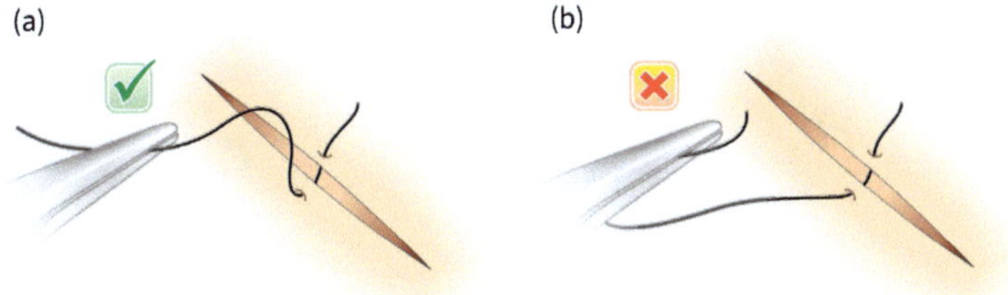

Figure 1.3.7 a. Prior to forming the loop for the first knot, the length of the thread grasped with the forceps (Jeweller's) must be approximately 1–2 cm. That will allow the formation of an optimum-sized loop and within the visual field. Grasping only a short length of the thread will lead to a small loop and will make it difficult to pass the tips of the needle holder through it, chasing the free end of the thread without disrupting the position of the vessels and the anastomosis. b. Grasping the thread from its end leaves too much useless thread length and a wide loop that is too difficult to control.

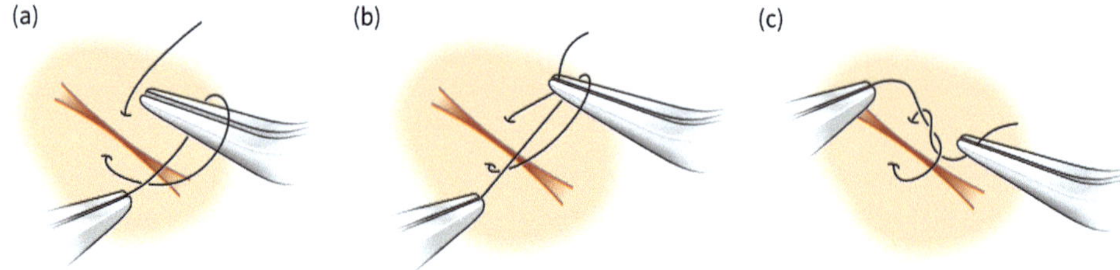

Figure 1.3.8 a. Form the loop and pass the needle holder through it, aiming to reach the free end of the thread. b. Once the loop is formed, the tips of the needle holder are passed through the loop and aim to catch the remaining free end of the thread. This has been left intentionally quite short in order to stick out (due to nylon memory), making it easier to grasp it. c. Once the free end is grasped with the needle holder, the two instruments must cross sides in order to form a square knot. The traction plane has to be perpendicular to the plane of the anastomosis in order for the knot to lie flat.

important to grasp the end of the thread; otherwise, the knot may trap part of the thread, causing frustration (Figure 1.3.8).

Bring the loop well into the tip of the needle holder and pull in a crossed manner at 90 degrees to the line of the anastomosis, in order to achieve a square knot (Figure 1.3.8). It is important to pull the thread and tie the knot with the precisely optimum tension that is required (Figure 1.3.9).

A loose knot will of course lead to anastomotic leak and will have to be replaced. However, a fundamental principle is to understand that the anastomotic sutures aim for a precise vessel wall alignment in all three dimensions only, and not for a tight compressive connection of the vessels. Tight sutures will cause *crumbling* of the inner walls (intima) and irregular projections in the lumen, predisposing to turbulent blood flow and thrombosis.

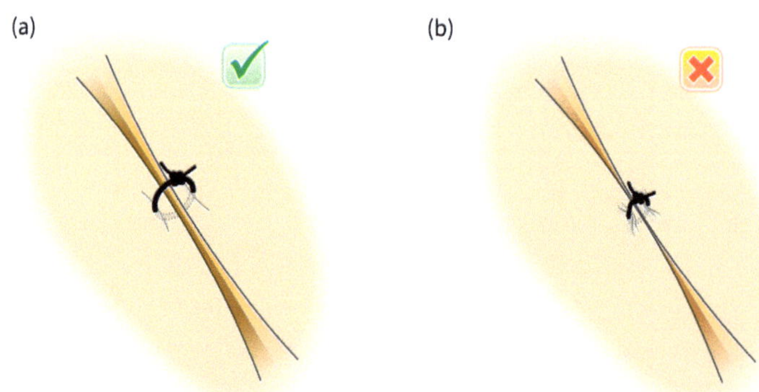

Figure 1.3.9 a. Optimum tension of the suture across the anastomosis leading to approximation and apposition of the opposed edges. b. Excessive tension crushes the edges and leads to the crumbling of the tissue and inner lumen irregularities that may cause turbulent blood flow and thrombosis.

Box 1.3.1 Key points in basic microvascular suturing

Microvascular surgery is all about finger movement.
The arms of the microvascular surgeon should be well rested with the elbows and wrists supported. All handling of the microvascular instruments is performed by finger motion.
The vessels should be positioned at the best possible plane.
Aim for a horizontal anastomosis rather than vertical. Entry and exit of the middle should be on a course perpendicular to the vessel wall. Passing of the needle should follow its curvature.
During passing and receiving of the needle, gentle counter pushing with the non-dominant handheld microvascular instruments or with the assistant facilitates better control.

The second half knot is easier; however, attention needs to be given to hold the loop and the short end of the stitch in a 90-degree plane to the anastomotic line, in order to achieve a square and flat knot.

During knot tying, the needle is safely placed within the periphery of the visual field and on a soft tissue but ideally inserted in soft tissue such as the sternomastoid muscle.

Techniques to overcome vessel calibre or thickness discrepancies (mismatch) are discussed in the relevant chapters.

Key points regarding basic microvascular suturing skills are highlighted in Box 1.3.1.

Technique—microvascular suturing principles

The microvascular suturing principles, which step further from the basic microvascular suturing skills, are discussed in detail in Chapter 8.2.

A brief summary of them is listed next and also presented in Box 8.2.1 (Chapter 8.2):

1. The vessel walls must be everted when suturing. To achieve this:
   - Gently grasp the adventitia close to the vessel end and pull so that the vessel edge is everted, or
   - Insert dilator forceps in the lumen and push outwards. This offers counter-resistance when the needle passes from out in.
2. Carefully plan and target the needle entry point.
3. Always pass the needle perpendicular through the vessel wall.
4. Through practice, aim to develop a sensitive fingertip tactile feedback sense. This helps to feel the 'give' when the needle penetrates through the vessel wall.
5. Never lose sight of the needle tip. Eversion of the vessel walls is important for this.
6. When the needle is through the first vessel, pull it out completely. Avoid passing the needle through the second vessel at once.
7. Carefully plan and target the needle exit point.
8. Always tie square knots.
9. Plan and space the sutures evenly.

1.4 **Microvascular anastomotic devices (MACD) or couplers**

Introduction

The venous coupler ring-pin system was first described in 1962. The technology was further developed in the late 1980s, early 1990s, in a system called the Microvascular Anastomotic Coupler System (Synovis Micro Companies Alliance, Birmingham, AL).

The technique is now widely utilized and is considered to be the standard of care for venous anastomoses by the majority of high-volume head and neck reconstructive units.

Indications and technique

The device is primarily designed for venous anastomosis as the venous vessel walls are relatively thin, pliable, and easily everted.

The MACD comes in a kit (Figure 1.4.1), that contains the main coupling device and two specially designed 'hockey-stick' shaped forceps, that permit gentle atraumatic

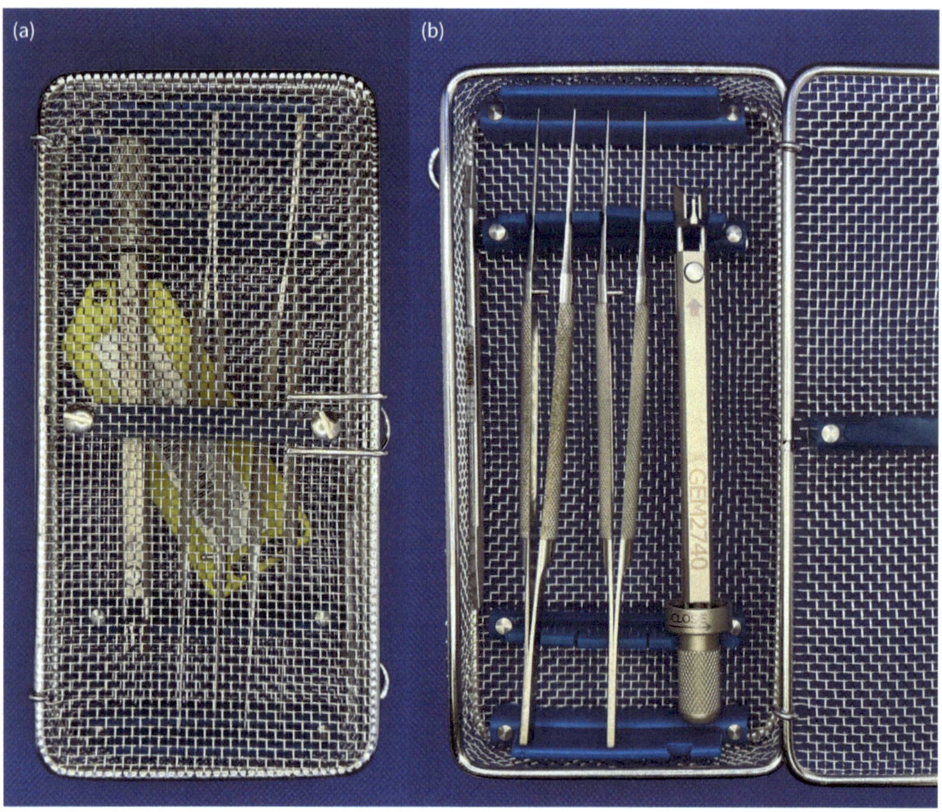

Figure 1.4.1 Microvascular anastomotic device (MACD) kit in case.
a. Closed.
b. Open.

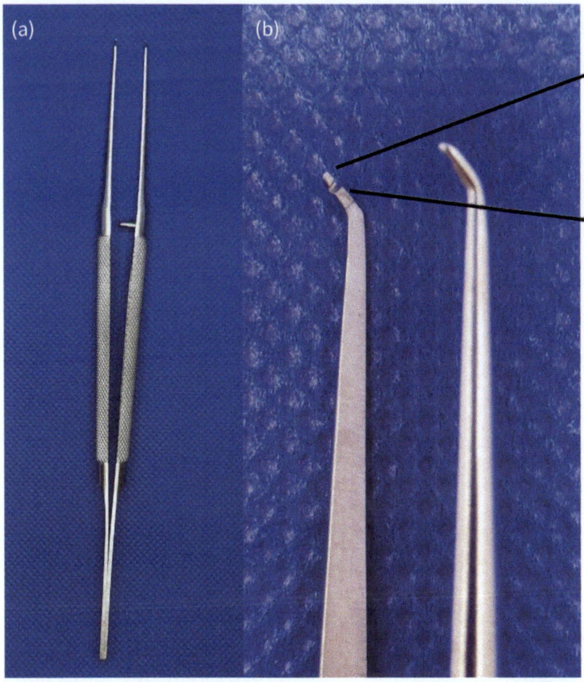

Figure 1.4.2 a. Hockey-stick forceps.
b. Tips of hockey-stick forceps, especially designed for atraumatic handling of thin vessel wall edges with an integrated hole, to allow vessel wall pressure against the tip of the pins for full thickness penetration.

handling of thin vessel edges and easy adaptation on the pins of the anastomotic rings (Figure 1.4.2).

The main coupler comprises a straight sterilizable handle at the end of which there is a lock mechanism that mounts the single-use frame with two opposing pin bearing rings (Figure 1.4.3).

The rings are made from high-density polyethylene and the pins are constructed from stainless steel. Available ring diameters range from 1.0 mm to 4.5 mm, at 0.5 mm increments and they come in single sterile packs (Figure 1.4.4).

Upon approximation, the pins of each ring are inserted into the holes of the other, creating a secure, watertight anastomosis.

The working principle relies on passing the vessel edges through the opposing rings and pinning the vessel wall through the pins after careful eversion of the vessel edge (Figure 1.4.5). When mounted on the ring pins, the vessel edges are averted by 90 degrees, allowing clear visualization of both lumens.

The pins come in predetermined fixed lengths and are not suitable for penetrating through thick-walled vessels and especially thick-walled arteries that contain a muscular media layer.

When both vessel ends are successfully mounted, then with rotation of a knob at the opposite end of the handle, the ring bearing frame gradually closes, approximating the rings until pins (friction-fit ring pins) interlock, completing the anastomosis.

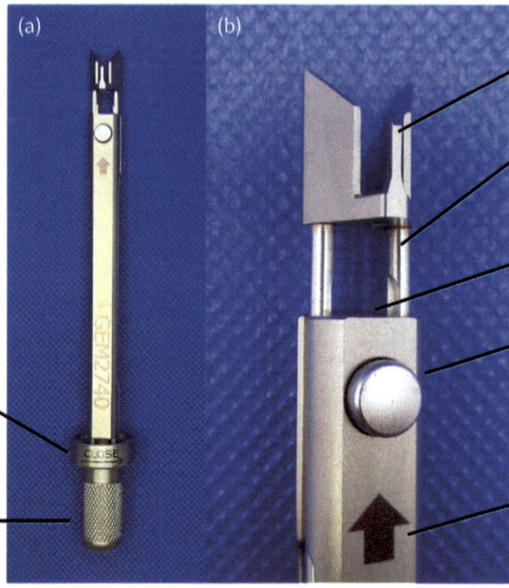

Figure 1.4.3 a. MACD device. Note the rotating/twisting node at the distal end. With clockwise rotation, the top-end placed frame gradually closes, bringing the anastomotic rings together and sealing the anastomosis. Further rotation brings the stylet forward, pushing outwards, and releasing the rings from the frame.
b. Close view of the front part of the anastomotic coupler device with markers indicating the utility of each component.

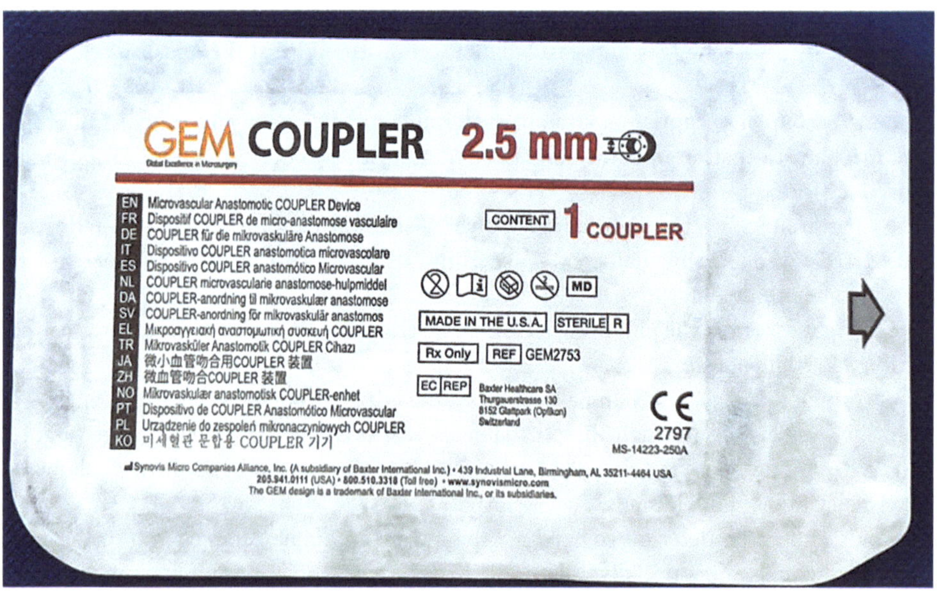

Figure 1.4.4 Indicative pack of a single-use 2.5 mm coupler.

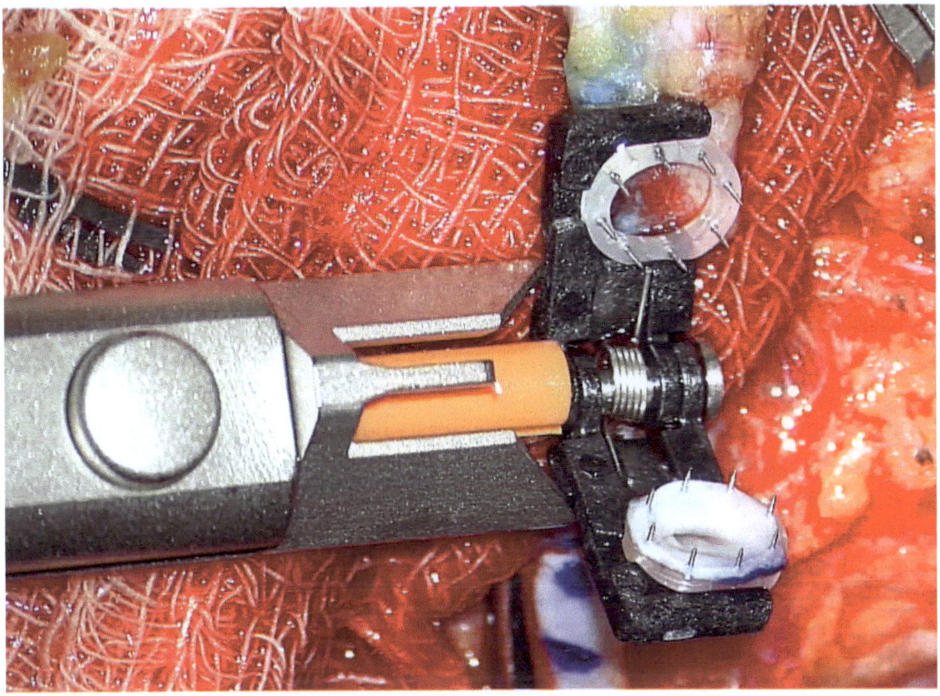

Figure 1.4.5 Clinical photograph showing the MACD device in use. On the bottom frame shown, the vein has already been everted and pinned on the lower ring. The upper ring is about to receive the vein which sits behind it. Note that between the pins of the free ring (upper), there are small holes in the rim of the ring. These correspond to the opposing pins. This design provides an interlocking mechanism; when the rings are opposed against each other, the pins adapt in the respective perforations, creating a watertight closed system.

Advantages, disadvantages and complications

Venous couplers have advantages in reducing operating time and improving the outcomes of anastomoses:

- Minimal vessel preparation in terms of adventitia excision is required as the design of the technique allows eversion of the vessel edge with visualization of the intima.
- *Stenting of the anastomosis:* Due to the coupled-ring system, the venous anastomotic site is prevented from venous wall collapse even under the rare circumstances of hypovolemia or compression (haematoma) acting as vascular 'stents' protecting the anastomotic area, which is prone to thrombosis in the first 48–72 hours while the intima endothelium is healing.
- *Reduction of operating time:* The overall operative time is reduced by approximately 2- to 3-fold compared to traditional hand-sewn anastomosis. The average time for an anastomosis using MACD is approximately five minutes, ranging from 3 to 10 minutes, which translates to reduced time of general anaesthetic (GA), beneficial primarily to the patient, but also cost-effective in resources utilization.

There is ample level 1a evidence supporting the use of MACD for venous anastomosis. Systematic reviews have demonstrated a thrombosis rate between 0.2% and 3.0% with patency rates of 98.5%. This is significantly better when compared to the hand-sewn technique.

In a systematic review by Wu et al. (see 'Further reading' at the end of the chapter), where MACD anastomoses in 8,955 cases were analysed, 11 patients developed postoperative extrusion and palpability of the couplers. This is a unique complication related to MACD and most often occurs when the anastomosis is performed at the external jugular vein (EJV), which is more superficial. However, after successful flap integration for over three weeks postoperatively, this has not been associated with flap failure. An extruded MACD can easily be excised and removed under local anaesthetic in the outpatient department.

Contraindications

A main contraindication is the end-to-side anastomosis, as it is not possible to pass the venotomy site inverted through the coupler device ring.

MACD are not indicated for thick-walled vessels. A point of attention is that if a vessel is of a relatively small calibre but contains thick-walled edges, passing through the ring may cause constriction of the lumen and predispose to thrombosis.

MACD cannot be used when the vessel calibre mismatch exceeds 2× the size of the coupler. The rings are of equal size and should be chosen based on the maximum diameter of the smallest calibre vessel to prevent tearing of the smaller vein. A vessel mismatch of 2- or above coupler sizes risks passing the larger vessel through a narrow ring, hence obstructing or completely obliterating the lumen.

The MACD used for arterial anastomosis is limited due to the vessel wall thickness. The arterial wall structure, including the muscular *tunica media*, renders the vessel significantly less pliable and difficult to evert. Frequently encountered in arterial anastomoses, calibre and thickness mismatch, and the high-pressure flow across the anastomosis are also points of concern regarding the suitability of MACD for arteries. These disadvantages become more prominent, especially for smaller-sized couplers, since the vessel edge has to pass through the inner hole of the ring prior to eversion, which causes an area of lumen constriction that predisposes for thrombosis in arterial anastomosis. Recent studies have reported successful outcomes in using MACD for arterial anastomoses; however, careful case selection is of paramount importance.

1.5 **Maintenance and back-up equipment**

All instruments must be carefully decontaminated (cleaned, disinfected, and sterilized) according to the manufacturer's instructions after their use. This process takes place in the designated sterile services department (SSD).

The fine, delicate tips of the microsurgical instruments must be protected at all times and must never be placed tip-first on the table or against hard surfaces.

The SSD team must ensure that the tips do not touch any other hard objects or the walls of the case.

The usual disinfectant solutions are haemolytic enzyme solutions, and the objects have to be submerged for a minimum of 30 minutes. This will dissolve any established blood clots. Following this, the instruments must be rinsed with water with particular attention to hinges, where a brisk jet of water under pressure may be indicated.

Sterilization is usually done in autoclaves. Prior to this, the instruments must be placed in their respective cases and secured appropriately, so that any vibrations or movement during handling and processing will not damage the fine working tips.

Minor damage to the tips can be corrected by specialists and under magnification. However, most usually any damage to the tip will render the instrument unfit for purpose and will require immediate replacement.

Occasionally, instruments in contact with electrical equipment such as diathermy or magnetized devices may become magnetized. In such situations, they may need to be treated with a de-magnetizer prior to further use.

Electrical equipment should be checked at regular intervals and maintained at the appropriate times.

Care of the microscope

The entire microscope should be checked by a specialized biomedical equipment technician at least twice a year and in accordance with the manufacturer's standards.

Before use it must be confirmed that the microscope is going to be plugged in power socket of appropriate voltage setting. It must also be ensured that the microscope is plugged into a power outlet which has a properly connected protective earth contact.

Following the use of the microscope, all glass surfaces including eye pieces and objective lenses need to be cleaned carefully with appropriate fabric and only use the cleansing solutions as per the manufacturer's advice.

The microscope head is usually protected by its own cover, which should be replaced each time after use.

After use, the team should clean and oil the wheels and the brakes of the microscope and remove any surplus oil when cleaning is finished.

It must be confirmed that all the mechanical connections are properly attached, and screw connections tightened, before and after every use of the microscope.

All cables and plugs must be maintained in good working condition.

If the microscope needs to be moved, it is important to ensure that the microscope is secured and the wheels are locked in the storage position.

Back-up equipment

It is important to always maintain a sterile back-up full set of instruments. Occasionally, instruments may be accidentally desterilized, dropped, or damaged during the procedure. Readily available sterile and packed replacement items or sets are important to salvage the situation.

A multitude of sterile and fully functional kits available is also important for cases of return to theatre for exploration and revision of the anastomosis in the immediate postoperative period, where the originally used equipment and instruments would have been sent to SSD.

Further reading

Acland RD. Microvascular anastomosis: a device for holding stay sutures and a new vascular clamp. *Surgery* 1974;75(2):185–7.

Acland RD. *Microsurgery Practice Manual*. London: Year Book Medical Publishers, 1980.

Acland RD. *Practice Manual for Microvascular Surgery*. St Louis, MO: C.V. Mosby, 1989: p. 134
Adam D, Broderick D, Kyzas P, Vassiliou L. Microvascular anastomotic coupler devices versus hand-sewn technique for arterial anastomosis: a systematic review. *Br J Oral Maxillofac Surg* 2021;59(5):524–33.
Ardehali B, Morritt AN, Jain A. Systematic review: anastomotic microvascular device. *J Plast Reconstr Aesthet Surg* 2014;67(6):752–5.
Barker EV, Enepekides DJ. The utility of microvascular anastomotic devices in head and neck reconstruction. *Curr Opin Otolaryngol Head Neck Surg* 2008;16(4):331–4.
Fried MP, Caminear DS, Sloman-Moll ER. The efficacy of absorbable suture for microvascular anastomoses. *Arch Otolaryngol Head Neck Surg* 1990;116(9):1051–4.
Gordon L. Advances in microsurgery. *Surg Technol Int* 1991;I:425–7.
Kiuchi T, Ishii N, Tani Y, Masaoka K, Suzuki A, Kishi K. The optimal color of background sheets for microsurgery. *Arch Plast Surg* 2017;44(2):175–6.
Li MM, *et al.* Utilization of microvascular couplers in salvage arterial anastomosis in head and neck free flap surgery: case series and literature review. *Head Neck* 2020;42(8):E1–7.
Maruccia M, *et al.* Microvascular coupler device versus hand-sewn venous anastomosis: a systematic review of the literature and data meta-analysis. *Microsurgery* 2020;40(5):608–17.
Wu GJ, Loewenstein SN, Mailey BA, Sasor S, Cook J, Hassanein AH. Unique complications of venous anastomotic couplers: a systematic review of the literature. *J Reconstr Microsurg* 2020;36(6):403–11.

2

Common flaps in head and neck reconstruction and considerations for flap selection

Fu-Chan Wei, Eleonora O.F. Dimovska, Nidal Al Deek, Leandros Vassilios F. Vassiliou, Panayiotis Kyzas, and Nicholas Kalavrezos

2.1 **Soft tissue flaps in head and neck reconstruction**

Introduction

This chapter describes the most commonly used soft tissue free flaps in head and neck reconstruction. There is an amplitude of flaps that provide fasciocutaneous skin paddles, myocutaneous skin paddles, or combination of fasciocutaneous perforator-based skin islands with surrounding muscle.

Fasciocutaneous flaps in principle are thinner and more pliable and can provide cover for defects spanning more than one subside due to their ability to contour easier.

Myocutaneous flaps are usually more inflexible to contour, however the benefit of those flaps is muscle and soft tissue bulk. Therefore, they are more suitable in obliterating deep defects such as extensive floor of mouth and subtotal or total glossectomy defects.

Finally, the jejunal flap is a naturally tubed flap ideal for oesophageal reconstructions especially for hypopharyngeal and oesophageal defects. In this subchapter each flap description provides basic anatomical information, techniques of harvest, and operating tips.

Radial forearm flap (fasciocutaneous)

Introduction

The anatomical study of the radial forearm flap was first published in Chinese in 1981. It was introduced to the world as the Chinese flap in an English publication in 1982 and has ever since served as a workhorse. The landmark paper for its use in oral cavity reconstruction goes back to 1986. The radial forearm flap owes its popularity on its versatility and relative easiness of harvest and microvascular anastomosis making it the flap of choice for multiple sites and sizes of defects.

Anatomy

The anatomy of the radial forearm flap is demonstrated in Figure 2.1.1.

- Artery—radial artery (2.5–3.5 mm)
- Vein—two venae-comitantes (VCs) (1–2 mm) +/– cephalic vein (2.5–4 mm)
- Pedicle length 15-22 cm
- Innervation—lateral and medial antebrachial nerves
- Common flap size 12 cm (4–30 cm) × 5 cm (4–15 cm) (1–2 cm width for primary closure)

Indications

- Tongue—partial and hemiglossectomies
- Floor of mouth
- Palate
- Pharynx/Larynx
- Lip
- Buccal mucosa
- External cutaneous resurfacing
- Osseocutaneous flap for small mandible/maxilla defects and total nose reconstruction
- Oro-cutaneous/oro-antral fistula closure

Advantages

- Thin and pliable skin paddle
- Long vascular pedicle
- Large calibre artery

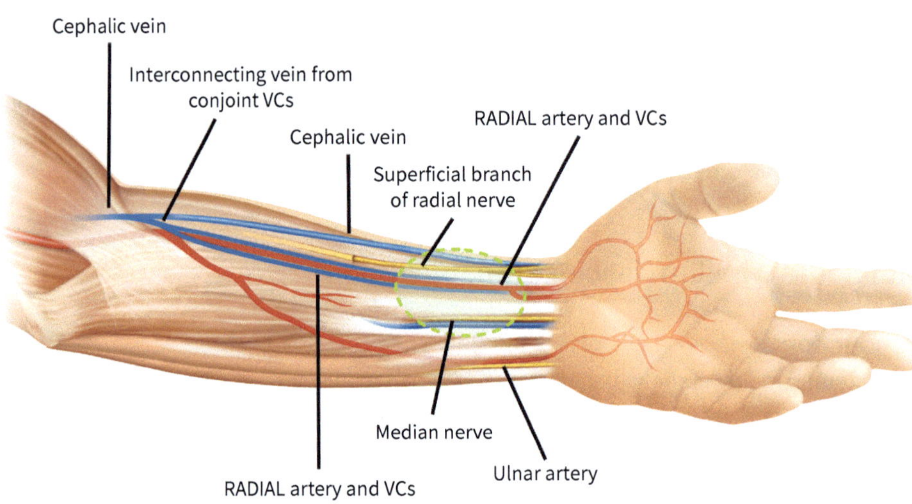

Figure 2.1.1 Schematic presentation of the Radial Forearm flap key anatomy. Note the relative positions of the radial artery and its accompanying VCs and the ulnar artery. In the region of the antecubital fossa the VCs join into a 'confluent' vein which in most cases continues to drain into the cephalic vein or the median cubital vein formulating a larger calibre vein (as further shown in Figure 2.1.2).

Adapted with permission from Raising of Microvascular Flaps: A Systematic Approach, 2nd Edition. Editors Wolff K.-D., Hölzle F.: Springer—Verlag Berlin Heidelberg; 2011. Chapter: Radial forearm flap 1–20, Page 10: Standard flap design.

Disadvantages

- Sacrificing major vessel to hand
- Aesthetically unpleasing
- Risk of donor-site sensory nerve injury
- Radius fracture in osseocutaneous flap

Harvest technique

Preoperative considerations

Imaging studies are not commonly required. An Allen's test should be performed to evaluate the capacity of the ulnar artery to singlehandedly supply the hand. The radial artery should be palpated for pulsatile strength to ascertain patency and good flow. A pulse oximeter on the thumb can provide confirmation of blood flow.

Flap markings

The location of the radial artery in the wrist and its path along the forearm is marked following palpation or using a handheld doppler; as are the paths of the superficial and cephalic veins. **It is important to mark the course of the cephalic vein as it runs superficially and if not tracked may inadvertently became injured when the main pedicle which runs deeper is chased.**

The width of the skin paddle is commonly kept within the border of the volar wrist (around 5 cm for a standard partial glossectomy defect). The width can be extended to the dorsal aspect to include the cephalic vein, and the length can extend proximally in the forearm if required.

Technique

The radial forearm flap is considered easy to harvest, which may lead to rushed harvest or delegation to a more inexperienced operator. Underestimating the venous anatomy of the flap may result in a difficult end-to-side microvascular anastomosis depended on a small vena comitans, effectively taking back the time gained by a 'quick' harvest. The technique described here details harvesting the flap including the cephalic vein and chasing the venous pedicle proximally in the antecubital fossa in order to harvest the vein that forms the confluence of the radial VCs and the cephalic. By harvesting this 'conjoint' vein that is often either the confluence of the deep venous system (conjoint VC) into the cephalic or median cubital vein (Figure 2.1.2) the flap stands the best chance of success with one only anastomosis—usually of a large calibre vein that drains both the deep and superficial vascular systems.

1. Patient is supine with the arm extended, under tourniquet control.
2. The harvest of the skin paddle is usually done in subfascial manner, although a suprafascial harvest can be utilized in order to minimize donor-site morbidity.
3. One could start the harvest from ulnar to radial when the skin paddle is large, however, starting with identifying the pedicle distally will prevent the risk of missing its inclusion in narrower skin paddles.
4. While elevating the skin paddle attention is given to maintain the paratenon that protects the tendons intact.
5. When raising the skin paddle—once the radial aspect of flexor carpi radialis (FCR) is reached on one side of the pedicle, and the ulnar aspect of the brachioradialis is reached

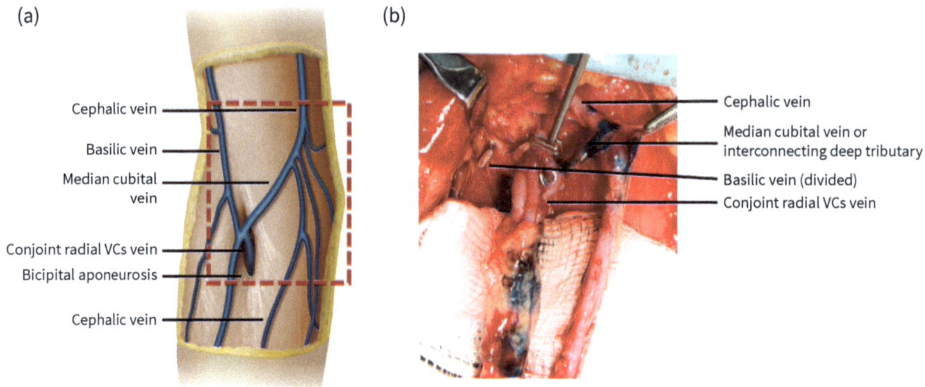

Figure 2.1.2 Venous anatomy in the antecubital fossa. a. Schematic presentation of the antecubital fossa venous anatomy. Note the two main superficial veins of the arm, namely the cephalic vein and the basilic vein. As the radial artery VCs emerge through the bicipital aponeurosis, they join into one confluent vein. The latter will further drain into the median cubital vein or directly into the cephalic vein. b. Antecubital fossa dissected for preparation of a radial forearm free flap. Note the conjoined radial VCs as they follow a separate course from the radial artery. The former drains into an interconnecting venous branch, which later drains into the cephalic system. The confluent cephalic vein can be harvested further proximally, providing one single large calibre vein that drains both the deep and the superficial systems and is easy to anastomose with MACD. Note that the confluent VCs were also draining into the basilic vein, which has been ligated and divided on the left side of the clinical photograph.

on the other, the conjoint fascia is incised taking the superficial layer of the fascia (with its containing vascular pedicle) with the flap, keeping the deep fascia intact to prevent bowstringing of the flexor tendons.

6. It is advised that the radial artery is not ligated and divided early. It is preferrable to expose the whole length of the pedicle ensuring normal anatomy, prior to committing to a definitive manoeuvre. In rare cases a median radial artery (Figure 2.1.3) is found which renders the flap unsuitable for use (see Varley et al. in 'Further reading'). Division of the pedicle distally in case of aberrant vascular anatomy may severely compromise the perfusion of the hand.
7. The cephalic vein (and other potential connecting superficial veins) are protected within in the fatty tissue harvested with the flap if included.
8. After the skin paddle is islanded, the incision is extended proximally opening the forearm:

When opening the forearm, the 'radial' skin flap is elevated at the level of the subcutaneous fat, deroofing the cephalic vein, and following it towards the antecubital fossa. It is practical to chase this important vein first protecting its integrity. Sometimes the cephalic vein runs slightly medially and careless opening of the forearm straight down to the muscle layer aiming to find the radial pedicle may injure the vessel.

The cephalic vein is followed proximally until its junction with the conjoint vein comitans formed by the confluence of the two radial VCs as it emerges through the bicipital aponeurosis. That gives the reassurance that the two venous systems, superficial and deep, are joining into a single vessel.

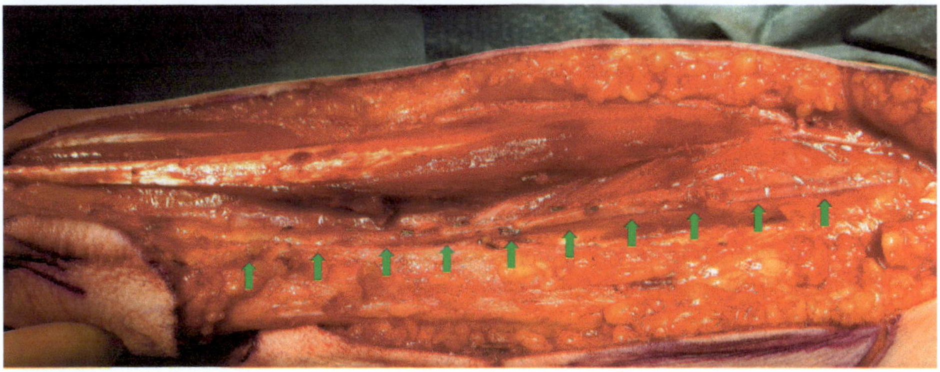

Figure 2.1.3 Abnormal radial pedicle. Note the abnormally thin calibre of the radial pedicle and its abnormal course (green arrows). The pedicle, instead of emerging from underneath the brachioradialis, passes over the flexor carpi radialis and pronator teres muscles. Chasing of the pedicle origin higher in the antecubital fossa revealed that it stemmed directly from the brachial artery. This anatomical variation is linked with palmar arch compromise in case of radial artery division. The pedicle had not been divided distally. Once the anatomical variation was recognized the flap was sutured back in its original position. This case highlights the importance of not committing to pedicle ligation and division until the whole anatomy has been appropriately validated.

9. The belly of the brachioradialis is exposed and reflected laterally uncovering the radial pedicle.
10. Returning back in raising the skin paddle, the superficial radial nerve, located in close proximity to the cephalic vein, is protected.
11. The flap is raised by ligating side and feeding branches.
12. Attention is given in mobilizing the pedicle from the undersurface of the branchioradialis tendon. This step requires the assistant to lift and carefully evert the tendon so that sharp dissection can be performed to free up the pedicle from the tendon. The proximal part of the superficial radial nerve will be encountered here as it emerges from underneath the brachioradialis.
13. The continued flap elevation can now be performed by holding the flap with the operator's non-dominant hand and dissecting out and ligating inferior perforators with the dominant hand.
14. The pedicle is dissected in a standard fashion until the antecubital fossa. At this level the radial artery dives deep towards its origin from the brachial artery while the VCs join in one confluent VC, which later drains into the main cephalic or median cubital vein (Figure 2.1.2). There are many other veins draining into this 'hilum' and should be very carefully dissected and ligated effectively isolating one venous path from the two VCs into one confluent vein that drains both superficial and deep systems. The recurrent radial artery branch may be seen and if interfering with the venous dissection can be ligated and divided. In this step, which requires focus and meticulous dissection, the arterial component of the flap is separated from the venous, and the flap is ready for disconnection.
15. The tourniquet is released, and perfusion of the hand and flap is checked.
16. Prior to disconnection, the flap is left to rest in its natural position and its perfusion is checked. At this point, it is crucial to mark with ink the superior aspect of the pedicle in its whole length. This step will prove useful during the inset and microvascular vessel

Box 2.1.1 Tips for harvesting the RFFF flap

- In order to recognize early any rare radial artery aberrant anatomy, it is recommended that the whole forearm is fully opened to ensure normal radial artery course prior to ligation and division of the radial artery distally.
- We recommend dissection of the venous system in the anti-cubital fossa proximal to the VCs in order to harvest a single large calibre vein, draining both the deep system (VCs) and the superficial (cephalic vein) and to maximize flow.

preparation, to guide the correct orientation of the pedicle and the avoidance of torsion or kinking, especially through the tunnel.

Important tips on harvesting the radial free forearm flap (RFFF) are highlighted in Box 2.1.1.

Technical modifications

Including the radius bone

A length of bone from the radial styloid to the insertion of the pronator teres can be harvested. Due to the segmental blood supply, multiple osteotomies can be performed without vascular compromise to the bone. One should however be mindful of the increased risk of future fractures, particularly in older patients and post-menopausal women; a patient group in which this osseous flap should not be the first line choice.

Including tendon

Tendon of choice is the palmaris longus (PL). This can be used as a fascial sling for e.g. mouth/ lip reconstruction.

Including nerve

The lateral antebrachial cutaneous nerve can be harvested and is easily included in the flap, as it lies in close proximity to the cephalic vein.

Donor-site management

- Skin graft, preferably full-thickness
- Local flap coverage, (perforator base or randomly based hatchet flap)
- 2-Stage reconstruction. Dermal substitute and negative pressure wound therapy followed by skin grafting

Tips for harvest

- Distal to proximal harvest, with radial artery identification and fixation to skin paddle first, to prevent separation.
- Leaving a longer stump distal to the ligating clip, which can be pulled to facilitate upward traction of the flap during initial raise.
- A 'boat-like' rather than box-like radius harvest reduces fracture risk of the remaining radius.

- Bone grafting (from e.g. the iliac crest) and locking plates for fixation of the remaining radius can reduce future fracture risk.
- Two separate skin paddles can be harvested on distal perforators and proximal septal skin vessels medial to the brachioradialis.

Latissimus dorsi flap (myocutaneous)

Introduction

The latissimus dorsi (LD) flap was initially described in 1906, but didn't come into regular use until the late 1970s. It was initially used as a myocutaneous or muscular flap, and later refined as a perforator flap termed the thoracodorsal artery perforator flap (TDAP). For the head & neck area, the flap can be used in either composition, commonly as a muscle flap for scalp cover and as a fasciocutaneous perforator flap for large intraoral defects.

Anatomy

The anatomy of the LD flap is demonstrated in Figure 2.1.4.

- Artery—thoracodorsal artery 3 mm (2–4 mm)
- Vein—thoracodorsal vein 3.5 mm (range 2–5 mm) (Venae comitantes secondary)
- Pedicle length 8.5 cm (6.5–15 cm)
- Innervation—thoracodorsal nerve for motor innervation
- Flap size—length 18–35 cm, width: 7–20 cm (up to 9 cm for primary closure)

Indications

See Figure 2.1.5.

- External cutaneous—muscle with skin graft for scalp, or wide face (cheek) defects.
- Large intraoral defects—as a perforator flap
- Facial re-animation—innervated muscle flap (uncommon donor site)
- Extensive maxillary defects.
- Mandible reconstruction in selected cases.

Advantages

- Easy and speedy harvest with consistent anatomy
- Long pedicle and large diameter vessels
- Skin paddle can be designed in several directions: horizontal, vertical, or oblique
- Possibility to harvest a chimeric flap based on branches from the subscapular system

Disadvantages

- Long scar
- Donor-site seroma is common
- Donor-site weakness and/or pelvic instability in vulnerable patients (crutch-dependent, poor mobility)

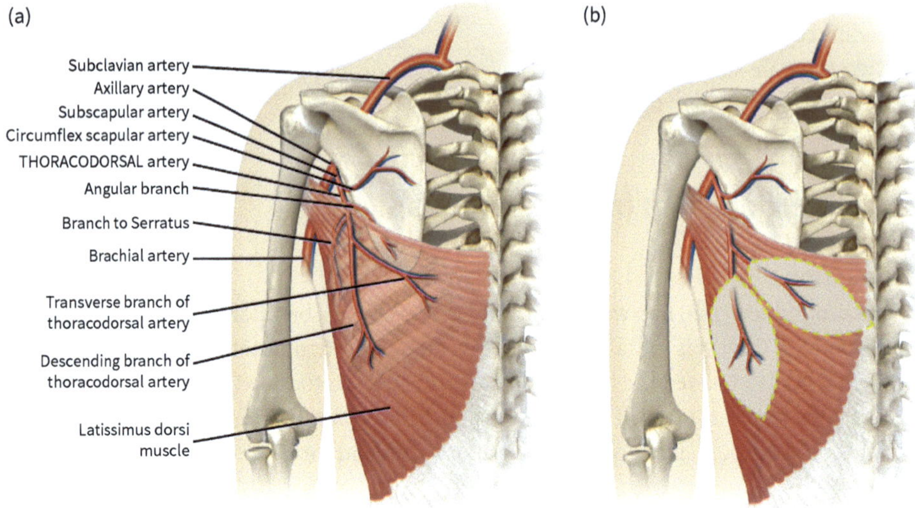

Figure 2.1.4 Schematic presentation of the latissimus dorsi flap key anatomy. a. Main vascular anatomy and topography of latissimus dorsi and its blood supply. Note the subclavian artery as it emerges in the axillary fossa as the axillary artery. The latter supplies the circumflex subscapular artery and the thoracodorsal artery, which is the main nutrient artery of the latissimus dorsi free flap. Note that further distally the thoracodorsal artery will give off the angular branch and the branch to the serratus muscle prior to continuing its intramuscular course and dividing in the transverse branch and the descending branch. b. The consistent anatomy and topography of the front transverse and descending branches of the thoracodorsal artery allow versatility in the flap design and orientation of the skin paddles in order to fit better the reconstructive requirements of each case.

Harvest technique

Preoperative considerations

Advanced imaging is not required. Handheld Doppler is used for perforator location if a perforator flap is planned. This is not required for musculocutaneous flaps as long as skin paddle is designed overlying the muscle. The thoracodorsal artery is close to the hard being located quite centrally and unlikely to be affected by atherosclerosis in contrast to more peripherally based vessels.

Flap markings

The borders of the latissimus muscle, the scapula, and the iliac crest are marked out. The incision for access is drawn vertical from the posterior axillary fold down to the medial border of the iliac crest. This incision is modified in the case of adding a skin paddle. A skin paddle should ideally be placed at the lateral border of the muscle in order to capture most perforators from the underlying vertical division of thoracodorsal artery.

Technique

1. Patient is in lateral decubitus position on a bean bag, with the arm in an arm gutter abducted at 45 degrees.

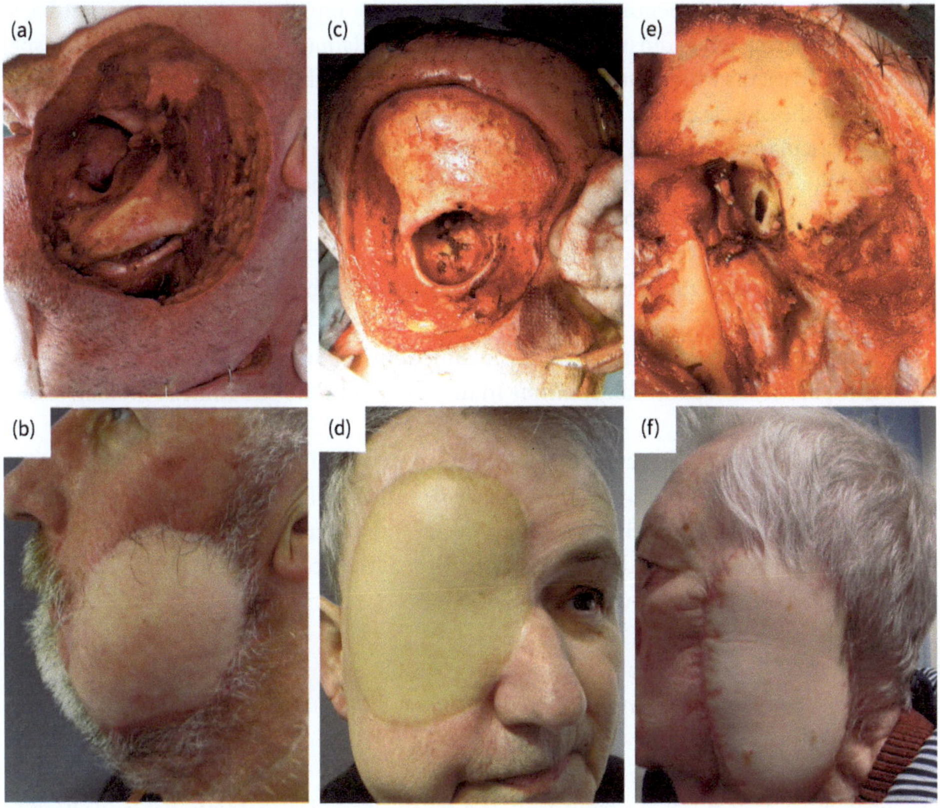

Figure 2.1.5 Clinical applications of the latissimus dorsi free flap. Note the large surface cover and part provided by this flap. a. Wide complementary through-and-through resection of the left cheek for dermatofibrosarcoma. b. Reconstruction with folded (bi-paddle) latissimus dorsi) providing inner and outer skin cover. c. Wide upper face soft tissue resection, including orbital exenteration for a Merkel Cell Carcinoma. d. Latissimus dorsi healed, providing excellent cover and obliteration of the orbital cavity with its muscular component (six-month postoperative photograph). e. Wide left temporal and parotid region resection including total pinnectomy for an extensive malignant parotid tumour invading skin. f. Reconstruction of the whole defect with a latissimus dorsi free flap (six-month postoperative photograph).

2. The incision is made and the skin flaps are elevated to expose the superior aspect of the LD. It is important if possible to elevate the skin in a suprafascial fashion, leaving the fascia that envelops the muscle intact.
3. The lateral border of the muscle is identified and lifted off the underlying serratus anterior. **Identifying the lateral border of the LD muscle is an important step as this defines the plane.** There is usually an avascular connective tissue plane separating the muscle for the serratus anterior and via correct identification of the plane the dissection can progress quickly almost in a 'blunt dissection' fashion.
4. The skin paddle is islanded and the borders of muscle are freed from their cranial, medial, and lateral part prior to incising the caudal portion and starting the elevation.

5. Tucking sutures 'suspending' the skin paddle to the muscle are important in order to avoid shearing stress during the elevation that can damage the microcirculation, especially in patients with high body mass index and thick subcutaneous layer.
6. Elevate the muscle caudal to cranial until the axilla and pedicle is reached.
7. The vascular pedicle will be identified in the undersurface of the flap as it is raised cranially. Usually the vascular hilum and the take-off of both the vertical and horizontal branches of the thoracodorsal pedicle can be visualized.
8. Dissect up to a desired pedicle length and diameter, ligating any branching vessels. The branches to the serratus anterior and the angular branch to the scapular tip are recognized and divided.
9. Ligate the thoracodorsal nerve unless planned for use in an innervated flap. The vascular pedicle dissection can continue in the axilla until the circumflex scapular vessels are reached.
10. Prior to disconnection the flap is left to rest in its natural position and its perfusion is checked. At this point it is crucial to mark with ink the superior aspect of the pedicle in its whole length. This step will prove useful during the inset and microvascular vessel preparation, to guide correct orientation of the pedicle and avoidance of torsion or kinking especially through the tunnel.

Technical modifications

- *Utilizing the subscapular artery system—Chimeric options (Scapula, split skin paddles, serratus)*

The subscapular system holds a truly great and reliable vascular anatomy that lends itself to several modifications and tissue inclusions. For complex 3D head & neck defects, this is one of the most diverse chimeric flap options. Along with the LD muscle, one can include scapular and parascapular skin paddles from the circumflex scapular artery, lateral scapula based on periosteal branches from the circumflex scapular artery, scapular tip based on the angular artery and serratus muscle based on the serratus branch. One can even split the LD muscle in two based on the descending and the horizontal branches of the thoracodorsal artery.

Including rib

The 9th or 10th can be harvested with the latissimus as a composite flap. About 12 cm of length can be taken

Endoscopic and robot-assisted harvest for muscle only with the benefit of shorter scars.

Donor-site management

- Large seromas are common. Subcutaneous quilting sutures and suction drains gradually changed from suction to passive mode over 2-3 weeks can be useful.

Tips for harvest

- One can either begin the harvest by dissecting out the muscle, or by identifying the pedicle in the posterior axillary fold first.

- Vertical design of the skin paddle is more useful in flap inset for head and neck reconstruction.
- Extend the pedicle length by including the subscapular artery, or by designing the skin paddle further distally on the back and dissect the vertical division intramuscularly until desired length.
- If harvesting a chimeric flap, identify the subscapular artery and delineate all branches to account for anatomical variations and confirm the possibility of your chimeric plan.
- Properly identify the thoracodorsal artery prior to ligating the serratus branch to avoid confusing them.
- When elevating the muscle from caudal to cranial, beware not to get into the wrong plane. Changing to a lateral to medial elevation after initial caudal approach can be advantageous to avoid accidentally ending up including other muscles, such as the serratus posterior.

Anterolateral thigh flap (perforator-based fasciocutaneous)

Introduction

Song et al. published the first report of the anterolateral thigh flap in 1984. It was, however, not until the landmark paper by Wei et al. in 2002 that the flap became a widely used workhorse flap for multiple indications. Further to this, studies have delineated the nerve supply of the area, which today facilitates innervated transfers of both muscle and skin from the area.

Anatomy

The anatomy of the anterolateral thigh flap is demonstrated in Figure 2.1.6.

- Artery—descending branch of lateral femoral circumflex artery (LFCA), 1.5-2.5 mm
- Venae comitantes, 2–3 mm
- Pedicle length 9–13 cm
- Innervation—motor nerve to vastus lateralis or lateral femoral cutaneous nerve (sensory).
- Flap size—mid-anterior thigh to mid-lateral thigh, commonly: 8×22 cm for primary closure

Indications

- External cutaneous defects
- Buccal-facial through-en-through defects
- Subtotal glossectomies with extensive floor of mouth
- Midface/Maxillary defects
- Laryngeal and pharyngeal defects
- Scalp and skull base

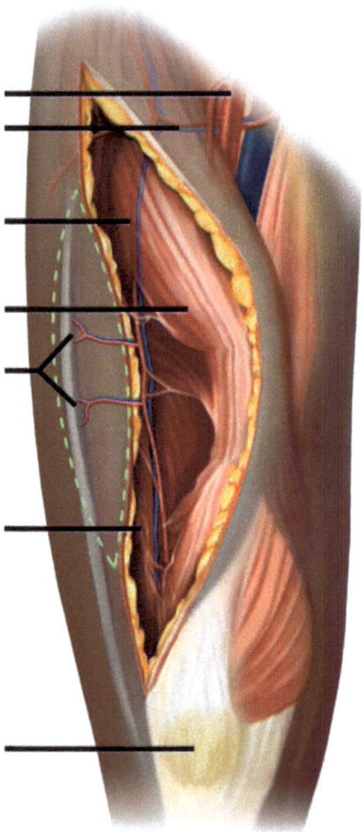

Figure 2.1.6 Schematic presentation of the anterior lateral thigh flap (ALT) key anatomy. Note at the top, the femoral artery as it emerges under the inguinal ligament. The femoral artery gives off the lateral circumflex femoral artery (LCFA), which provides the descending branch. The latter is the main nutrient artery (pedicle) of the ALT flap. Note the rectus femoris muscle retracted medially to expose the ALT pedicle, which provides cutaneous or myocutaneous perforators supplying a large area of thigh skin.

Advantages

- Long pedicle
- Large calibre vessels
- Chimeric properties
- Can be thinned or raised suprafascially.
- Multiple flap harvest at different time points.
- Innervated free functioning muscle transfer.

Disadvantages

- Variable flap thickness (thicker proximally, thinner distally)
- Occasionally long intramuscular dissection
- Donor-site numbness in cases of cutaneous nerve damage.

Harvest technique

Preoperative

Imaging is not required as handheld doppler is adequate for perforator localization. Ultrasound or CT can however be used.

Flap markings

A line connecting the lateral patella and the anterior superior iliac spine. This line marks the intermuscular septum between the vastus lateralis and the rectus femoris. Most perforators are found within 3 cm of the midline and in the inferolateral quadrant. A skin paddle of a maximum of 8×22 cm is drawn around the midline.

Technique

1. The medial margin is incised through fascia and down to muscle.
2. Elevate the skin flap from medial to lateral to identify the perforators coming through the vastus lateralis (VL) muscle.
3. Open the intermuscular septum and identify the descending branch of LFCA.
4. Perform the intermuscular dissection from distal to proximal to connect the perforator with the descending branch of LFCA.
5. Dissect the pedicle up to a desired length/diameter, maximally to its origin at the profunda femoris.
6. Prior to disconnection the flap is left to rest in its natural position and its perfusion is checked. At this point it is crucial to mark with ink the superior aspect of the pedicle in its whole length. This step will prove useful during the inset and microvascular vessel preparation, to guide correct orientation of the pedicle and avoidance of torsion or kinking especially through the tunnel.

Technical modifications

Including muscle

The vastus lateralis can be included as a composite flap or as a combined flap—islanded on its on pedicle—the distal run off of the LFCA. The muscle can also be harvested on its own.

Including nerve

One can include the lateral femoral cutaneous nerve (LFCN), which runs within the skin paddle suprafascially, or the motor nerve to the vastus lateralis, which runs with the vascular pedicle.

Donor-site management

- Primary closure
- Local flap closure (randomly based or perforator based)

Tips for harvest

- Use self-retractors or fish-hooks to retract the RF medially to facilitate exposure of the pedicle during dissection.
- Use a small double-ended retractor to elevate the pedicle during harvest to facilitate elevation from its inferior surface and ligation of inferior muscular perforators
- In cases of unsuitable perforator within the ALT territory, the flap can be converted to an anteromedial thigh perforator flap by utilizing a superior and medial perforator, or a tensor fascia lata perforator flap by using a transverse branch.

Profunda artery perforator flap (perforator-based fasciocutaneous)

Introduction

The profunda artery perforator (PAP) flap was introduced in 2001 and is supplied by predominantly musculocutaneous perforators through the adductor magnus muscle, but occasionally arise through the semitendinosus or semimembranosus. A septocutaneous course between the semimembranosus and gracilis has also been observed.

Anatomy

- Artery—medial branch of the profunda femoris artery, 0.8–2 mm
- Vein VCs, 2–2.5 mm
- Pedicle, up to 13 cm
- Innervation, none
- Flap size 7×10 cm for direct closure

Indication

- External cutaneous defects
- Tongue +/- floor of mouth
- Midface/Maxillary defects
- Buccal mucosa

Advantages

- Less obvious donor-site scar
- No sensory nerve sacrifice at the donor site
- Wide diameter vessels
- Pliable tissue

Disadvantages

- Pedicle is long but often around 9 cm
- Skin paddle size is dependent on patient characteristics, but is usually limited in size
- Not ideal as a chimeric flap
- Can produce contour deformity or wound dehiscence since the donor site is under constant stretch
- Damage to the gracilis muscle during perforator dissection in some cases

Harvest technique

Preoperative considerations

Handheld doppler is used to identify perforator location and course.

Flap markings

A vertical skin paddle is designed with the medial edge of its long axis on and parallel to the gracilis, to ensure preventing a too anterior placement. Its lateral margin is designed according to pinch in order to ensure primary closure. A transverse skin paddle is marked with the patient standing. It's designed with the superior edge of its long axis 1 cm superior to the inferior gluteal crease. Its inferior border is designed according to pinch and availability of tissue. Its anterior tip extends maximally to the anterior edge of the gracilis and its posterior tip does not extend beyond the lateral border of the inferior gluteal crease.

Technique

1. Patient is in supine, frog-leg position, and a transverse or vertically oriented skin paddle is designed incorporating the perforator location on the posteromedial thigh.
2. The flap is harvested anterior to posterior (for both skin paddle designs).
3. The dissection starts by incising down to, and through gracilis muscle fascia, then proceeds posteriorly to identify targeted perforator, once found it proceeds as in every perforator dissection.
4. The perforator is dissected through the adductor magnus muscle, the gracilis is reflected medically, until adequate length and diameter is achieved.
5. Prior to disconnection the flap is left to rest in its natural position and its perfusion is checked. At this point it is crucial to mark with ink the superior aspect of the pedicle in its whole length. This step will prove useful during the inset and microvascular vessel preparation, to guide correct orientation of the pedicle and avoidance of tortion or kinking especially through the tunnel.

Technical modifications

- Harvest could be performed from an anterior direction or from a posterior direction.
- Small piece of the adductor magnus, or the gracilis can be included.

Donor-site management

- Primary closure is always preferred and a skin paddle is designed accordingly to ensure this.

Tips for harvest

- Its best for the operator to be positioned across the table from the donor site (on right side for left PAP flap) for better posture.
- Lithotomy position, when possible, ensures the most comfortable access to flap territory.

Jejunal flap (mucosal flap—segmental blood supply)

Introduction

The free jejunal flap was first described in 1959, transferred to a pharyngo-oesophageal defect. The second or third loop is used as a free flap.

Anatomy

The anatomy of the jejunal flap is demonstrated in Figure 2.1.7.

- Artery—jejunal artery 1.5–3 mm diameter
- Vein—jejunal veins 2–4 mm diameter
- Pedicle—up to 20 cm

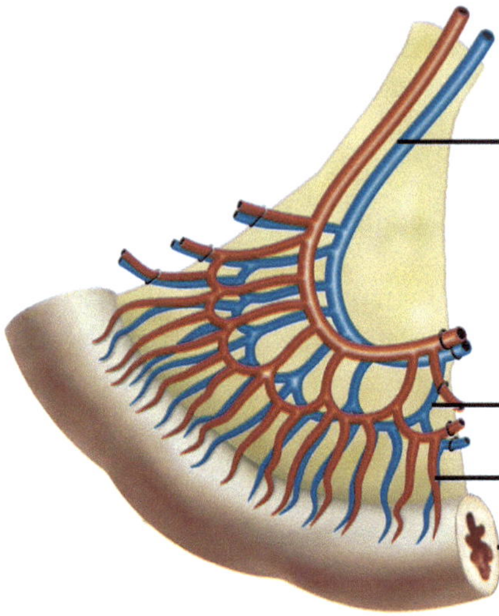

Figure 2.1.7 Schematic presentation of the jejunal flap key anatomy. The figure demonstrates a jejunum segment that can be used for circumferential (tube) reconstruction of oesophageal defects. Note the segmental blood supply of the jejunum, which relies on vascular arcades (loops) that may have one or two orders prior to supplying vasa rectus blood vessels that nourish the jejunum.

- Innervation—none
- Flap size—7–25 cm in length

Indications

- Oesophagus
- Hypopharynx

Advantages

- The tubed structure and good diameter makes it ideal for pharyngeal and oesophageal reconstructions.
- The accompanying mesentery can provide additional soft tissue bulk/cover.
- Lubricated and peristaltic.
- Robust blood supply with the large diameter vessels.

Disadvantages

- Requires entry into the intra-abdominal space.
- Limited ischaemia time tolerance.
- Fistulas/leaks in this type of reconstruction carry high morbidity.

Harvest technique

Preoperative considerations

No vascular studies are required, however a thorough history to reveal contraindications such as inflammatory bowel disease is vital. Bowel preparation is performed the night before surgery.

Flap markings

A standard midline laparotomy incision is marked.

Technique for harvest

- Patient is in a supine position and a midline laparotomy is performed to access intraperitoneal space.
- The transverse colon and stomach are retracted to expose the small intestine and the ligament of Treitz.
- The small bowel is traced approximately 40–60 cm from the ligament of Treitz, where supply from the second or third branch from the superior mesenteric artery (SMA) is found.
- An adequate length of jejunum is excised after placing bowel-clamps on either side, ensuring the most proximal of possible vascular pedicles from the SMA is supplying the segment.
- The accompanying mesentery at either side of the chosen vascular pedicle is carefully ligated off/freed.
- The resulting defect in the small bowel is closed by primary anastomosis.

Technical modifications

- Harvest can be performed open or laparoscopic (the standard nowadays).
- Can be inset double-barrelled, i.e. folded and connected proximally to match a larger required diameter.

Donor-site management

- The abdomen is closed as per standard fashion.

Tips for harvest

- Transillumination of the mesentery with a flashlight reveals the vasculature for safe division.
- Peristaltic motion from the intrinsic autonomic nervous system remains and thus one must inset in an antegrade fashion.
- Mark either the proximal and distal end of the jejunum with sutures to ensure you perform an anastomosis to the hypopharynx/oesophagus in the correct peristaltic direction.
- Supercharging the pedicle jejunal flap for oesophageal reconstruction could minimize complications rate.

2.2 Bone flaps in head and neck reconstruction

Introduction

The chapter discusses the most commonly used bony flaps in head and neck reconstruction namely the fibula flap, the scapula flap and the deep circumflex iliac artery (DCIA) flap. Its subchapter describes the basic anatomical information, the technique of harvest as well as tips for easier harvest and avoidance of complications.

The operator needs to know that bony flaps harvest subject the patient to higher peri-operative and postoperative stress and careful patient and case selection is required based on thorough anaesthetic and preoperative assessment taking into account the parameters discussed in Chapter 2.4.

Fibula flap

Introduction

The fibula free flap (FFF) was introduced by Taylor and Ham in 1975. It was first used for mandibular reconstruction in 1989. It has evolved to become the workhorse flap for bony mandibular reconstruction. With modern 3D planning techniques it can be combined with condylar component for temporomandibular joint replacement (Figure 2.1.1).

Anatomy

The anatomy of the fibula flap is demonstrated in Figure 2.2.2.

- Artery: Peroneal artery (1.5–2.5 mm diameter)
- Vein: Two VCs (2–4 mm diameter)
- Pedicle length: 2–6 cm (largely depends on the bone segment length)
- Innervation: Lateral sural nerve
- Flap size: 26 cm length of bone in an adult. Max 14×32 cm skin (3–4 cm width allows primary closure)

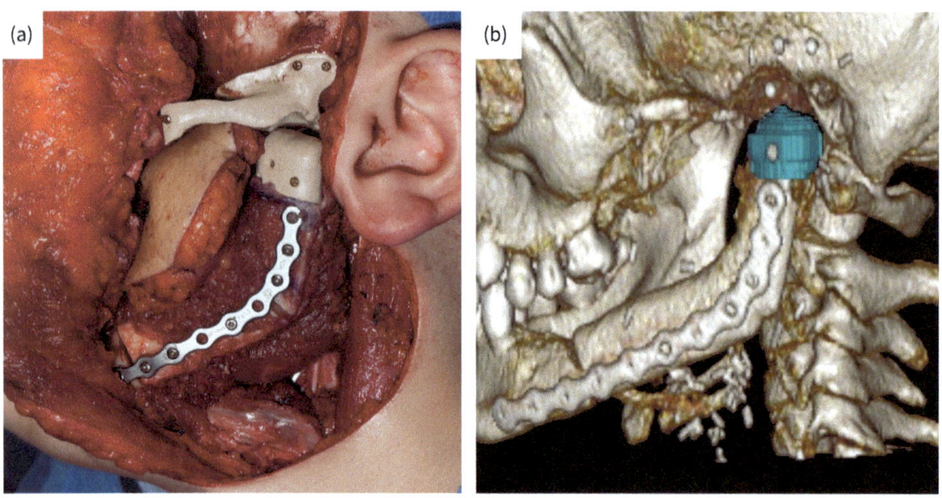

Figure 2.2.1 Left-sided total hemi-mandibulectomy including condylar disarticulation and temporo-mandibular joint articular resection for osteosarcoma. a. Note the fibula flap contoured and in position with the skin paddle for intraoral cover. Prior 3D planning and 3D printing has allowed the construction of a custom-made TMJ implant. Note the condylar component fixed to the fibula. b. Postoperative CT scan demonstrating the fibula free flap with the condylar component in place and the precision of contouring and inset of the flap.

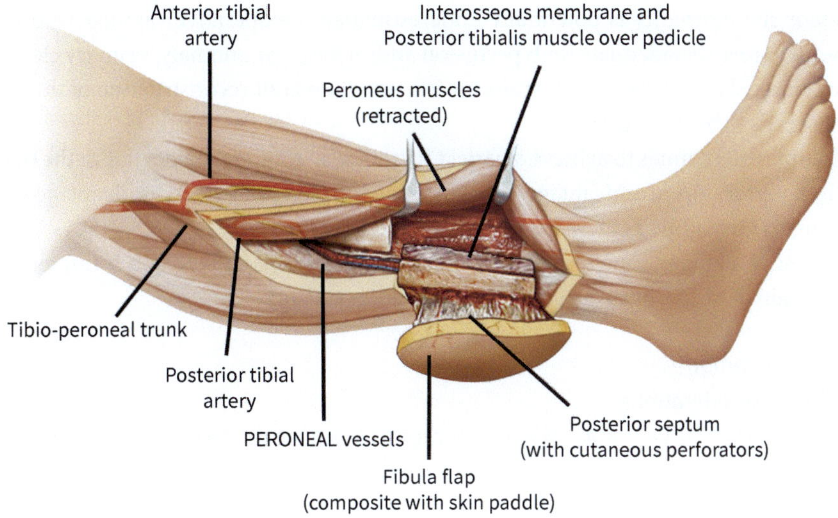

Figure 2.2.2 Schematic presentation of the fibula flap key anatomy. Note at the lower leg, the fibula flap osteotomized and mobilized, carrying the posterior septum that transverses the cutaneous perforators and the respective skin paddle (composite osseocutaneous fibula flap). More proximally and past the popliteal fossa, note the tibio-peroneal trunk that bifurcates into posterior tibial and peroneal vessels. The anterior tibial artery comes off the popliteal artery more proximally. This is the typical lower leg three-vessel run-off configuration. Note that in the lower leg, the anterior tibial artery can often be very close and almost behind the anterior septum (crura); hence dissection deeper to the anterior (superior) fibula free edge has to be careful in order to avoid its inadvertent injury.

Adapted with permission from Raising of Microvascular Flaps: A Systematic Approach, 2nd Edition. Editors Wolff K.-D., Hölzle F.: Springer—Verlag Berlin Heidelberg; 2011. Chapter: Fibula flap 105–30, Page 115: Arteries of the lower leg and Page 127: Flap raising completed.

Indications

- Mandible defects
- Maxillary defects
- Orbital and periorbital subunits

Advantages

- Long vascularized bony segment
- Robust periosteal blood supply that enables survival of osteotomized segments
- Wide diameter pedicle
- Potential to include both skin and muscle with the bone (usually harvested as osseomyocutaneous flap)

Disadvantages

- Steep learning curve for the technique of harvest and inset. This has now improved with the introduction of patient-specific planning and 3D printing.

- Donor site morbidity is potentially underestimated. Preoperative vascular studies are useful to reveal inadequate limb perfusion and/or vascular anomaly. Primary closure is discouraged as compartment syndrome is a risk. Skin graft reconstruction of the donor side needs to be meticulous.
- Multiple osteotomies to achieve a perfect mandibular contour can devitalize the bone.
- Distal perforators are advantageous to ensure a longer pedicle, but disadvantageous for a longer skin paddle as there is a risk of proximal necrosis.
- Harvest of a longer bone segment will shorten the pedicle—the length is limited up to the origin of the peroneal artery at the tibioperoneal trunk.

Harvesting technique

Preoperative considerations

A CT angiography (CTA) or an MR angiography (MRA) must be performed to evaluate the anatomy of the tibioperoneal trunk, the vessel patency, and the perfusion of the lower limb.

The majority of population (88%) has normal vascular anatomy of the lower limb. However vascular variations (absent anterior tibial artery 3.8%, absent posterior tibial artery 1.6%, peroneal artery magna 0.2%, absent peroneal artery <0.1% and long tibioperoneal trunk <0.1%) may be encountered rendering the fibula inappropriate for harvesting.

A CTA is preferable in diabetic patients, where it can reveal microcalcifications; this may point out towards selecting another bony flap. A hand-held Doppler is used prior to commencing the procedure, to identify the perforators and help orient the skin paddle.

A CTA is useful in 3D planning, as this type of imaging in contrast to magnetic resonance is suitable for virtual planning software.

Flap markings

The head of the fibula, and the lateral malleolus are the landmarks for the flap harvesting procedure. A straight line drawn between those two landmarks indicates the position of the intermuscular septum. Perforators are found at approximately 5 cm, 10 cm, and 15 cm cranial from the lateral malleolus and most commonly along the posterior fibula margin.

The skin component

1. Patient is positioned supine, with the leg flexed at the knee. The use of a tourniquet on the thigh is optional and up to the surgeon's preference. If is used, it must not stay inflated for over 90 minutes. Use of half or folded bean bag can provide stable support the leg in the desired position. A pulse oximeter can be placed on the toe to monitor perfusion. It is also advised that the dorsal aspect of the foot is left exposed from the drapes to allow palpation of the dorsalis pedis pulse.
2. The skin paddle is incised anteriorly, using a defensive approach. Suprafascial dissection is carried out until the tendon of the peroneus longus is reached, at which point the fascia is incised and the dissection continues in a subfascial level.
3. The fascia is reflected and dissected towards the posterior crural septum (between the peroneus muscles and the soleus). Perforators are identified and marked with

methylene blue. Most surgeons would consider an alternative flap in the absence of reliable septocutaneous perforators.

4. The dissection begins by incising the anterior crural septum. This allows entry into the anterior compartment and by release of the peroneal muscles from the fibula bone. It is important to note that when passing from the lateral to the anterior compartment the direction of dissection has to change pointing sharply downwards once the anterior border of the fibula is met. This is because of the shape of the anterior fibula surface where the bone bows in sharply passed the anterior border rim (Figure 2.2.3). Continuation of the direction of the dissection deep to the anterior crura pointing medially without inwards curving might risk injuring the anterior tibial vessels, especially in patients with thin legs.
5. Detachment of the extensor muscles off the anterior surface of the fibula will lead to the interosseous membrane. The anterior compartment is dissected away, protecting the deep peroneal nerve and the anterior tibial vessels (ATv). It is useful to visualize the anterior tibial artery pedicle, ensuring that this remains protected especially prior to the osteotomies.

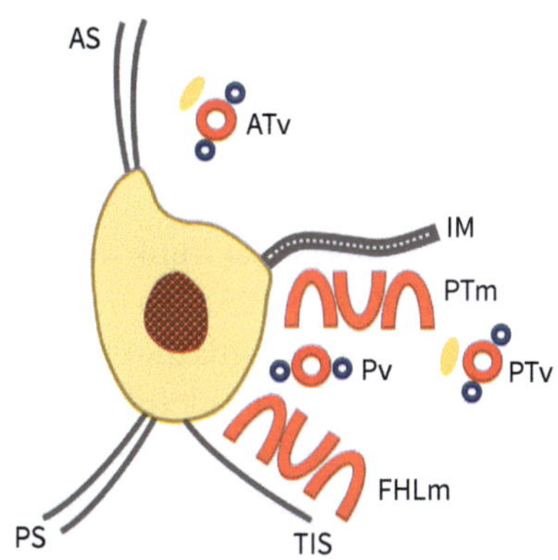

Figure 2.2.3 Cross-sectional topography of fibula flap anatomy. Note the shape of the fibula bone and especially the anterior (superior) free bone edge that sharply dives in, past the anterior septum towards the anterior muscle compartment. The anterior tibial vessels (ATv) are variably but closely related to the deep aspect of the anterior septum. Hence the operator at this point after dividing the anterior septum must change the direction of the dissection, aiming deep (posteriorly) in order to remain intimate to the bone surface and avoid the ATVs. As the dissection continues and immediately beneath the interosseous membrane (IM) the operator will encounter the chevron muscle fibres of the posterior tibial muscle (PTm). The latter need to be divided in order to deroof the superior aspect of the peroneal vessels (PV). Completion of flap mobilization requires division of the flexor hallucis longus muscle (FHLm). Once this is achieved, division of the transverse intermuscular septum (TIS) is required. For the inexperienced operator, this fibrous membrane may cause confusion with the posterior septum (PS). The two are completely separate facial layers, the posterior septum which contains the perforators and supports the skin paddle once it has been mobilized can be retracted superiorly and held together with a bony flap in order to allow division of the TIS and partial harvest of the soleus muscle if required.

6. Prior to the bone osteotomies, a periosteal elevator is inserted in a subperiosteal plane, to protect the underlying vascular pedicle. Around 6 cm of fibula bone must be spared at its cranial end and about 6–8 cm at the lateral malleolus, to ensure stability of the ankle joint. The introduction of the piezoelectric saw has revolutionized the bone osteotomies, ensuring maximum protection of the adjacent soft tissues.
7. Once the bone osteotomies have bene completed, bone holding clamps are applied at each end of the fibula to allow traction and external rotational movement to facilitate dissection.
8. The interosseous membrane in incised to reveal the tibialis posterior muscle and its characteristic chevron-like appearance. The peroneal pedicle lies between tibialis posterior and flexor hallucis longus. The pedicle is carefully unroofed and dissected.
9. The distal end of the peroneal pedicle is prepared for ligation. It is advised that at this stage and when a tourniquet is not used that the pedicle is temporarily clamped and the perfusion of the foot is assessed. Palpation of the dorsalis pedis and posterior tibial artery and normal saturations from the pulse oximeter attached to the big toe provide the operator with the assurance to proceed with division of the pedicle. Often the peroneal artery distally gives off a communicating branch. The operator must be aware of this to avoid confusion. It is strongly advised that the anterior tibial pedicle is visualized in its plane on the lateral aspect of the extensors and above the interosseous membrane prior to proceeding to the definitive move of ligating the peroneal artery distally. The operator must be absolutely confident and certain of the anatomy at this point.
10. The pedicle is followed to the tibioperoneal trunk. Identification of the posterior tibial nerve medial to the pedicle signifies proximity to the posterior tibial main pedicle and the dissection must proceed carefully towards the bifurcation.
11. In order to fully mobilize the flap the skin paddle has to be completely dissected via the 'back-cut'. The posterior margin of the skin paddle is incised through the deep fascia, taking care to protect the lesser saphenous vein and lateral sural nerve, which are reflected away.
12. The soleus muscle is dissected off the skin paddle and the posterior crural septum. Intramuscular cutaneous perforators through soleus could in theory be used as a back-up.
13. The flap is elevated by releasing the last underlying fascial attachment. The pedicle is then followed proximally and skeletonized in preparation for disconnection. The flap is left to rest in as natural position as possible and its perfusion is checked. At this point it is crucial to mark with ink the superior aspect of the pedicle in its whole length. This step will prove useful during the inset and microvascular vessel preparation, to guide correct orientation of the pedicle and avoidance of torsion or kinking especially through the tunnel.
14. Prior to detaching the flap, and in order to reduce ischaemia time, any preplanned osteotomies can be performed with the use of 3D-printed guides.

Important tips in harvesting the FFF are highlighted in Box 2.2.1.

Box 2.2.1 Tips for harvesting the FFF flap

- In order to ensure maximum safety for foot perfusion, use a saturation probe on the first toe (ATA), and also through palpation of the dorsalis pedis prior and after clamping the peroneal vessels.
- It is recommended to clamp the peroneal vessels distally prior to division in order to ensure stable and constant perfusion of the foot as described above.
- The peroneal vessels are always DEEP (beneath) to the interosseous membrane. The distal leg anatomy close to the ankle joint can occasionally be confusing. The first pedicle encountered may be the anterior tibial vessels. Appropriate tests both anatomical and perfusion based need to be taken prior to deciding to ligate and divide the peroneal vessels as described above.
- Having de-roofed and exposed the peroneal vessels all the way up, proximally, and when performing the back cut of the osseocutaneous FFF, note that the transverse intramuscular septum (TIS) can be safely divided. This can occasionally cause confusion for the operator. The transfers intramuscular septum (TIS) is separate to the posterior septum that harbours the peroneal perforators.

Technical modifications

- *Muscle transfer*

The soleus muscle can be included in the flap, should there is a need for bulk. One can spare the supplying branch to the soleus coming off the peroneal artery, seen at its proximal end during the final step of the fibula harvest. The disadvantage of its inclusion is a resulting short pedicle, and increased donor site complications.

The flexor hallucis longus (FHL) can also be included with the fibula bone as it derives its main blood supply from the peroneal artery, and it is so closely linked to the peroneal system that this transfer is effortless and causes the least donor site morbidity (compared to soleus muscle transfer).

- *Two skin paddles*

A superior and inferior skin paddle can be designed if one includes the main superior peroneal septocutaneous perforator. This allows soft tissue coverage of complex intraoral and extraoral defects. However, it reduces the possible pedicle length.

- *Prefabrication/Prelamination*

Modern 3D methodologies allow prefabrication with dental implants and even artificial dermis for 'jaw in a day' reconstructions, mainly for non-cancerous diagnoses (See Vassiliou et al in further reading).

Donor site management

- Smaller skin paddles can allow for primary closure (up to 4 cm width); however, skin grafting is preferred to avoid tight closure and subsequent compartment syndrome. A split-thickness skin graft from the ipsilateral thigh is the preferred option; the leg is stabilized in an orthopaedic boot to minimize skin graft mobility.

Tips

- Commonly harvesting approach is anterior to posterior. A posterior to anterior approach is also possible.
- More than two osteotomies are discouraged when the length of one or more segments is less than 3.5 cm.
- In the absence of septocutaneous perforators, the surgeon should consider alternative soft tissue flap options.

Deep circumflex iliac artery flap (DCIA)

Introduction

The anatomy of the deep circumflex iliac artery (DCIA) and its ability to supply the iliac bone, the internal oblique muscle, and the overlying skin, was established by Taylor in 1979.

Anatomy

The anatomy of the DCIA flap is demonstrated in Figure 2.2.4.

- Artery: DCIA (1.5–3 cm diameter)
- Vein: Deep circumflex iliac vein (2.5– 3 mm diameter)
- Pedicle length: Up to 7–8 cm, heavily dependent on body habitus
- Innervation: None
- Flap size: 15×6 cm bone, 8×20 cm skin paddle

Indications

- Mandible defects
- Maxillary defects

Advantages

- Good bone height to support dental implants.
- Good contour for mandibular reconstruction.
- Excellent shape for high maxillary defects—facial projection

Disadvantages

- Short vascular pedicle
- Bulky skin paddle

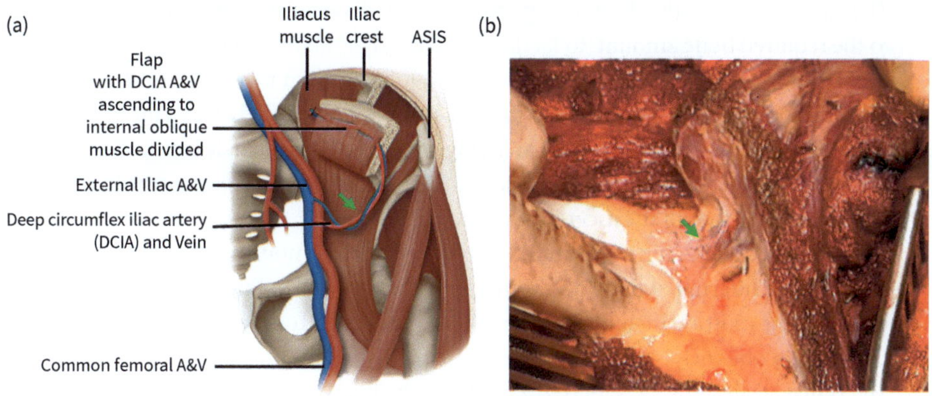

Figure 2.2.4 Presentation of the deep circumflex iliac artery (DCIA) flap key anatomy. a. Schematic presentation of the iliac crest and the relevant blood supply for harvesting a DCIA flap. Note the external iliac vessels that provide the DCIA that courses initially on the medial aspect of the iliacus muscle prior to entering it. The pedicle can be located approximately a centimetre below and medially to the anterior superior iliac spine (ASIS). The flap can be contoured to match the defect. The flap can contain part of the internal oblique muscle as the DCIA vessels continue into the ascending branch that enters and supplies the internal oblique muscle. b. Interoperative photograph showing the DCIA pedicle entering the iliacus muscle that supplies the DCIA flap. Note that the tranversus abdominus and internal oblique muscles (above) have been divided to provide access to the pre-peritoneal area in order to identify and dissect the DCIA vessels to their origins.

- Relatively high donor site morbidity, including hematoma, hernia formation, pain, waist deformity
- More suitable for lateral mandibular defects and anterior chin defects

Harvesting technique

Preoperative considerations

Advanced imaging is not necessary. PSP 3D planning is advisable to minimize lateral gluteus muscles dissection.

Flap markings

Landmarks include the anterior superior iliac spine, the inguinal ligament, and the femoral vessels at the mid-inguinal point. The skin incision line is placed 2 cm medially and parallel to the iliac crest for myo-osseous flaps. If an osseomyocutaneous flap is planned, a skin ellipse centred over the iliac crest is designed. The proximal end is marked out 2 cm superior to the inguinal ligament.

Technique

1. The patient is in a supine position, with a sandbag under the hip.
2. The external oblique muscle is exposed and incised—care must be taken to separate muscle fibres to avoid bleeding and aid closure. The plane between external and internal oblique is easily defined. The internal oblique muscle is exposed in its entirety.

3. The lateral aspect of the ilium is exposed by sharp dissection of the gluteus muscles, up to the required bone amount, to facilitate insertion of the PSP/3D guide.
4. The DCIA pedicle is always constant, and it's located 1 cm medially and 1 cm deep to the anterior superior iliac spine (ASIS). The pedicle is identified by careful dissection of the internal oblique muscle in that area (Figure 2.2.4b). The pedicle is traced towards its origin at the iliac (or the femoral) vessels. Care must be taken to identify any possible anatomic variations of the ascending branch.
5. The internal oblique muscle is marked to the required amount and incised. The plane between the internal oblique and transversalis is not well defined; the fascia overlying transversalis must be included, as the ascending branch travels between the fascia and the internal oblique.
6. The transversalis muscle is incised 2 cm from the iliac crest, to reveal the preperitoneal fat. A cuff of iliacus is also taken to ensure the DCIA is included, as it travels between transversalis and iliacus.
7. The bone osteotomies are performed according to the preoperative plan.
8. Prior to disconnection the flap is left to rest in its natural position and its perfusion is checked. At this point it is crucial to mark with ink the superior aspect of the pedicle in its whole length. This step will prove useful during the inset and microvascular vessel preparation, to guide correct orientation of the pedicle and avoidance of torsion or kinking especially through the tunnel.

Technical modifications

Multiple osteotomies

The used bone receives its blood supply through the inner table, and therefore, the outer table could be severed longitudinally given that the periosteum of the inner table and the iliacus transferred with the bone remains intact. The inclusion of the above-mentioned size-able perforating branches can aid in planning the osteotomies, so that each segment receives a perforator when possible.

Donor site management

Donor site closure must be meticulous, in a multilayer fashion. The iliacus is sutured to transversalis and a propylene mesh is used to cover the internal oblique defect, anchored on the ilium bone to prevent hernias. Suction drains are used, and an infusion catheter is inserted for analgesia.

Tips

- The lateral cutaneous nerve of the thigh, which is divided in the harvest, can be resutured to limit morbidity from the harvest.
- When a skin paddle is needed, it is helpful to expose the pedicle more proximally to locate the DCIA and the superficial circumflex iliac artery (SCIA). If the SCIA and DCIA do not share a common trunk, one can opt for an alternative skin flap like ALT.

Alternatively, one can consider including the cutaneous perforators that travel through all three abdominal wall muscles. This will result in significant bulk.

- Inclusion of a superficial vein is recommended when a skin flap based on the SCIA is planned, as the superficial circumflex iliac vein (SCIV) can be very small in diameter.
- The perforating branches that perforate the iliacus to supply the bone can be skeletonized to minimize the muscular cuff and therefore the bulk of the bone, and also to minimize the donor site morbidity following the transfer of a large chunk of the iliacus muscle along with a large bone segment.

Scapula flap

Introduction

Saijo was the first to describe a composite osseocutaneous flap based on the circumflex scapular artery (CSA), whereas Swartz has previously described the composite osseocutaneous flap based on the thoracodorsal vessels and the tip of the scapula bone.

Anatomy

The anatomy of the scapula flap is demonstrated in Figure 2.2.5.

- Artery: Circumflex scapular artery (2–3 cm diameter), thoracodorsal artery (1–2 cm diameter)
- Vein: Circumflex scapular vein (3–4 cm diameter), thoracodorsal vein (1–2 cm diameter)

If both systems are to be used, then the subscapular artery and vein can be utilized; however, the very short length of the subscapular pedicle (2 cm) and the mismatch with donor neck vessels make its utility difficult.

- Pedicle length: Up to 5–6 cm for the CSA, over 15 cm for the TD
- Innervation: Thoracodorsal nerve
- Flap size: 12×3 cm bone, 14×24 cm skin paddle

Indication

- Mandible defects
- Maxillary defects
- When soft tissue requirement is a priority over bone reconstruction

Advantages

- Consistent anatomy and easy dissection
- Good contour for palate/maxillary reconstruction
- Pedicle length in case of TD—scapula tip flap
- Robust vessel quality
- Low donor site morbidity

Disadvantages

- Short vascular pedicle if CSA is selected
- Thin bone—difficult dental rehabilitation
- Two-team approach very difficult

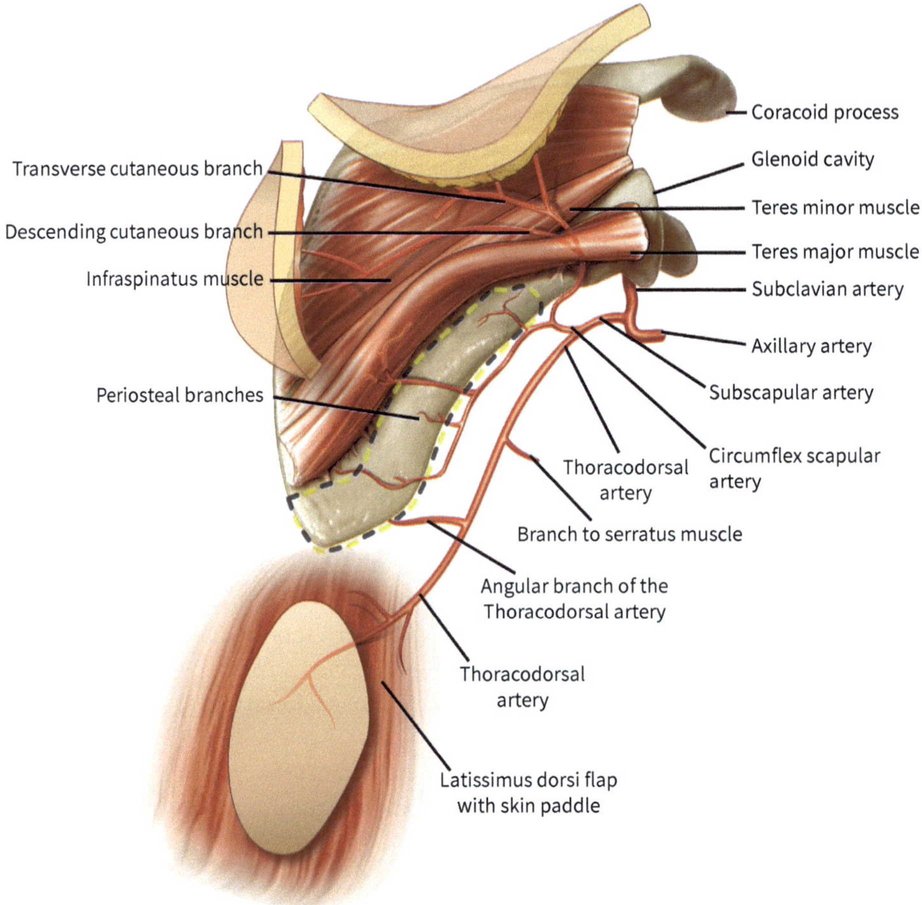

Figure 2.2.5 Schematic presentation of the scapular flap key anatomy. Note the main scapular bone anatomy including the glenoid cavity. For a composite scapular flap, a skin paddle can be included. The latter can be supplied by either the transverse or descending subcutaneous branches of the circumflex scapular artery. Note that the latter transverses through the triangular space (boundaries are the teres major, the teres minor, and the long head of the triceps muscle). When harvesting a scapula flap, upon identification of the most superficial area of the circumflex scapular artery the teres major has to be divided to provide access for dissection of the vascular pedicle further proximally. Note that the subscapular artery divides into the circumflex scapular artery and also the thoracodorsal artery that continues distally and also provides another significant blood vessel (angular branch) that supplies the lower part of the scapula bone (tip of the scapula). A more composite flap (mega-flap) can be harvested with the inclusion of the thoracodorsal artery that can also provide muscle and cutaneous component (myocutaneous paddle).

Adapted with permission from Raising of Microvascular Flaps: A Systematic Approach, 2nd Edition. Editors Wolff K.-D., Hölzle F.: Springer-Verlag Berlin Heidelberg; 2011. Chapter: Scapular Flap 81–104, Page 101: Vascular anatomy of the osteocutaneous scapular flap.

Harvesting technique

Preoperative considerations

The most important preoperative consideration is to decide which pedicle to utilize. This will depend on the required bone length and whether osteotomies need to be performed. A straight segment of bone up to 8 cm can safely be supplied by the angular branch and the TD pedicle, whereas longer segments and/or requirement of osteotomies require taking the CSA. One could consider taking all of the lateral border of the scapular bone by incorporating both vascular pedicles and dissecting up to and including the SA or by considering separate anastomoses for both pedicles. Advanced imaging is not necessary. PSP 3D planning is advisable.

Flap markings

Landmarks include the lateral border of the scapula and the triangular space, which transmits the CSA. This is identified with the use of a hand-held Doppler prior to the start of the procedure.

Technique

1. The patient is positioned in the lateral decubitus position, with the arm extended on an arm gutter, to allow access to the axilla.
2. For a TD-scapula tip flap, the skin paddle is centred over the latissimus dorsi muscle, aiming to incorporate both the horizontal and the vertical cutaneous branches. For a CSA flap, the skin paddle is usually centred over the course of the transverse cutaneous branch of the CSA, although parascapular skin paddles incorporating the descending cutaneous branch can also be considered.
3. Following skin incision, the most important step is to identify and outline the interface between the latissimus dorsi muscle and the teres major muscle. Sharp dissection of the fascia overlying the teres major will safely lead into the triangular space.
4. For a TD-scapula tip flap, the latissimus dorsi muscle is dissected in a similar fashion as the soft tissue flap (Figure 2.2.6). Care must be taken not to divide the branch to the serratus anterior until the angular branch is identified, as this can arise from the branch to the serratus anterior in 48%.
5. Once the TD pedicle and the angular branch are dissected, the teres major muscle is detached from the scapula bone and the preplanned osteotomies are made.
6. For a CSA flap, the pedicle must be identified and dissected in the triangular space. This often requires division of the teres major, which needs to be repaired during donor site closure.
7. The periosteal CSA branches are protected by including an adequate cuff of subscapularis to the bone osteotomy. The cutaneous paddle needs to be carefully dissected, allowing mobility, but there is no need to be skeletonized up to the CSA.
8. Prior to disconnection the flap is left to rest in its natural position and its perfusion is checked. At this point it is crucial to mark with ink the superior aspect of the pedicle in its whole length. This step will prove useful during the inset and microvascular vessel preparation, to guide correct orientation of the pedicle and avoidance of torsion or kinking especially through the tunnel.

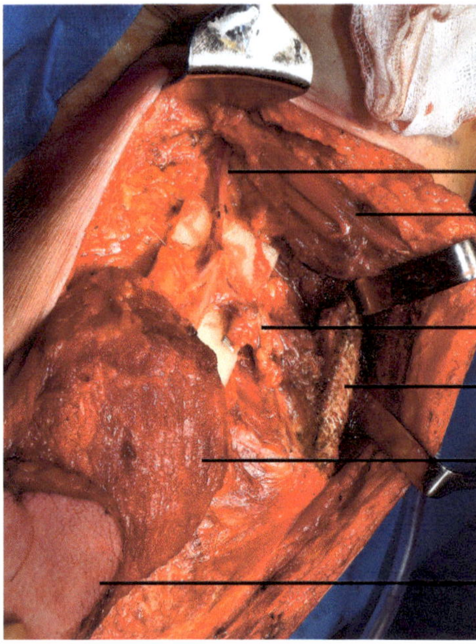

Figure 2.2.6 Intraoperative photograph of composite latissimus dorsi and scapula tip flap. Note at the top, the thoracodorsal artery is dissected. At the top right part of the clinical photograph, the teres major muscle has been retracted superiorly, and the lateral edge of the scapula has been exposed. The latter is nourished by the angular branch of the thoracodorsal artery (dissected). The composite flap contains a sizeable part of the latissimus dorsi flap (muscle component) and a myocutaneous island containing a skin paddle for reconstruction of a large lower face defect.

Multiple osteotomies

Osteotomies are possible when the CSA system is utilized, but they shouldn't be more than one and every effort should be made to preserve the periosteum.

Donor site management

Donor site closure includes repair or resuspension of the teres major. Suction drains are used, and an infusion catheter is inserted for analgesia.

Tips

- The TD-angular chimeric flap is easier to harvest and will suffice for most cases.
- An adequate soft tissue cuff is required around the scapula tip to protect the angular branch.
- The CSA gives substantial branches to the teres major that require control and ligation.
- Adequate exposure is key regardless of which pedicle is to be utilized.

2.3 Body habitus and anatomical considerations: Appropriate choice of flap

Introduction

The selection of the most appropriate free flap differs from patient to patient and depends on the body habitus and other anatomical considerations. Optimum choice of flap in terms of pliability, size, and volume is critical for a functional and aesthetic outcome.

The flap of choice should be selected carefully based on defect-specific parameters as well as donor site assessment and patient-specific criteria.

Defect parameters: Size—site(s)—depth

The general principle of reconstruction is to 'replace like with like'. Large size (over T3 stage) oral and head neck defects can be categorized as follows:

- Predominantly surface +/– composite
- Predominantly depth +/– composite
- Complex three-dimensional

Predominantly surface +/– composite defects

The first type is predominantly 'wide' surface defects and may extend to include different subsites of the oral cavity and/or the oropharynx. These are, for example, defects deriving from ablation of T3 or larger tumours encompassing, for example, the retromolar trigone, palatoglossal fold, lateral pharyngeal wall, and lateral floor of mouth or tongue. In this scenario, large (in surface) but pliable flaps are required. This can be achieved by fasciocutaneous flaps. A radial forearm free flap is the workhorse in soft tissue oral reconstruction, but it may not be able to provide adequate width to cover the defect. An ALT flap may be more appropriate. In relatively thin patients, a latissimus dorsi may be pliable enough to be contoured to match the defect. Additionally, regional flaps such as the supraclavicular island flap (SCAIF) carry less morbidity and still achieve the goal.

Predominantly depth +/- composite defects

The second type of defects refers to 'high-volume ablative defects'. In such a case, and if the patient is of slim body type, then musculocutaneous flaps may add an extra layer of cover (muscle layer) and still remain flexible and pliable enough to provide cover for essentially more than one anatomical subsite.

It is always important to prioritize reconstruction of the floor of the mouth and midline areas such as the base of the tongue or oral tongue defects, as these are areas at risk of resulting in communication between the oral cavity and neck, which can be significantly troublesome. Oral–neck communication can result in delayed healing or cutaneous fistulas, vascular complications (even carotid blowout), or functional problems.

High-volume defects, especially those involving midline structures such as through and through floor of mouth defects, subtotal or total glossectomies, and resections involving most of the tongue, require flaps that provide bulk and robust volume aside from surface cover. To this end, the selection process should be directed more towards musculocutaneous flaps, such as:

- Latissimus dorsi flap
- Rectus abdominis flap
- ALT flap, including part of the vastus lateralis

A pectoralis major flap may always be considered, especially in patients who aren't medically fit enough for free flap reconstruction.

Complex three-dimensional defects

- Complex three-dimensional defects, especially those incorporating intraoral and extraoral components are difficult to treat. For those large fasciocutaneous or osseocutaneous flaps, the skin paddle can be split into two separate islands, one used to close the intraoral defect and one for the external skin. Alternatively, a 'thick' myocutaneous flap with a split-thickness skin graft can be used. In these cases, it is preferable to inset the skin paddle intraorally and split skin graft the extraoral defect. The opposite will cause intraoral scar contracture of the muscle and long-term trismus—aside from the fact that it is difficult to immobilize a skin graft intraorally.
- Another solution for complex three-dimensional head neck defects is multicomponent free flaps, such as the latissimus dorsi and scapula 'mega-flap' or the tripartite deep circumflex iliac artery (DCIA) flap. The first incorporates a myocutaneous skin paddle based on the thoracodorsal vessels and a bony component based on the scapular angular pedicle or the scapular circumflex pedicle. The latter is an osseomuscular flap encompassing the bony ilium with a variable portion of the internal oblique muscle, plus a fasciocutaneous skin island based on the associated cutaneous perforator.
- Dual flap reconstruction to cover extensive defects often is required and may include predominantly one osseocutaneous flap for skeletal reconstruction plus a second fasciocutaneous or myocutaneous flap for surface cover. In practice, this could include complex low face defects of the mandible, skin, and tongue, or three-dimensional midface defects including facial skin. Dual flap reconstruction increases the duration of surgery, it adds morbidity, and is not appropriate for compromised patients. We do not advocate this approach if the defect can be addressed with a single flap (either an LD or an ALT flap).

Individualized patient-specific reconstruction planning

Nowadays with the advancements of medical imaging and 3D planning and printing technology patient-specific reconstruction planning is becoming the norm. The process mainly refers to executing bone-associated reconstructions by preoperative detailed planning of the exact osteotomies on the defect site and on the flap donor site to allow precise match of the bony flap into the defect with predictable cosmetic outcomes. The process is facilitated through 3D-printed cutting guides and a prefabricated reconstruction plate that reduce operative time and guarantee a seamless direct fit of the flap into the defect. The process is further supplemented with guides facilitating dental implants insertion and even immediate application of a dental rehabilitation suprastructure as described by Vassilliou et al. in 'Further reading'.

Body habitus

It is important to assess the patient globally and not just determine the type of reconstruction based on the scans or the 'textbook' recommendations. Every patient has a different build. For example, a posterior maxillary reconstruction in a patient with medical conditions not fit for microvascular free transfer could be easily achieved with a pectoralis major flap if the patient has a short neck and a long torso (for this scenario and depending on the bony maxillary defect, an obturator would also be a valid reconstructive option).

It is important to carefully assess the build of the patient to decide for the most appropriate reconstruction.

ALT flap

The anterolateral thigh flap is a versatile flap that can provide large 'surface' cover and also bulk, depending on:

1. The patient's build and body habitus
2. The harvest technique
3. Whether part of the vastus lateralis is harvested.

It is crucial to examine the patient's lower limbs when an ALT flap is considered.

Appropriate case selection, harvesting technique and reconstructive planning with the ALT flap can achieve a 'dome' creation (Figure 2.3.1) of the new construct, enabling contact of the food bolus between the roof of the mouth and neo-tongue, crucial for the functionality of the neo-tongue.

In such scenarios, if the base of tongue and the hypoglossal nerve(s) are preserved, this can provide sufficient support and 'shielding' of the glottic area during the oro-pharyngeal phase of swallowing.

The presence of dominant fasciocutaneous perforators differs between different ethnic backgrounds and this must be considered in the preoperative planning, as demonstrated by Peirong Yu in 'Characteristics of the anterolateral thigh flap in a Western population and its application in head and neck reconstruction' (see 'Further reading').

The ALT flap is a perforator flap and effectively the profusion of the skin component relies on one or two delicate perforator vessels. The risk of skin paddle necrosis increases with the length of the perforator required, as it travels between tissue layers before reaching the dermal microcirculation. To this end, an ALT flap may be an excellent choice for a large soft tissue defect on a relatively slim patient, in a defect that requires spanning over one or two anatomical subsites of the oral cavity.

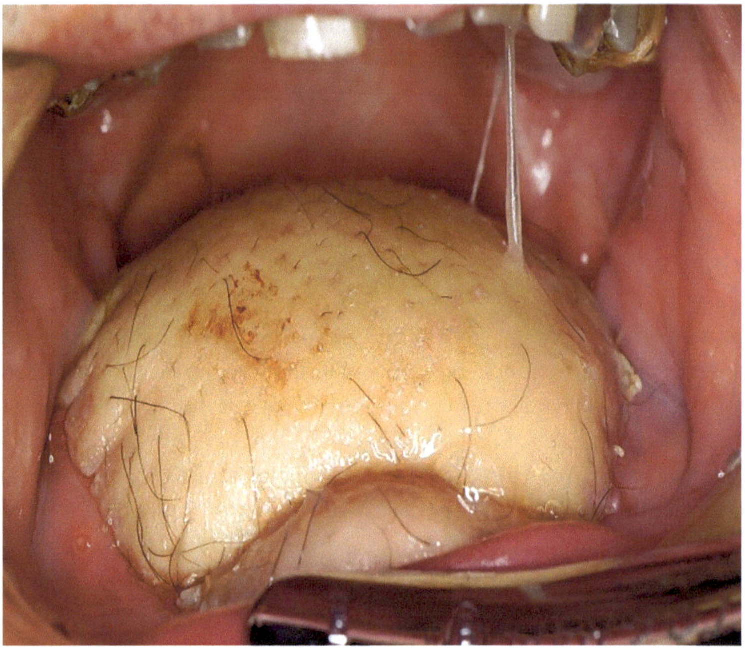

Figure 2.3.1 Subtotal glossectomy reconstructed with an ALT flap and good swallowing function. Note the 'dome' shaped neo-tongue that enables *'tongue-to-roof of mouth'* contact.

An ALT flap offers ample pliability and versatility, providing an excellent reconstruction. However, the opposite is true in a patient whose thigh is of a large diameter: A fasciocutaneous subfascially harvested ALT flap, even sparing the vastus lateralis component, may be too bulky or difficult to inset and may be predisposed to ischaemia of the skin paddle as the perforator flap may be subject to kinking or pressure.

Different harvesting techniques have been described to allow differential thickness of the ALT skin paddle. While subfascial (below plane of deep fascia) harvest offers maximum perforator protection, suprafascial (above plane of deep fascia) and even superficial fascia (just below plane of superficial scarpa fascial) harvest techniques have been described to obtain a thinner ALT flap (see Tuluy et al. in 'Further reading').

Latissimus dorsi flap

A latissimus dorsi flap is an appropriate flap for subtotal or total glossectomies or complex 'high-volume' defects that incorporate areas of the tongue or different combinations of floor of mouth, tongue, buccal, palatal, and oropharyngeal areas. The LD flap is relatively pliable and on an average body habitus patient, it provides multiple layers of tissue cover (muscle, subcutaneous fat, and skin).

As discussed in the ALT flap rection—a careful study of the patient's individual anatomy is key for the correct flap selection.

A latissimus dorsi flap can easily be used for total glossectomy reconstruction. However, for optimum results, the surgeon must follow a specific flap inset technique: The muscle is sutured alongside the U-shaped remaining edge of the glossectomy defect on the vallecula and is suspended over the mandibular alveolar ridge, suturing the muscle to the buccal gingival mucosal edges. This allows the subcutaneous fat and skin to protrude above the level of the mandible, passively and freely. This technique provides a good dome-shaped reconstruction which resembles the native tongue and can recreate the lingual sulcus on each side lateral to the epiglottis, which diverts saliva and secretions onto the gutters lateral to the laryngeal inlet and, thus, protects the patient from the risk of aspiration. Although this approach is not clearly evidence-based, the current concept is that this technique may also lead to a higher quality speech in patients who have undergone subtotal or total glossectomies.

The muscle component of the LD flap provides adequate bulk for obliteration of the submandibular space, thus reducing the risk of oral–neck communication.

When one considers an LD free flap, it is important to assess the torso of the patient. Patients with high body mass index (BMI) are at risk of carrying a too thick subcutaneous component that will effectively make the latissimus dorsi too difficult to contour and may inadvertently result in excessive intraoral bulk, reducing the airway space, and resulting in delayed decannulation or discomfort. In such cases, a muscle-only LD flap or an alternative option (such as an ALT flap or a pedicled pectoralis major flap, if less bulky) can be considered. Once again, the flap selection process must be thorough, comprehensive and holistic, taking into account all parameters such as stage of disease, body habitus/build, and the possibility of postoperative radiotherapy. A pectoralis major flap may be subjected to gravitational effect, contraction, and radiotherapy-induced fibrosis with poor long-term functional outcomes.

2.4 **Comorbidities and age in head and neck free-flap surgery**

Introduction

The reconstructive surgeon should pay serious consideration to the age and comorbidities of the patient when deciding on the reconstructive plan.

A high level of prediction of possible complications and careful planning is required prior to an appropriate choice of suitable reconstruction. Never deviate from the primary endpoints of head and neck surgery which is adequate tumour resection with clear margins (an R0 resection) and a viable reconstruction. Important goals are a relatively uncomplicated recovery and hospital discharge, within the timeframe required to allow adjuvant treatment to assume without delays.

It is a common pitfall that often complex reconstruction plans are selected involving osseo-cutaneous flaps and dental implants. These reconstructions may increase the complexity of the primary operation and the length of recovery and may predispose to postoperative complications.

For advanced-stage tumours in medically compromised patients, the oncological treatment plan involves at least tumour-directed treatment such as radical surgery including reconstruction followed by radiotherapy. Careful preoperative assessment will avoid surpass the capacity of the patient's physiological reserves. Surgeons should always be reminded not to put their own surgical ambition before the benefit to the patient—the goal must be that the patient receives appropriate care, customized and tailored to their needs.

Comorbidities and head and neck reconstruction

The American Society of Anaesthesiologists (ASA) has produced a widely used classification system of a patient's overall physical status (PS) as shown in Table 2.4.1. This is a helpful guide for the surgeons and anaesthetists to grade the patients' overall health. Head and neck major surgery can be performed in the first three grades of the ASA scale (I to III) obviously with appropriate adjustments and precautions for ASA II and III patients.

The following paragraphs describe the most common major medical conditions encountered in head and neck surgery and their impact on the choice of reconstruction plan.

Cardiac disease

Effect on patient

H&N cancer patients are prone to cardiac events due to their smoking and alcohol history, which increases the risk of hypertension and atherosclerosis. A perioperative cardiac event results in high mortality postoperatively, both at short and long term, and additionally increases the length of stay.

Effect on free flap

Prolonged surgery and carotid baroreceptor insult during neck dissection increase the risk of haemodynamic instability intraoperatively. Patients are often administered more fluids rather than vasopressors to correct hypotension, despite evidence supporting the use of vasopressors (particularly metaraminol) in free flap surgery. Volume replacement has been found to increase flap failure when administered in excess of 5.5 litres and thus restricted and goal-directed fluid therapy with the aim of keeping mean arterial pressure above 60 mmHg, is frequently advocated in enhanced recovery pathways.

- *Issues in the postoperative period*
  - Hypotension and cardiovascular events
  - Cardiac arrhythmia
  - Fluid overload and pulmonary oedema

- *Key management*
  - Goal directed fluid management
  - Monitor symptoms of cardiac events
  - Close communication with cardiologists

Respiratory disease

Effect on patient

Respiratory disease due to smoking can influence the patient's postoperative recovery and rehabilitation, due to pneumonia and prolonged tracheostomy need. Prevention of fluid overload to reduce the risk of pulmonary oedema is important.

Effect on free flap

Actual flap compromise has not been proven; however, smoking is known to have a pro-coagulative, pro-thrombotic, and vasospasm effect. Smoking particularly influences wound

Table 2.4.1 American Society of Anaesthesiologists (ASA) Physical Status (PS) classification system of a patient's overall health and ASA-approved examples Reproduced with permission from Committee on Economics, 'Statement on ASA Physical Status Classification System'. American Society of Anesthesiologists (ASA). Anesthesiology Open 1(1):p e0002, January 2026. Last Amended: January 9th, 2026 (original approval: October 15, 2014). Available at https://www.asahq.org/standards-and-practice-parameters/statement-on-asa-physical-status-classification-system

ASA PS Classification	Definition	Adult Examples, Including, but not Limited to:	Pediatric Examples, Including but not Limited to:	Obstetric Examples, Including but not Limited to:
ASA I	A normal healthy patient	Healthy, non-smoking, no or minimal alcohol use	Healthy (no acute or chronic disease), normal BMI percentile for age	
ASA II	A patient with mild systemic disease	Mild diseases only without substantive functional limitations or end organ involvement. Current smoker, social alcohol drinker, pregnancy, obesity (30<BMI<40), well-controlled DM or HTN, mild lung disease, CHF NYHA Class 1, mild cognitive dysfunction, isolated mild/moderate obstructive sleep apnea with compliance with CPAP as prescribed.	Asymptomatic non cyanotic congenital cardiac disease, well controlled dysrhythmias, asthma without exacerbation, well controlled epilepsy, non-insulin dependent DM, abnormal BMI percentile for age, mild/moderate OSA, oncologic state in remission, autism with mild limitations, malignant hyperthermia risk (family history or patient with history)	Normal pregnancy,* well controlled gestational HTN, diet-controlled gestational DM
ASA III	A patient with severe systemic disease	Substantive functional limitations; One or more moderate to severe diseases. COPD, morbid obesity (BMI ≥40), active hepatitis, compensated cirrhosis, alcohol dependence or abuse, functional implanted pacemaker, moderate reduction of ejection fraction or CHF NYHA class 2 or 3, ESRD undergoing regularly scheduled dialysis, history (>3 months) of MI, CVA, TIA, PE, or CAD/stents, significant cognitive dysfunction, isolated severe OSA regardless of CPAP compliance or any severity of obstructive sleep apnea with CPAP noncompliance. Poorly controlled DM or HTN with or without end organ dysfunction.	Uncorrected stable congenital cardiac abnormality, asthma with exacerbation, poorly controlled epilepsy, insulin dependent diabetes mellitus, morbid obesity, malnutrition, severe OSA, oncologic state, renal failure, muscular dystrophy, cystic fibrosis, history of organ transplantation, brain/spinal cord malformation, symptomatic hydrocephalus, premature infant PCA <60 weeks, autism with severe limitations, metabolic disease, difficult airway, long term parenteral nutrition. Full term infants <6 weeks of age.	Preeclampsia with or without severe features, gestational diabetes poorly controlled or with complications or high insulin requirements, a thrombophilic disease requiring anticoagulation.

(*continued*)

Table 2.4.1 Continued

ASA PS Classification	Definition	Adult Examples, Including, but not Limited to:	Pediatric Examples, Including but not Limited to:	Obstetric Examples, Including but not Limited to:
ASA IV	A patient with severe systemic disease that is a constant threat to life	Recent (<3 months) MI, CVA, TIA or CAD/stents, ongoing cardiac ischemia or severe valve dysfunction, severe reduction of ejection fraction or CHF NYHA class 4, shock, sepsis, DIC, ARDS, ESRD not undergoing regularly scheduled dialysis, uncompensated cirrhosis, severe cognitive dysfunction	Symptomatic congenital cardiac abnormality, congestive heart failure, active sequelae of prematurity, acute hypoxic-ischemic encephalopathy, shock, sepsis, disseminated intravascular coagulation, automatic implantable cardioverter-defibrillator, ventilator dependence, endocrinopathy, severe trauma, severe respiratory distress, advanced oncologic state.	Preeclampsia with severe features complicated by HELLP or other adverse event, peripartum cardiomyopathy, uncorrected/ decompensated heart disease.
ASA V	A moribund patient who is not expected to survive without the operation	Ruptured abdominal or thoracic aneurysm, massive trauma, intracranial bleed with mass effect, ischemic bowel in the face of significant cardiac pathology or multiple organ/system dysfunction	Massive trauma, intracranial hemorrhage with mass effect, patient requiring ECMO, respiratory failure or arrest, malignant hypertension with hypertensive crisis, decompensated congestive heart failure, hepatic encephalopathy, ischemic bowel or multiple organ/system dysfunction.	Uterine rupture, amniotic fluid embolism
ASA VI	A declared brain-dead patient whose organs are being removed for donor purposes			

*Although pregnancy is not a disease, the parturient's physiologic state is significantly altered from when the woman is not pregnant, hence the assignment of ASA PS II for a woman with uncomplicated pregnancy.

**The addition of "E" denotes Emergency surgery: (An emergency is defined as existing when delay in treatment of the patient would lead to a significant increase in the threat to life or body part).

ARDS, acute respiratory distress syndrome; ASA, American Society of Anesthesiologists; BMI, body mass index; CAD, coronary artery disease; CHF NYHA, congestive heart failure, New York Heart Association classification; COPD, chronic obstructive pulmonary disease; CPAP, continuous positive airway pressure; CVA, cerebrovascular accident; DIC, disseminated intravascular coagulation; DM, diabetes mellitus; ECMO, extracorporeal membrane oxygenation; ESRD, end-stage renal disease; HELLP, hemolysis, elevated liver enzymes, low platelets; HTN, hypertension; MI, myocardial infarction; OSA, obstructive sleep apnea; PCA, post-conceptual age; PE, pulmonary embolism; PS, physical status; TIA, transient ischemic attack healing and leads to donor site complications. Smoking cessation for a minimum of 4 weeks prior to surgery has been found to decrease postoperative complications such as pneumonias and wound healing problems.

- *Issues in the postoperative period*
  - Risk of pneumonia
  - Risk of donor site complications

- *Key management*
  - *Encourage pre- and postoperative smoking cessation.*
  - *Chest physiotherapy for all patients*
  - *Fluid balance control to prevent pulmonary oedema.*

Peripheral vascular disease

Comorbidities are known to play a key role in the choice of flap. For example, a patient with significant risk factors such as significant years of smoking, alcohol, and excess use is at risk of peripheral vascular disease. To this end, the choice of a free fibula flap may be precarious.

It is important to note that angiographic studies such as an MRA, CTA or an ultrasound doppler may not be able to pick up a relatively early, or otherwise not established atherosclerotic disease. It would be detrimental to plan a fibula flap on a vascular-compromised patient and find yourself in a situation where a flap is ready for anastomosis only to realize that the vessel (and particularly the intima) are severely compromised due to vascular disease and the flap doesn't perfuse or develops ischaemia and arterial failure shortly after surgery

Diabetes

- *Effect of patient*

Diabetes presents an increased risk for surgical postoperative infections, particularly wound problems such as dehiscence. Diabetes often co-exists with a high body mass index (BMI), hypertension, and atherosclerosis, and may predispose for peripheral vascular disease. Albeit not a contraindication to free flap surgery, this combination of comorbidities does increase the risk for postoperative cardiac complications.

- Effect on free flap

No direct negative impact on the microsurgical anastomosis has been found, but the presence of atherosclerosis can narrow and damage the arterial vessel wall. The anastomotic technique requires meticulous attention and avoiding crushing the vessel with forceps or with scissors to prevent separation of the vessel wall layers (particularly the intima) is key. In addition, generalized atherosclerosis can impact the donor site. For example, free fibula harvest can result in ischaemic complications of the donor limb.

- *Issues in the postoperative period*
  - Wound dehiscence
  - Wound infection
  - Medical cardiac complications

- *Key management*
  - o Optimize diabetic control preoperatively.
  - o Close collaboration with diabetic nurse for peri-operative glucose control
  - o CTA preoperatively in patients with suspected severe atherosclerosis
  - o Consideration of a more 'central' bony donor site (ie scapula) instead of a lower extremity

Cirrhosis

- *Effect on patient*

H&N patients with cirrhosis have significantly increased morbidity compared to non-cirrhotic patients. With a greater risk for hypotension, hypovolemia, and hypoxia, they are at an increased risk of hepatic ischaemia and thus exacerbated cirrhosis-associated complications. Cirrhotic liver disease affects the coagulation cascade, metabolic, and immunological processes. An increased bleeding potential will risk haemodynamic and electrolyte imbalance, due to the loss of intravascular volume and the need for blood transfusions. A mismanaged fluid balance can lead to renal failure, in fluid deficiency, or cardiorespiratory compromise, in overload. Furthermore, excessive blood transfusions can cause further clotting abnormalities, in addition to hyperkalaemia and hypothermia that lead to arrythmias.

- *Effect on free flap*

No impact on flap failure is described, but there is an increased risk of postoperative haematoma. As such, patients would require further surgery, which would risk anaesthetic insults such as hypotension and possible fluid overload if using volume to correct hypotension. Furthermore, excessive fluid administration (in particular over 5.5 litres) has been found to be an independent predictor of major surgical and medical complications. Wound healing could also be compromised due to the downregulated protein synthesis and malnutrition that can compromise the immune system in cirrhotic patients.

- *Issues in the postoperative period*
  - o Fluid balance
  - o Coagulation disturbance
  - o Immune-compromise and wound healing issues
  - o Malnutrition
- *Key management*
  - o Close collaboration with gastroenterologist, haematologist, dietitian
  - o Cirrhosis is a relevant contraindication for free flap surgery

Age

Age is frequently a significant factor that can influence the reconstructive planning. Both the incidence and number of comorbidities increase in the elderly. This is one of the reasons behind the higher prevalence of medical complications encountered in the early postoperative period in these patients. However, several studies demonstrated how age alone fails to correlate with postoperative morbidity, mortality, and quality of life, and thus a more detailed evaluation of a patient's comorbidities and performance status, irrespective of age, is warranted. Indeed, the success in complex free flap surgery is multifactorial, and (importantly) depends on a patient's ability to recover and rehabilitate in order to achieve the expected functional and quality-of-life outcomes. The challenge in determining appropriateness of such surgery lies in balancing the assessment of patient's motivation and individual physiological and psychological reserve, taking into account the disease and the surgical capability of achieving expected reconstructive outcomes.

The young (<50 years)

Key concerns

Head and neck cancers (HNC) in this age group are uncommon and account for less than 5% of patients. Prognosis is good, which is perhaps less surprising considering the lower likelihood of comorbidities (and multiple comorbidities) and a higher prevalence of oral tumour sites, which are linked to better survival and superior quality of life.

Outcomes

This patient group are offered aggressive treatment, which could account for their improved prognosis. This group is found to have a lower prevalence of alcohol and tobacco use, which further explains the low incidence and better outcomes in these younger patients.

The older (50–70 years)

Key concerns

Head and neck cancers are most common in this age group, and this is partly due to the increase of the human papilloma virus (HPV)-related oropharyngeal cancer. Despite the favourable outlook on HPV-related H&N cancers, their location in the oropharynx means that the first-line treatment is non-surgical (i.e. radiotherapy). Surgery is reserved as a salvage option, which in the context of post-radiotherapy, leads these patients to require more debilitating resections and challenging reconstructions. This has significant implications on speech, swallowing, and quality of life.

Outcomes

Most studies evaluating patients below and above the age of 50 years agree on a similar survival outcome. This could be due to the better prognosis associated with HPV-related H&N cancers in the older group.

The very old (>70 years)

Key concerns

As well as primary H&N cancers, this group will encounter tumour recurrences. The elderly is more prone to cardiovascular and respiratory morbidity. These comorbidities, coupled with recurrent cancers present a particularly difficult scenario; as one would have to balance the aggressiveness of the surgical approach with the availability of surgical options and the possibility to improve or preserve quality of life. The donor-side selection for reconstruction has been found to be associated with the incidence of medical complications. Mandibulectomies, laryngectomies, and total glossectomies have been found to negatively impact health-related quality of life the most, as they impact psycho-social function, but most importantly, they influence postoperative respiratory recovery.

Cardiac deterioration can equally ensue. In the elderly, this can result from fluid mismanagement and/or electrolyte imbalance. Fluid administration and nutrition should therefore be goal-directed and closely monitored (see Chapter 3).

Delirium is also an important postoperative phenomenon, exacerbated by prolonged operative time and blood transfusions (disturbing fluid and electrolyte balance), preoperative respiratory morbidity, mandibular reconstructions and tracheostomy need, and alcohol abuse.

Outcomes

Despite the increased risk for postoperative medical complications, the right reconstruction for the right elderly patient can lead to a successful outcome and a good quality of life. One should consider tumour stage alongside comorbidities when counselling patients for the appropriate reconstruction.

Table 2.4.2 summarizes the age categories and treatment planning approaches.

Performance and frailty

The patient's age should not be seen in isolation as a criterion for treatment planning. A more holistic assessment including performance and frailty offers a better insight into the potential physiological tolerance for major surgery, recovery time, and possible complications, and predicted length of hospital stay.

The widely used performance status and the most popular frailty scale are shown in Table 2.4.3 and Table 2.4.4, respectively.

Table 2.4.2 Age and comorbidities summary on head neck reconstruction approach

Ages	Key concerns	Risk factors	Suggested approach
The young <50	Multiple comorbidities uncommon	Impact of smoking and drinking is less common. Some may have HPV-related cancers with a better prognosis. Many may require complex reconstructive surgery for benign disease (odontogenic tumours)	Likely eligible for a complex approach
The older 50–70	Multiple comorbidities can be present	HPV-related cancers with better prognosis	Selective approach based on comorbidities
The very old >70	Multiple comorbidities Recurrent disease Previously operated and/or irradiated neck Potentially poor preoperative quality of life (QoL); difficult to improve	Recurrences more common	Balanced/prioritized approach

Table 2.4.3 Performance status scale

Performance status (ECOG/WHO score)
0 Fully active, able to carry on all pre-disease performance without restriction
1 Restricted in physically strenuous activity, but ambulatory and able to carry out work of a light and sedentary nature (e.g. light housework, office work)
2 Ambulatory and capable of all self-care but unable to carry out any work activities. Up and about more than 50% of waking hours
3 Capable of only limited self-care, confined to bed or chair more than 50% of waking hours
4 Completely disabled. Cannot carry on any self-care. Totally confined to bed or chair
5 Dead

Adapted with permission from Oken MM, Creech RH, Tormey DC, Horton J, Davis TE, McFadden ET, Carbone PP. Toxicity and response criteria of the Eastern Cooperative Oncology Group. *Am J Clin Oncol.* 1982 Dec;5(6):649–55.

Table 2.4.4 Clinical frailty scale

Clinical frailty scale
1. Very fit—People who are robust, active, energetic, and motivated. These people commonly exercise regularly. They are among the fittest for their age.
2. Well—People who have no active disease symptoms but are less fit than category 1. Often, they exercise or are very active occasionally, e.g. seasonally.
3. Managing well—People whose medical problems are well controlled but are not regularly active beyond routine walking.
4. Vulnerable—While not dependent on others for daily help, often symptoms limit activities. A common complaint is being 'slowed up' and or/being tired during the day.
5. Mildly frail—These people often have more evident slowing and need help in high-order instrumental activities of daily living (IADLs) (finances, transportation, heavy housework, medications). Typically, mild frailty progressively impairs shopping and walking outside alone, meal preparation, and housework.
6. Moderately frail—People need help with all outside activities and with keeping house. Inside, they often have problems with stairs and need help with bathing and might need minimal assistance (cuing standby) with dressing.
7. Severely frail—Completely dependent for personal care, from whatever cause (physical or cognitive). Even so, they seem stable and not at high risk of dying (within 6 months).
8. Very severely frail—Completely dependent, approaching the end of life. Typically, they could not recover even from a minor illness.
9. Terminally ill—Approaching the end of life. This category applies to people with a life expectancy <6 months, who are not otherwise frail.

Adapted with permission from Moorhouse P, Rockwood K. Frailty and its quantitative clinical evaluation. *J R Coll Physicians Edinb.* 2012;42(4):333–40.

Major head and neck surgery including free-flap reconstruction should not be encouraged in patients with a performance status of 3 and above and/or frailty score of 5 and above, with necessary adjustments in patients scoring high on each scale (see Cuccolo et al. in 'Further reading'). For patients scoring high in either scale, if treatment is carried out for tumour ablation a simplified and non-free-flap reconstructive option might be appropriate.

Conceptual considerations

Free flaps could theoretically be divided into 'low-resistance' systems (soft tissue flaps with large calibre vessels, i.e. radial forearm free flap, latissimus dorsi flap) and 'high-resistance' systems (composite bony flaps). High-resistance flaps should be selected primarily in patients with cardiovascular fitness adequate to maintain perfusion pressure to power the flap. The judgement requires an eye of experience and a global, holistic assessment of the patient. It is important for the surgeon to be reminded that the reconstruction should be guided by what benefits the patient and not the surgeon's ambition.

When assessing the patient, even if there are no recorded comorbidities and the ASA grade is low risk (such as 1 or 2), age is an important factor that should be taken into account.

An 80-year-old patient with no significant comorbidities or risk factors could score relatively low on frailty score. This may mislead that is fit for free flap reconstruction. However, different free flaps carry different metabolic demands and although this kind of patient may do well with a fasciocutaneous free flap reconstruction, a high metabolic demand and high-resistance flap such as an osseocutaneous flap may fail, predisposing the patient to return to theatres, postoperative complications, and prolonged stay.

Patients with reduced physiological reserves may display signs of slow flap hypoperfusion and progressive ischaemia that often is not attributed to microvascular surgery technical problems. These patients may return to theatre only to find that the arterial anastomosis is technically sound, and there is no presence of thrombosis or occlusion; the issue is in the microcirculation and the perfusion pressure to the flap (Type B failures as described in Chapters 12, 13.4, and 14.4).

The gold standard for reconstructing a lateral mandibulectomy defect is an osseocutaneous flap including dental implants. This solution would be a perfectly reasonable choice for a young person with no comorbidities and especially for defects following resections of benign odontogenic tumours. However, on a relatively elderly patient with multiple comorbidities and a baseline compromised dentition this might be viewed as an unnecessary overtreatment.

A choice of a reconstruction plate covered by a musculocutaneous flap is a far less morbid procedure, linked with a less complicated recovery with far more predictable results and length of stay, and certainly less metabolic stress. For a patient of this background, dental rehabilitation is often not possible or wise, as it requires a significantly riskier procedure and might lead to deviation from the primary end point, which is adequate oncological treatment. The long-term functional outcome with a soft tissue flap on a lateral mandibulectomy defect can be acceptable but with a far lesser cost in terms of complications and recovery for patients not fit enough for more complex reconstructive surgery. An article published by Chang et al. from the Texas MD Anderson Cancer Centre (see 'Further reading') further analyses this topic.

These important aspects that contribute in flap selection are highlighted in Box 2.4.1.

Box 2.4.1 Important aspects in selecting the flap of choice

- Careful assessment of the patient's medical status, physiological reserves, and stamina to withstand major surgery is a paramount component in the appropriate flap selection process.
- Each patient theoretically has a finite maximum tolerance for major surgery. For a patient with limited reserves and major ablations compromise in terms of surgical stress can be achieved by simplifying the reconstructive plan.
- In patients with limited total physiological reserves, a complex reconstruction with a composite flap may predispose to type B failure (see Chapters 12, 13.4, and 14.4).

2.5 Strategies to minimize free flap complications: Flap design and pedicle planning

Introduction

In this chapter we mention a few tips and advice from experience to avoid pedicle positioning related issues that may impact on the viability and success of the anastomosis. These few tips of flap design, inset, and pedicle management that derive from experience.

Flap design

Flap design refers to addressing the defect in terms of shape, orientation, components (and their inter-relationship), placement of perforation(s) within the tissue and decision for the donor site.

In the setting of a two-team simultaneous operating, 'intra-harvest flexibility' is key, in case of change in the extent of defect. One should, e.g. refrain from dividing potential muscular branches and cutting all the borders of the skin paddle, until the final defect is observed and measured. This approach will occasionally preserve the option for a combined or chimeric composition of the flap.

The location of the flap harvest at the donor site is important in terms of pedicle length, positioning of the tissue around a perforator and adapting the design in relation to tissue thickness. The anterolateral thigh (ALT) flap can for example be designed more distally or more proximally on the thigh, depending on the bulk of tissue needed. A more distal placement will be useful for patients with more subcutaneous fat, as this will be less more distally in the thigh.

Innovative hand-made templates from various materials can aid in customizing the flap design. Furthermore, novel augmented reality and virtual planning tools can enhance precision in planning; preoperatively, by examining vascular topography and possible options for tissue inclusion, and intraoperatively by confirming tissue perfusion.

Flap inset

The 'make or break' of a head and neck (H&N) reconstruction is truly the flap inset. The complex defect-configuration demands not only the correct tissue, but also its correct placement, thereof highlighting the crucial intra-harvest approach of maintaining flexibility in tissue design and tissue inclusion until tumour ablation is completed.

Careless design and inset can cause inadequate obliteration of dead space and inadequate coverage of tissues and fixation plates, which subsequently can lead to leaks, infected collections, fistula formation, and metalwork exposure. In addition, functional and aesthetic deterioration can ensue, with an external unbalanced appearance of either exaggerated hollowing or bulk, or internal bulk and tethering of structures causing inability to maintain oromandibular function.

The effect of postoperative radiotherapy will undoubtedly affect the reconstruction, causing fibrosis and reduced tissue perfusion. The resulting volume loss and tissue contracture can cause trismus and malocclusion, which subsequently will impact speech, swallowing, and the overall oromandibular function. As such, being familiar with how different tissues respond to radiotherapy is crucial in order to maximize their potential, and choose tissue type and tissue placement correctly.

Passing the flap through the tunnel

The vast majority if not all head neck reconstructive cases involve a tunnel through which the flap pedicle transits into the neck, for the donor vessels to meet the recipient ones. The tunnels vary in length (floor of mouth, tongue, mandibular reconstructions require relatively short tunnels, whereas maxillary and upper face defects result in long tunnels), and tissue laxity (floor of mouth, tongue, maxillary reconstructions involve a bony tunnel wall due to the mandible).

As it is described in Chapter 7.1 the tunnel needs to be spacious and straight and allow passive passage of the flap pedicle into the neck.

During flap inset, the flap has to be passed through the tunnel and into the site of the defect with extreme care and utilizing a methodical technique that will minimize the risk of pedicle kinking, stretching, or twisting within the tunnel.

Pedicle management and crucially passing the flap through the tunnel is as important as the technical proficiency needed for the microsurgeon to accomplish the anastomosis.

The second biggest cause of flap failures and when this is not due to anastomotic technical error, is related to substandard pedicle management the majority of which have to do with tunnel issues.

This technique is described in detail and illustrated in Chapter 7.1.

Soft tissue inset

The soft tissue component of a reconstruction is the most vital to prevent complications such as fistulas and plate exposure and can severely affect functional rehabilitation if inset wrongly or when subjected to radiotherapy.

Muscle is known to lose substantial amount of volume (about a third) due to denervation and after radiotherapy, compared to fasciocutaneous flaps as adipose tissue tend to maintain its volume (despite radiotherapy induced fat attenuation). As such, muscle only flaps are suitable for a scalp or hard palate resurfacing, whereas fasciocutaneous flaps would be more suitable for external or internal defects requiring less bulk, or in a combination with muscle for significant dead space defects.

One should be aware of the 'sagging effect' of soft tissue flaps, which one should try to mitigate, either with immediate facial slings or secondary revisions. Soft tissue flaps can be de-epithelialized and tucked under a skin flap to improve contour or folded to ensure compartment separation. One should aim for a watertight closure and separation between the skull base and nasal cavity, nasal and oral cavity, oral cavity, and neck. In doing so, compression of the pedicle should be avoided at all costs.

Bony inset

Bony flaps present a steep learning curve for inset; particularly as subsequent dental rehabilitation demands adequate depth of bone in the vertical plane. Selecting the laterality of the donor side is crucial, as the side harvested will determine the recipient site's external or internal position of the skin paddle, and the medial or lateral placement of the pedicle.

Traditional teaching favours an ipsilateral anastomosis by advocating the contralateral fibula for a skin paddle needed for intraoral resurfacing, and an ipsilateral fibula for a skin paddle needed for external coverage. This approach does however limit the surgeon, and in fact, either fibula can be used for either side—as long as there is a generous size of skin paddle that can be turned either way—bearing in mind the requirement for anastomosis to the contralateral neck vessels.

It is important to plan the appropriate inset of both the soft tissue and bony component of a composite flap, taking into account the exit point of the vascular pedicle.

Novel virtual planning tools (PSP/3D) have been developed to increase precision in osteotomies and body contact, but their current limitation is in predicting the soft tissue component.

In term of postoperative radiotherapy, bony tissue is at risk of non-union and osteoradionecrosis, and as such minimal periosteal stripping should be performed.

Additionally, to minimize complications with bony flaps, the number of osteotomies should be kept to the minimal number required, while the length of the segment is kept at the maximum length possible to ensure viable bone. The primary objective is bone viability, and all contour deformities could be corrected by secondary osteotomies, when needed.

In our practice and to avoid ischaemia time and development of microthrombi in the bony Haversian canals we recommend suspension of the bony flap with one or two screws followed by immediate anastomosis. The rest of the bony and soft tissue inset is completed after both anastomoses have been performed.

Pedicle positioning

Handling the pedicle

The best course of the pedicle to the neck can vary depending on the inset of the flap, and it is important to test one's options by moving the neck in various directions prior to anastomosis. For oral reconstruction, one should aim to tunnel the pedicle below the mandibular border or through the floor of the mouth in a wide tunnel. Avoid twisting by marking the pedicle as described by Ardehali et al. in 'Further reading', ensuring meticulous haemostasis and dividing compressing structures such as the digastric muscle. The pedicle should form a gentle curve avoiding acute angle formation and ideally one should separate the individual vessels substantially in order to account for the different locations of the recipient artery and vein.

Furthermore, performing the arterial anastomosis first will enable one to visualize the curve of the vessels in their engorged status, and thus be able to alter their position to avoid kinking (particularly in the vein) with better accuracy; and ensure good outflow in the chosen vein. The sequence of anastomosis varies among surgeons; however this has no impact on flap survival.

Key points

- Preserve options for muscle inclusion and various skin paddle designs until tumour ablation is completed and the defect is examined.
- Choose the correct tissue for the given site, defect and effect of radiotherapy, including the patient's anticipated postoperative oromandibular function and prognosis.
- Perform flap inset before anastomosis.
- Test the pedicle for malposition prior to anastomosis by altering neck positions.
- Choose the path of the pedicle to the neck to be that of least tension/torsion/compression.
- Perform arterial anastomosis first to remedy malpositioned vessels and ensure good venous outflow.

Further reading

Angrigiani C, Grilli D. Latissimnus dorsi musculocutaneous flap without muscle. *Plast Reconstructive Surg* 1994;96:1608–14.

Ardehali B, Mehrara B, Cordeiro P, Mosahebi A. Painting the pedicle: a twist-proof marking method. *J Reconst Microsurg* 2011;3:207–8.

Bhama P, Patel S, Khan U, Bhrany A, Futran, N. Head and neck free flap reconstruction in patients older than 80 years. *J Reconstr Microsurg* 2014;30:523–30.

Blanchard P, *et al.* Outcomes and prognostic factors for squamous cell carcinoma of the oral tongue in young adults: a single-institution case-matched analysis. *Eur Arch Oto-rhinol* 2017;274:1683–90.

Bardsley JL, Staple TW. Variations in branching of the popliteal artery. *Radiology* 1970;94:581–7.

Chang EI, Hanasono MM, Butler CE. Management of unfavorable outcomes in head and neck free flap reconstruction experience-based lessons from the MD Anderson Cancer Center. *Clin Plast Surg* 2016;43:653–67.

Chang S-M, Hou C-L, Xu D-C. An overview of skin flap surgery in the mainland China: 20 years' achievements (1981 to 2000). *J Reconstr Microsurg* 2009;25:361–7.

Chen H-C, *et al.* Guidelines for the optimization of microsurgery in atherosclerotic patients. *Microsurgery* 2006;5:356–62.

Cohen WA, *et al.* Health-related quality of life following reconstruction for common head and neck surgical defects. *Plast Reconstr Surg* 2016;138:1312–20.

Coskunfirat OK, Chen H, Spanio S, Tang Y. The safety of microvascular free tissue transfer in the elderly population. *Plast Reconstr Surg* 2005;115:771–5.

Crawford JE, *et al.* Postoperative delirium in patients with head and neck oral cancer in the West of Scotland. *Br J Oral Maxillofac Surg* 2021;59(3):353–61.

Cuccolo NG, Sparenberg S, Ibrahim AMS, Crystal DT, Blankensteijn LL, Lin SJ. Does age or frailty have more predictive effect on outcomes following pedicled flap reconstruction? An analysis of 44,986 cases†. *J Plast Surg Hand Surg* 2020;54(2):67–76.

Deek NA. Virtual surgical planning in fibula free flap reconstruction of head and neck defects: Advice to novice surgeons. *J Plastic Reconstr Aesthetic Surg* 2019;72:2069–70.

Deek, N. F. A., Tsao, C.-K. & Wei, F.-C. The surgeon's fist with the thumb up to guide the design and inset of the osteoseptocutaneous fibula flap in mandibular reconstruction. *Plast Reconstr Surg* 2017;140:1259–62.

Deek NFA, Wei F-C, Kao H-K. Free tissue transfer to head and neck lessons learned from unfavorable results—experience per subsite. *Clin Plast Surg* 2016;43:621–30.

Densky J, *et al.* Risk factors associated with postoperative delirium in patients undergoing head and neck free flap reconstruction. *JAMA Otolaryngology Head Neck Surg* 2019;145:216–21.

Dimovska EOF, Clibbon JJ, Moncrieff MDS, Heaton MJ, Figus A. Microsurgical reconstructions for head and neck cancers in elderly aged >80 years: an analysis of surgical outcomes and quality of life. *Ann Surg Oncol* 2016;23:1684–92.

Divo MJ, Martinez CH, Mannino DM. Ageing and the epidemiology of multimorbidity. *Eur Respir J* 2014;44:1055–68.

Dort JC, *et al.* Optimal perioperative care in major head and neck cancer surgery with free flap reconstruction: a consensus review and recommendations from the Enhanced Recovery After Surgery Society. *JAMA Otolaryngology Head Neck Surg* 2016;143:292.

Driessen C, *et al.* Usefulness of a template-based anterolateral thigh flap for reconstruction of head and neck defects. *Microsurg* 2020;40:776–82.

Eley KA, Young JD, Watt-Smith SR. Epinephrine, norepinephrine, dobutamine, and dopexamine effects on free flap skin blood flow. *Plast Reconstr Surg* 2012;130;564–70.

Eley KA, Young JD, Watt-Smith SR. Power spectral analysis of the effects of epinephrine, norepinephrine, dobutamine and dopexamine on microcirculation following free tissue transfer. *Microsurg* 2013;33:275–81.

Ettinger KS, *et al.* Higher perioperative fluid administration is associated with increased rates of complications following head and neck microvascular reconstruction with fibular free flaps. *Microsurg* 2017;37:128–36.

Fagin AP, Gelesko S, Wax MK, Petrisor D. Morbidity and functional outcomes with head and neck free flap reconstruction in patients aged 90 years or older. *J Oral Maxil Surg* 2017;75:1549–54.

Germann G, Reichenberger M. Latissimus dorsi flap. In: *Flaps & Reconstructive Surgery* (eds. Wei F-C, Mardini S). Oxford: Elsevier, 2016: pp. 446–63.

Gilroy JS, Morris CG, Amdur RJ, Mendenhall WM. Impact of young age on prognosis for head and neck cancer: a matched-pair analysis. *Head Neck* 2005;27:269–73.

Grammatica A, *et al.* Free flaps for advanced oral cancer in the 'older old' and 'oldest old': a retrospective multi-institutional study. *Frontiers Oncol* 2019;9:604.

Huang W, *et al.* Reconstruction of through-and-through cheek defects involving the oral commissure, using chimeric flaps from the thigh lateral femoral circumflex system. *Plast Reconstr Surg* 2002;109:433–41.

Hwang L, Natividad EM, Ellis M. Fibula flap harvest: How leg selection impacts inset for mandible defects. *Microsurg* 2017;37:459–60.

Inbal A, *et al.* The 'origami' composite free fibula flap for complex defects of the mandible, floor of the mouth, and tongue. *J Oral Maxil Surg* 2015;73:1617–26.

Joseph TA, Upton J. Radial forearm flap. In: *Flaps and Reconstructive Surgery* (eds. Wei F-C, Mardini S). Oxford: Elsevier, 2016: pp. 321–338.

Kao H-K, *et al.* The impacts of liver cirrhosis on head and neck cancer patients undergoing microsurgical free tissue transfer: an evaluation of flap outcome and flap-related complications. *Oral Oncol* 2009;45:1058–62.

Karamanos E, Walker R, Wang HT, Shah AR. Perioperative fluid resuscitation in free flap breast reconstruction: when is enough enough? *Plastic ReconstrSurg* 2020;8:e2662.

Kass JL, *et al.* Intraoperative hypotension and flap loss in free tissue transfer surgery of the head and neck. *Head Neck* 2018;40:2334–9.

Kearns M, Ermogenous P, Myers S, Ghanem AM. Osteocutaneous flaps for head and neck reconstruction: a focused evaluation of donor site morbidity and patient reported outcome measures in different reconstruction options. *Archives Plastic Surg* 2018;45:495–503.

Kelly AM, Cronin P, Hussain HK, Londy FJ, Chepeha DB, Carlos RC. Preoperative MR angiography in free fibula flap transfer for head and neck cancer: clinical application and influence on surgical decision making. *AJR Am J Roentgenol* 2007;188(1):268–74.
Khan MN, *et al.* Association of body mass index with infectious complications in free tissue transfer for head and neck reconstructive surgery. *JAMA Otolaryngology Head Neck Surg* 2017;143:574.
Lassig AAD, *et al.* The effect of young age on outcomes in head and neck cancer. *Laryngoscope* 2013;123:1896–902.
Liu Y, Di Y, Fu S. Risk factors for ventilator-associated pneumonia among patients undergoing major oncological surgery for head and neck cancer. *Front Med* 2017;11:239–46.
Mills E, *et al.* Smoking cessation reduces postoperative complications: a systematic review and meta-analysis. *Am J Med* 2011;124:144–54.e8.
Millwala F, Nguyen GC, Thuluvath PJ. Outcomes of patients with cirrhosis undergoing non-hepatic surgery: risk assessment and management. *World J Gastroenterol* 2007;30:4056–63.
Moorhouse P, Rockwood K. Frailty and its quantitative clinical evaluation. *J R Coll Physicians Edinb* 2012;42(4):333–40.
Mosahebi A, *et al.* Reconstruction of extensive composite posterolateral mandibular defects using nonosseous free tissue transfer. *Plast Reconstr Surg* 2009;124:1571–7.
Nagele P, *et al.* Postoperative myocardial injury after major head and neck cancer surgery. *Head Neck* 2011;33;1085–91.
Nouraei SAR, *et al.* Incidence and significance of myocardial injury after surgical treatment of head and neck cancer. *Laryngoscope* 2007;117:1581–7.
Oken MM, et al. Toxicity and response criteria of the Eastern Cooperative Oncology Group. *Am J Clin Oncol* 1982;5(6):649–55.
Olsson P, *et al.* Haptics-assisted virtual planning of bone, soft tissue, and vessels in fibula osteocutaneous free flaps. *Plastic Reconstr Surg—Global Open* 2015;3:e479.
Peters TTA, *et al.* Free flap reconstruction for head and neck cancer can be safely performed in both young and elderly patients after careful patient selection. *Eur Arch Oto-rhino-l* 2015;272:2999–3005.
Rinker B. The evils of nicotine. *Ann Plas Surg* 2013;70:599–605.
Sakakibara A, *et al.* Long-term effects on volume change in musculocutaneous flaps after head and neck reconstruction. *J Reconstr Microsurg* 2018;35;235–43.
Serletti JM, Higgins JP, Moran S, Orlando GS. Factors affecting outcome in free-tissue transfer in the elderly. *Plast Reconstr Surg* 2000;106:66–70.
Silverman DA, *et al.* Evaluation of bone length and number of osteotomies utilizing the osteocutaneous radial forearm free flap for mandible reconstruction: An 8-year review of complications and flap survival. *Head Neck* 2016;38:434–8.
Soutar D, McGregor, I. The radial forearm flap in intraoral reconstruction: the experience of 60 consecutive cases. *Plast Reconstr Surg* 1986;78:1–8.
Stone HB, Coleman CN, Anscher MS, McBride WH. Effects of radiation on normal tissue: consequences and mechanisms. *Lancet Oncol* 1986;4:529–36.
Suchyta M, Mardini, S. Innovations and future directions in head and neck microsurgical reconstruction. *Clin Plast Surg* 2017;44:325–44.
Tam K, Ghazizadeh S, Abemayor E, John MA. Introduction: Leaps and bounds. In: *Novel Therapies in Head and Neck Cancer: Beyond the Horizon* (eds. St. John MA, Park N-H). Cambridge, MA: Academic Press, 2020: pp. 1–15.
Tang NSJ, Ahmadi I, Ramakrishnan A. Virtual surgical planning in fibula free flap head and neck reconstruction: a systematic review and meta-analysis. *J Plastic ReconstrAesthetic Surg* 2019;72:1465–77.
Torina PJ, Matros E, Athanasian EA, Cordeiro PG. Immediate bone grafting and plating of the radial osteocutaneous free flap donor site. *Ann Plas Surg* 2014;73:315–20.
Tsai C-H, *et al.* Postoperative morbidity in head and neck cancer ablative surgery followed by microsurgical free tissue transfer in the elderly. *Oral Oncol* 2012;48:811–16.
Tuluy Y, Bali ZU, Ünsal MÖ, Parspancı A, Yoleri L, Çiçek Ç, Filinte GT. Comparison of the thickness of free anterolateral thigh flap in different fascial planes: clinical results of subfascial and superficial fat flap. *Arch Plast Surg* 2023;50(6):601–9.

Üstün GG, Aksu AE, Uzun H, Bitik O. The systematic review and meta-analysis of free flap safety in the elderly patients. *Microsurgery* 2017;37(5):442–50.
Varley I, Wales CJ, Carter LM. The median artery: its potential implications for the radial forearm flap. *J Plast Reconstr Aesthet Surg* 2008;61(6):693–5.
Vassiliou LV, Sinha D, Dawood A, Kalavrezos N. Vascularized free fibula flap oral rehabilitation using tissue engineered mucosa: report of 3 cases. *J Craniomaxillofac Surg* 2022;50(6):485–92.
Vieira L, Isacson D, Dimovska EOF, Rodriguez-Lorenzo A. Four lessons learned from complications in head and neck microvascular reconstructions and prevention strategies. *Plastic Reconstr Surg—Global Open* 2021;9(1):e3329.
Wei F-C, Deek NFA, Cheng M-H, Lin C-H. The triangle of unfavorable outcomes after microsurgical head and neck reconstruction planning, design, and execution. *Clin Plast Surg* 2016;43:615–20.
Weinzweig N, Jones NF, Shestak KC, Moon HK, Davies BW. Oromandibular reconstruction using a keel-shaped modification of the radial forearm osteocutaneous flap. *Ann Plas Surg* 1994;33:359–70.
Wilson JL, et al. Avoiding complications. In *Flaps and Reconstructive Surgery*. (eds. Wei F-C, Mardini S). Oxford: Elsevier, 2016: pp. 323–32.
Wolff K.-D., Hölzle F. *Raising of Microvascular Flaps: A Systematic Approach*, 2nd edition. Berlin Heidelberg: Springer-Verlag, 2011.
Yu P. Characteristics of the anterolateral thigh flap in a Western population and its application in head and neck reconstruction. *Head Neck* 2004;26(9):759–69.
Zhang F, *et al*. Effect of sequence, timing of vascular anastomosis, and clamp removal on survival of microsurgical flaps. *J Reconstr Microsurg* 2002;18:697–702.

3

Anaesthetic considerations for head and neck free-flap reconstructive surgery

Danielle Ormandy, Leandros Vassilios F. Vassiliou, Panayiotis Kyzas, and Nicholas Kalavrezos

3.1 Preoperative assessment, airway assessment, and planning

Introduction

Comprehensive preoperative assessment, optimization when possible, and strategic airway management planning are significant factors of success in major head neck surgery. In an ideal setting a qualified anaesthetist, who regularly performs anaesthesia for major head and neck operations should be in the clinic jointly reviewing the patients preoperatively, alongside the surgical team.

Preoperative assessment

The aims of preoperative assessment are the following:

- Identification of patients with potentially difficult airways.
- Stratification of perioperative risks.
- Management of comorbidities.
- Optimization of patient's physiology prior to major surgery.

Identifying and optimizing reversible elements of disease early is crucial to improving surgical outcomes.

Head and neck cancer patients often present with a high burden of comorbid disease. A large proportion of this cohort of patients smoke and drink to excess and are thus predisposed to cardiorespiratory, peripheral vascular, and liver disease. In addition, a poor nutritional status, whether associated with excess alcohol intake or as a direct result of the physical presence of the tumour and/or its related pain, is not uncommon. Preoperative malnutrition independently correlates with poor wound healing, infection, and an increased risk of postoperative complications. It is therefore imperative the patient has early specialized dietician input.

Patients with a high level of alcohol dependency should be considered for active in-patient withdrawal treatment, allowing also time for nutritional and electrolyte optimization.

Standard preoperative investigations should include the following:

Baseline bloods

Electrocardiography (ECG) and COVID-19 status, as a minimum.

If the patient has risk factors and/or symptoms of cardiorespiratory disease, lung-function tests, and an echocardiogram should be requested. If available, Cardio-pulmonary exercise testing (CPET) provides a dynamic measure of the cardiovascular, respiratory, and circulatory physiology that can be extrapolated to perioperative survival. A low Anaerobic Threshold (AT) is associated with a poor outcome postoperatively, and high risk is suggested when the AT is <11 mL/kg/min. It is worth noting that these tests are not definitive but should be used in the context of the clinical picture to guide preoperative discussions, risk stratification, optimization plans, and determine the level of postoperative care.

An important role of the anaesthetic preoperative assessment is to take into consideration all patients' comorbidities, performance status, and physiological parameters and provide advisory context in the surgical plan. A comprehensive anaesthetic assessment may be able to gauge the patient's physiological reserves to withstand major surgery or depict risks for postoperative cardiac or respiratory complications and offer valuable input in adjusting the surgical plan as discussed in Chapter 2.4.

Airway assessment

The incidence of difficult airways in head and neck cancer is higher than in the general surgical population. A comprehensive evaluation of the patient's airway, including a review of any previous anaesthetic records and imaging is imperative to formulate the safest airway management plan.

A thorough medical history should be taken to identify any medical conditions associated with airway difficulty (Box 3.1.1).

Previous treatment with radiotherapy results in a fibrotic airway associated with stiff, non-compliant tissue, which can make both face mask ventilation and laryngoscopy difficult. **A previously documented difficult airway should always be taken seriously irrespective of the experience of the anaesthetist involved.** The patient should be questioned specifically on signs or symptoms of potential airway obstruction: Changes to the voice, dysphagia, orthopnoea, dyspnoea at rest, drooling, and stridor may indicate airway compromise.

A clinical examination of the airway should be undertaken to establish a detailed knowledge of the tumour location, type, size, and impact of the pathology on the airway. An initial examination of the gross anatomy may help predict difficult facemask ventilation. Airway assessment should include an assessment of mouth opening, Mallampati classification (Figure 3.1.1), Mandibular Subluxation (Calder score), Thyromental distance, length and thickness of the neck, and neck extension.

Predictors of difficult bag-mask ventilation and direct laryngoscopy are included in Table 3.1.1.

Box 3.1.1 Medical conditions associated with a difficult airway

Medical conditions associated with a difficult airway
Previous head and neck surgery or radiotherapy
Obesity
Obstructive sleep apnoea
Rheumatoid Arthritis
Ankylosing spondylitis
Pituitary tumours (Acromegaly)
Scleroderma
Thyroid disease
Previous cervical spine surgery

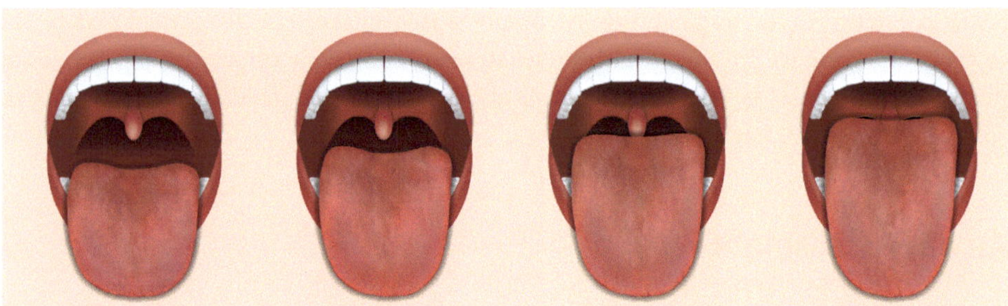

Figure 3.1.1 Mallampati classification: a pictorial guide of pharyngeal structures seen when assessing the airway.

Table 3.1.1 Predictors of difficult bag-mask ventilation and direct laryngoscopy

Difficult mask ventilation	Difficult direct laryngoscopy
Presence of beard	Reduced mouth opening/Trismus
Gross facial abnormalities	Mallampati grades 3 to 4
Micrognathia	Decreased mandibular protrusion
Obesity	Neck radiation changes
Male gender	Previous head and neck surgery
Edentulous	Decreased thyromental distance
Decreased mandibular protrusion	Reduced/Fixed neck movement
Mallampati grades 3 to 4	Tongue fixation (tumour invasion)
Neck radiation changes	Abnormal anatomy secondary to pathology

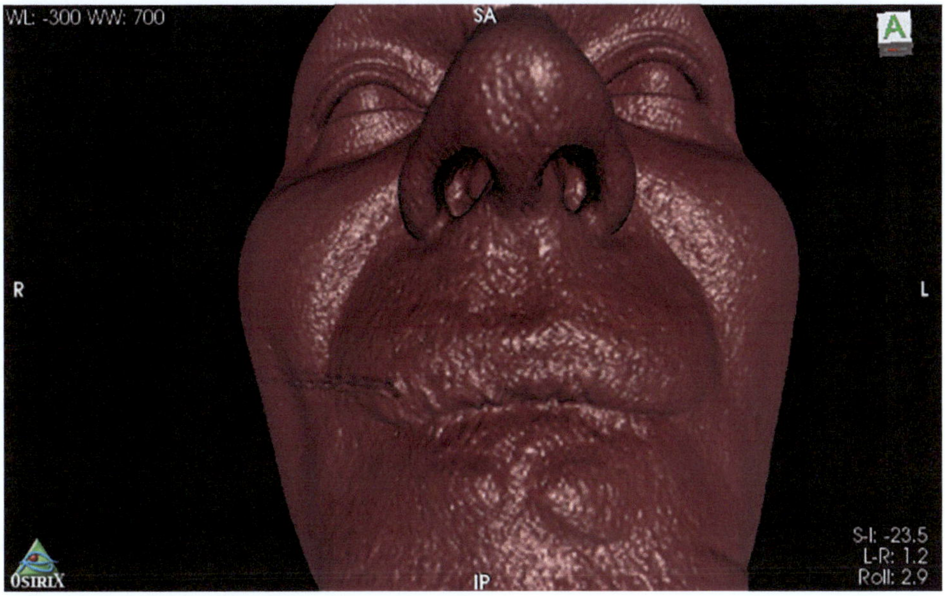

Video 3.1.1 Virtual laryngoscopy.
See this video online by searching for this book's title or ISBN at https://academic.oup.com/
Reproduced courtesy of Leandros Vassiliou, Manchester University NHS Foundation Trust, Manchester, UK.

Clinical examination should be supplemented with a review of any available radiological imaging and if availability allows, a flexible nasendoscopy. A review of any radiological investigations will typically provide detailed information on the anatomical location and extent of the tumour, any involvement of secondary tissues and critically, whether there is any distortion or narrowing of the airway.

Awake flexible nasendoscopy (FNE) gives a dynamic assessment of the upper airway and larynx and is useful in identifying those patients that require an awake intubation technique.

CT scanning with 3D reconstruction and virtual endoscopy is a relatively new concept within anaesthetics. It allows a more comprehensive airway assessment, improving the ability to fully assess head and neck tumours and any extension and/or encroachment on the airway (Video 3.1.1). Virtual laryngoscopy studies can be generated by importing Digital Imaging and Communications in Medicine (DICOM) files of the patient's preoperative scan into specialized 3D imaging software platforms such as the OsiriX®.

The strategy for airway management, including the postoperative airway plan, should be formulated in conjunction with the surgeon in a multidisciplinary team discussion.

Airway management plan

The strategy for airway management should be discussed with the operating surgeon(s) preoperatively and must include a postoperative airway plan.

The optimal airway management approach depends on the location of the tumour, the proposed surgical procedure, the patients' signs and symptoms and the acuity of the situation. In the majority of patients undergoing elective head and neck resections with free-flap reconstruction, there is time to fully appraise all airway options and formulate the safest airway management plan. A plan should only be devised after a thorough history and examination, including reviewing any radiological imaging and if appropriate, performing an FNE.

The following questions should be answered prior to induction of anaesthesia:

- Is facemask ventilation likely to be possible after induction of anaesthesia?
- Is laryngoscopy and intubation likely to be difficult?
- Is an awake technique more appropriate?
- Is emergency front of neck access (FONA) feasible?

When difficulty in bag-mask ventilation and tracheal intubation is predicted, or has been previously experienced, awake tracheal intubation is indicated. An awake technique affords the benefit of maintenance of airway patency, continued spontaneous ventilation, and thus oxygenation, and protection against aspiration during intubation.

Awake tracheal intubation is performed, after adequate toplicalization with local anaesthetic, using a flexible fibreoptic scope or a video-laryngoscope. If sedation is used, this should not compromise the patient's airway patency or ventilation: Remifentanil Target-Controlled Infusion is an excellent drug for this setting.

Ultimately, the chosen technique for awake tracheal intubation should be one that the operating anaesthetist is familiar with and offers the greatest chance of first pass tracheal intubation. Where awake tracheal intubation is not possible, an awake tracheostomy should be strongly considered.

Surgical Tracheostomy

A surgical tracheostomy is essential for the postoperative period after extensive reconstructive surgery when swelling and oedema can compromise the airway.

It is preferable to perform the tracheostomy at the beginning of the surgery under controlled conditions. This has several important advantages:

- It provides a secure airway,
- it improves surgical access to the operating site,
- it reduces dead-space improving ventilation and importantly,
- carrying out the tracheostomy at the start of surgery means that any immediate tracheostomy-related complications can be identified, and rectified, safely in theatre.

An elective tracheostomy may feel for many an unnecessary invasive procedure which may increase the morbidity of a head and neck major operation and also inflict or induce risks for postoperative airway complications.

An elective tracheostomy also means that postoperatively the patient has to be admitted and nursed in a level 3 environment. This in an era of shortages in an intensive care unit, may pose restrictions in service provision and the volume of patients that can be treated electively.

It is our opinion that an elective tracheostomy does not only offer a postoperatively secure airway and guards the patient from complications such as bleeding in their airway, haematoma, or oedema. The presence of a tracheostomy also allows for advanced respiratory management and lung toilet and lavage.

A significant portion of head and neck cancer patients have co-existing respiratory diseases such as chronic obstructive pulmonary disorder (COPD). Moreover, a prolonged head and neck operation predisposes the patient to postoperative lower respiratory tract infections. For these reasons, the presence of a tracheostomy helps with respiratory management and mitigation of pneumonia.

Anecdotally tracheostomy is also associated with (splinting) the position of the neck. This is quite crucial in the first 72 hours for the anastomosis to be established. The absence of the tracheostomy may predispose the patient to neck movements and flexion that may kink the early vessel pedicle anastomosis predisposing for free-flap compromise.

For these reasons in our practice, we have a low threshold on performing elective tracheostomy for head and neck major ablation and reconstruction.

The advocates of delayed extubation propose that a patient remains intubated by an oral or nasal tube overnight postoperatively following which an airway assessment is performed prior to extubation.

The counter argument is that following head and neck major surgery the patient is at risk of airway compromise due to bleeding, haematoma, or oedema. All three of these can occur in a window frame over three days, especially the postoperative oedema which peaks 72 hours postoperatively. Hence, a secure airway for less than 24 hours postoperatively doesn't completely cover for the immediate high risk postoperative period and a tracheostomy would be the preferrable safety option.

The argument of elective tracheostomy versus delayed extubation has been explored in over 700 patients in a study published by Myatra et al. The authors conclude that strict case selection is required prior to the decision for a delayed extubation.

The criteria that could render this option safe are no neck dissection or a unilateral neck dissection, tumour size (T1/T2), no preoperative radiation therapy (difficult airway and difficult reintubation if required), the absence of extensive surgical resection and primary closure or fasciocutaneous flap only.

These criteria summarize that delayed extubation can be considered for patients with a relatively small resection and flaps that don't tend to significantly become oedematous postoperatively, such as bony flaps or flaps with a muscular component. In addition to that we would advocate that any midline structure resection that would involve the tongue, floor of mouth, or oropharynx would require an elective tracheostomy.

Delayed extubations can be considered for lateralized resections such as alveolectomies, small segmental mandibulectomies with no floor of mouth or oropharyngeal component and buccal or facial skin resections and parotidectomies. In those cases, the midline structures and effectively the tongue, oropharynx and laryngeal inlet remain relatively unaffected by the surgical procedure and therefore the airway anatomy is at a lower risk.

3.2 **Surgical tracheostomy**

Introduction

Our proposed tracheostomy technique includes a number of modifications/steps aiming to improve safety in the postoperative period. These have been described by Ormandy et al. in 'Tracheostomy suspension modified approach for securing the airway' (see 'Further reading').

Surgical technique

- The tracheostomy is performed via the open surgical technique (Figure 3.2.1) and aims to provide safety net features in case of accidental tracheostomy tube dislodgement.
- Removal of all the subcutaneous fat. In the immediate postoperative period, significant neck oedema is not uncommon. In case of accidental tracheostomy tube dislodgement or displacement in the first week, any remaining subcutaneous fat may be oedematous, hence obscuring the access into the tracheostomy window for the placement of a new tracheostomy tube.
- Meticulous intraoperative haemostasis and ideally tissue dissection via bipolar forceps.
- Division of the thyroid isthmus. It is strongly advocated that a thyroid isthmus is not displaced superiorly or inferiorly to the tracheostomy window. If not divided, in case

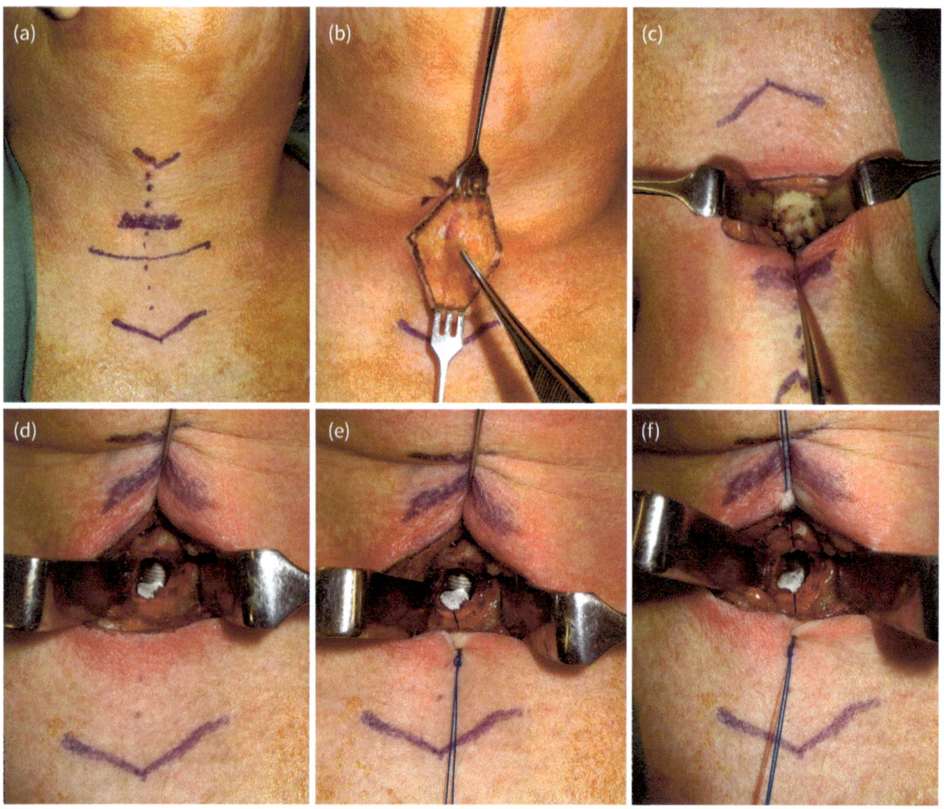

Figure 3.2.1 Tracheostomy technique. a. Surface markings. b. Incision and excision of subcutaneous fat. c. Exposure of the anterior tracheal wall after division of the thyroid isthmus. d. Tracheostomy window via partial removal of the anterior tracheal ring cartilage. It is important to avoid wide windows as this may cause tracheal stenosis and also risk tracheostomy tube dislodgement. It is advised to keep the window relatively small but use tracheal dilators to increase access prior to tube insertion. e. Rescue stitch in place—note that the knot is not tightened tightly to avoid distortion (forward kink) of the tracheal axis. The knot is placed on the skin surface with minimal tug, just enough to 'suspend' the trachea. f. For high-risk patients (short neck, high BMI, anticipated postoperative neck swelling/oedema, pectoralis major flap or bulky musculocutaneous flaps) additional rescue stitches are recommended.

of inadvertent tracheostomy tube dislodgement, the thyroid isthmus will automatically resume its original position, obstructing the tracheostomy window with highly vascular tissue, rendering any attempt at re-cannulation extremely difficult or impossible.

- Prior to opening the trachea and creating a window, the anaesthetist can be requested to deflate the endotracheal tube (ETT) tube's cuff, advance the ETT tube caudally and reinflate the cuff. This manoeuvre avoids inadvertent perforation of the cuff during the tracheal incision, yet allows seamless ventilation of the patient when the trachea above the inflated cuff is instrumented.
- Dissection of cartilaginous segment and formation of a formal tracheostomy window. This step, and in contrast to a 'tracheotomy' incision, ensures that an open window will remain patent, allowing prompt tracheal intubation in case of an emergency. The previously described Björk flap can prove dangerous, as during tracheal re-intubation, the tracheal 'flap' may inadvertently be pushed inwards, causing obstruction of the airway and inhibiting a tube insertion.
- The window should not be too wide (less than a third of the anterior cartilaginous circumference) to prevent postoperative tracheal stenosis, but can be dilated using tracheal dilators. A marginally narrower than the tracheostomy tube window also prevents accidental dislodgement, naturally 'clamping' the tube and preventing it from slipping out, especially at the cuff site.

Rescue sutures

In addition to the above, we advocate airway securing via one or more rescue sutures (Figure 3.2.1e and Figure 3.2.1f). The following consists of a thick nylon (Prolene) 0.0 on a round-bodied needle. The stitch should be passed around the inferior and superior cartilaginous tracheal rings. A round-bodied needle minimizes inadvertent cheese wiring through the tracheal cartilage.

The suspension of the trachea with a rescue stitch has important safety advantages:

- The tracheal window is brought closer to the skin, allowing direct visualization in case of emergency tracheal re-cannulation.
- The trachea is 'suspended' closer to the surface and traction of the rescue stitch provides countertraction and prevention of the trachea falling backwards during the pressure of a new tracheostomy tube insertion.
- In case of ventilation with a laryngeal mask, the rescue stitch suspends the trachea closer to the skin surface, preventing surgical emphysema.
- The presence of the rescue stitch prevents inadvertent creation of false passage during an emergency tracheal re-cannulation.

If the patient has a high-risk anatomy such as short, or/and increased size neck (high BMI), then placement of two or more rescue stitches (superior and inferior rings) is recommended. In an emergency, pulling of both rescue stitches not only brings the trachea closer to the skin surface and the operator, but also widens the tracheal window in an '*open fish mouth*' fashion to allow easier tracheal intubation.

The degree of postoperative neck swelling, making any attempt at tracheal re-intubation in case of emergency tube dislocation, should never be underestimated. Rescue stitches are

Box 3.2.1 Important tips for tracheostomy safety

- The tracheostomy window has to be of a carefully assessed size. Small windows may not allow the tracheostomy tube to pass. Wide windows may predispose to tracheostomy tube movement and dislodgement as well as tracheal stenosis.
- Rescue stitches are highly recommended as they can facilitate easier trachea re-cannulation in case of tracheostomy tube dislodgement. Loss of airway in a head and neck patient can be detrimental.
- In cases of tracheostomy tube dislodgement or emergency removal, intubation from the oral cavity may be extremely difficult. Rescue stitches facilitate pulling the tracheal window close to the surface and provide countertraction during re-cannulation, also avoiding introducing false passage.

especially recommended when postoperative difficult airways are anticipated such as in the following situations:

- Muscle and bone flap reconstruction. The flaps in the immediate postoperative period and for over one week develop significant oedema and subsequent neck swelling is not unusual. This is mainly due to compromised lymphatic drainage (free tissue transfer is based on arterial and venous anastomosis but no lymphatic vessels are anastomosed until integration with recipient time takes place).
- Postoperative neck collections (seromas, haematomas) may increase the distance between the skin surface and tracheal window making tracheal re-cannulation in the emergency setting extremely difficult.
- Loss of 'laryngeal suspension', such as in anterior segmental mandibulectomies, renders tracheal re-intubation extremely difficult. The trachea after the mandibular resection can no longer be controlled by simple airway management manoeuvres (jaw thrust, mandible tilt). The pressure of insertion of a new tracheostomy or ETT tube may push the trachea backwards risking formation of false passage and loss of airway.
- Pectoralis Major reconstruction. The muscle pedicle over the clavicle significantly raises the surface of the skin away from the tracheal window, making any subsequent attempt for re-cannulation extremely difficult in the absence of rescue sutures.

Important highlights in tracheostomy safety for patients undergoing major head and neck surgery are found in Box 3.2.1.

Post-tracheostomy nursing

Patients following head and neck major surgery carrying a tracheostomy should always be nursed postoperatively in wards staffed with 'airway trained' clinical teams.

A clear 'Airway Plan' must be documented in the postoperative notes by the surgeon and anaesthetist and communicated with the receiving team (intensive care unit).

The emergency tracheostomy management algorithm (Figure 3.2.2) is a synopsis of all the critical steps that need to be followed in the event of a tracheostomy-related complication.

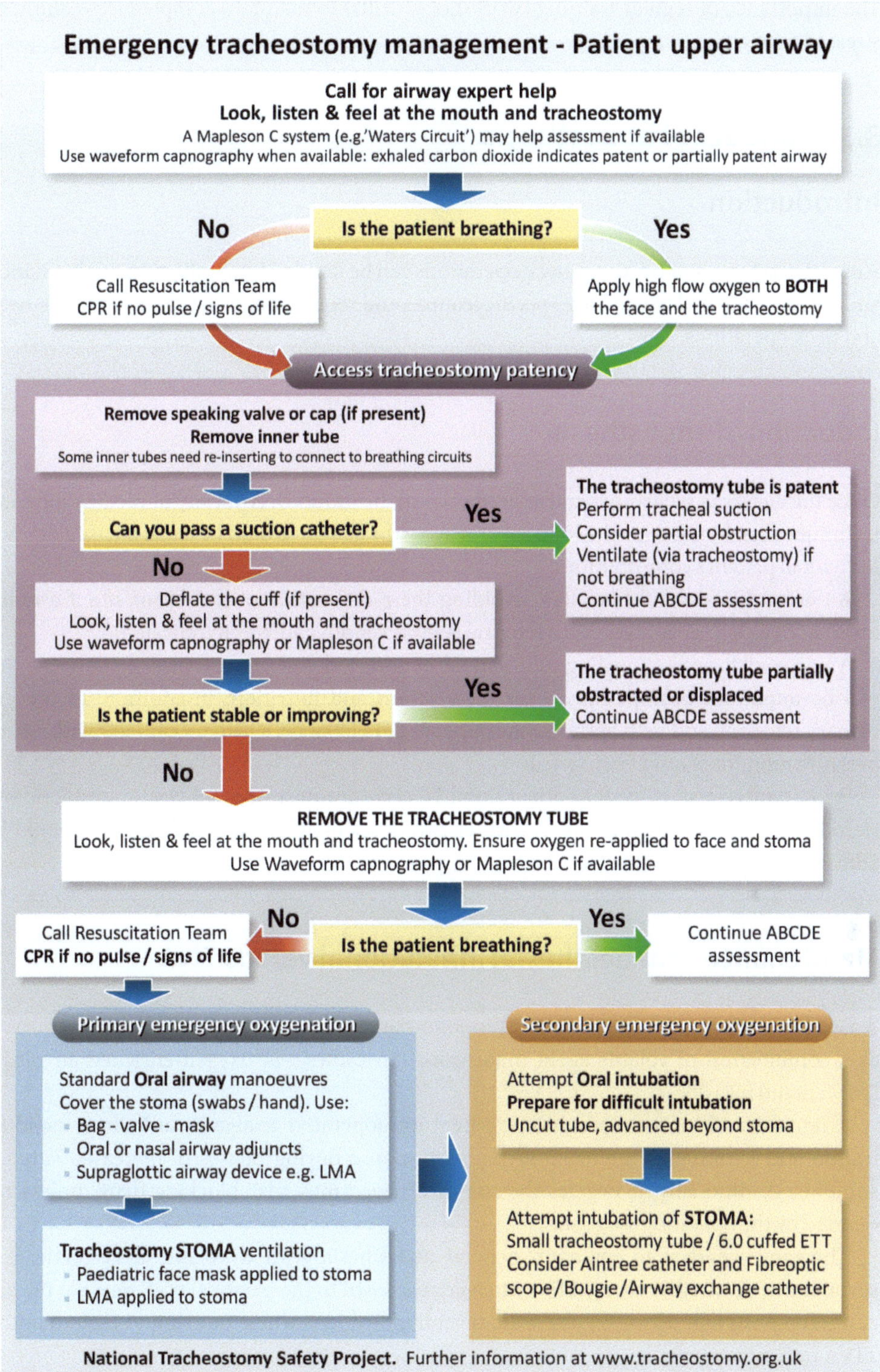

Figure 3.2.2 Emergency tracheostomy troubleshooting algorithm as demonstrated by the United Kingdom National Tracheostomy Safety Project.

Reproduced with permission from McGrath A, Bates L, Atkinson D, Moore JA. National Tracheostomy Safety Project: Multidisciplinary guidelines for the management of tracheostomy and laryngectomy airway emergencies. *Anaesthesia* 2012; 67: 1025–41.

The importance of regular training (workshops, drills) to maintain competences cannot be stressed enough.

3.3 Conduct of anaesthesia

Introduction

Anaesthesia for major head and neck operations can be divided into induction, maintenance, and emergence, all of which have specific features and requirements in practising major head and neck operations.

Induction of anaesthesia

Once the airway is secure, general anaesthesia can be induced. A variety of medications and techniques can be used for the induction of anaesthesia and should be chosen based on each individual patient's comorbidities.

An arterial line should be sited, avoiding the radial artery of the donor site if a radial forearm free-flap is planned, and a femoral central venous catheter if indicated.

A nasogastric enteral feeding tube should be inserted and secured prior to surgery; this will be important postoperatively for medications and nutrition. In addition, to prevent urinary retention and help optimize the patient's fluid balance, a urinary catheter with a temperature monitor should be inserted.

Prior to surgery starting, the patient should receive one dose of prophylactic antibiotic and steroids, usually dexamethasone. A further two doses of antibiotics and steroids should be administered at eight-hourly intervals.

Maintenance of anaesthesia: Inhalational versus TIVA

Anaesthesia may be maintained with propofol-based total intravenous anaesthesia (TIVA) or a combination of volatile agent inhalational anaesthetic in oxygen-enriched air plus a remifentanil infusion.

A remifentanil infusion provides excellent intraoperative analgesia and allows rapid titration and blunting of the haemodynamic response during phases of increased surgical stimulus. Additionally, it negates the use of a neuro-muscular blocking drug, unless requested by the operating surgeon.

Choosing whether to maintain general anaesthesia with a volatile anaesthetic, e.g. sevoflurane, or whether to use TIVA often comes down to the personal preference of the anaesthetic consultant. However, there are several indications where one should elect to utilize TIVA rather than volatile:

- Patients with malignant hyperthermia (MH) or MH susceptibility
- Patients with previous postoperative nausea and vomiting (PONV) or multiple risk factors for PONV

- Patients who are pregnant, particularly in the first trimester
- Patients with long-QT syndrome (QTc ≥ 500 ms)

Maintenance of anaesthesia: Physiological parameters

There are several critical stages during a major head and neck cancer resection and reconstruction with a free flap, whereby the anaesthetic management needs to be manipulated to achieve various cardiovascular parameters (see Chapter 3.4).

Insensible fluid and blood loss can occur from both the tumour resection and the flap donor site.

Intraoperative haemoglobin and haematocrit measurements help guide the need for blood transfusions. Cardiac output monitoring with stroke volume variation is useful in guiding intraoperative fluid therapy to optimize free-flap perfusion (see Chapter 3.4).

Urine output, arterial pulse pressures, haematocrit, base excess, lactate, and cardiac output monitoring trends should all be used simultaneously to guide the patient's fluid administration.

The patient's electrolytes and blood glucose should be monitored at regular intervals throughout the duration of surgery and corrected as necessary. It is not uncommon for patients with diabetes mellitus to require an insulin infusion intraoperatively.

Ventilation parameters should include lung-protective ventilation strategies (6 ml/kg) and be guided by the patient's arterial blood gases to maintain both normoxia and normocapnia. Hypoxia and hypocapnia lead to vasoconstriction, thus reducing microcirculation perfusion, while hypercapnia can cause sympathetic nervous system stimulation.

Emergence and extubation

Coughing, retching, and straining increase venous pressure, reducing flap flow, while hypertensive spikes risk the integrity of the newly formed anastomoses and the development of haematoma. Therefore, it is critical that patients have a smooth emergence from anaesthesia.

The presence of a new tracheostomy is uncomfortable for patients, causing coughing and irritation during both emergence and in recovery. To help mitigate this sensation, lidocaine can be sprayed down the tracheostomy via a mucosal atomizer device or alternatively, can be nebulized. Intravenous lidocaine (1/5 mg/kg) has been shown to reduce tracheal irritation and post-extubation coughing. In addition, good analgesia is essential.

To facilitate a smooth emergence, a low-dose remifentanil infusion with an effect site target of 1–1.5 ng/ml can be continued. This helps obtund cardiovascular reflexes and reduces agitation and coughing.

Antiemetics

Prior to waking, all patients should receive aggressive prophylaxis for PONV. A multimodal approach is best utilized, consisting of ondansetron 4 mg IV (5-HT_3 antagonist), dexamethasone 8 mg IV, and a third antiemetic agent if the patient is at high risk for PONV, such as cyclizine 50 mg IV (H1-receptor antagonist) or prochlorperazine 12.5 mg IM (D2-receptor antagonist). Regular antiemetics should be prescribed postoperatively, with additional 'breakthrough' antiemetics should they be required.

3.4 Practical anaesthetic management and monitoring

Introduction

Major head and neck surgery poses significant physiological and metabolic stress. The role of an Anaesthetist is important in addressing the patient's systemic demands throughout the operation. Anaesthetic induction, management of the airway, choice of vascular access, and continuous monitoring with proactive resuscitation through the different phases of the operation (ablation, reconstruction, anastomosis) are of paramount importance.

The airway

The majority of head and neck operations require the patient to be positioned supine with a 15–20-degree head-up tilt, with the head at the opposite end to the anaesthetic machine, therefore access to the airway by the anaesthetist is limited.

A joint airway plan should be decided preoperatively to ensure the safety of the patient intraoperatively and postoperatively while considering the surgical access required.

Long ventilator tubing and capnography lines are required. Difficult airway equipment should be immediately available.

Vascular access

Venous access sites can be limited due to multiple surgical sites (head neck, flap donor site, skin graft site, tourniquets, drapes) and patient positioning; therefore, all intravenous lines should be well secured with the appropriate length infusion sets. For major resections, large-bore venous access is essential.

Prior to the induction of anaesthesia and at the team brief, a detailed discussion regarding the appropriate placement of intravascular catheters between the anaesthetist and the surgeon must take place. Intravenous catheters, arterial lines, or central venous catheters should not be placed at flap donor sites or areas that may be subjected to flexion, pressure, or obstruction during the procedure due to patient positioning, drapes, or other equipment.

A central venous catheter in the femoral vein should be considered for large resections, lengthy procedures, patients with poor peripheral access or those patients who may require longer-term perioperative access.

Monitoring requirements

Standard monitoring includes:

- ECG monitoring, often positioned away from the surgical site
- Non-invasive blood pressure cuff
- Pulse oximetry for oxygen saturations
- Neuromuscular monitoring
- Capnography
- Invasive arterial monitoring is required to allow the optimization of arterial pressure and regular arterial blood gas sampling
- Cardiac output monitoring, using pulse contour analysis, is recommended to assess fluid balance and optimize cardiac output
- Temperature, both peripheral and core, should be monitored as discussed earlier
- Urine output is monitored to guide fluid administration and organ perfusion

Cardiac output monitoring

Cardiac output can be monitored by many techniques: the gold standard remains the pulmonary artery catheter (PAC); however, the most commonly used techniques are pulse contour analysis and the oesophageal Doppler.

Pulmonary artery catheter: The PAC is seen as the 'gold standard' in measuring cardiac output and is what all other modalities are validated against. It involves placing a special catheter with a thermistor at the tip into a pulmonary artery via the right atrium and right ventricle. In addition to cardiac output parameters, it also provides pulmonary artery pressures, left-sided filling pressures, and mixed central venous oxygen saturations. It carries a high risk of serious complications, including pulmonary haemorrhage, pulmonary infarct, arrhythmias, and thromboembolism. Due to the invasiveness and risks of complications from this method, it is now mainly reserved for patients having cardiothoracic surgery, particularly recipients of cardiac and/or lung transplants.

Pulse contour analysis: The two main systems in place that utilize pulse contour analysis are the PiCCO® and LiDCO® systems (Figure 3.4.1). Pulse contour analysis uses algorithms, modified by inputting the patient's parameters (age, gender, height, weight), to analyse the patient's arterial pressure waveform. This produces a set of measured variables and derived variables, dependent on the system used. The LiDCO® monitor provides the following parameters:

- Stroke volume (SV): the volume of blood ejected from the left ventricle with each systolic contraction.
- Cardiac output (CO): the amount of blood pumped through the circulatory system in one minute, calculated by multiplying SV and heart rate (HR).
- Systemic vascular resistance (SVR): is the resistance to flow in the systemic circulation.
- Oxygen delivery (DO_2): represents the delivery of oxygen to tissues and is calculated by multiplying CO with oxygen concentration.

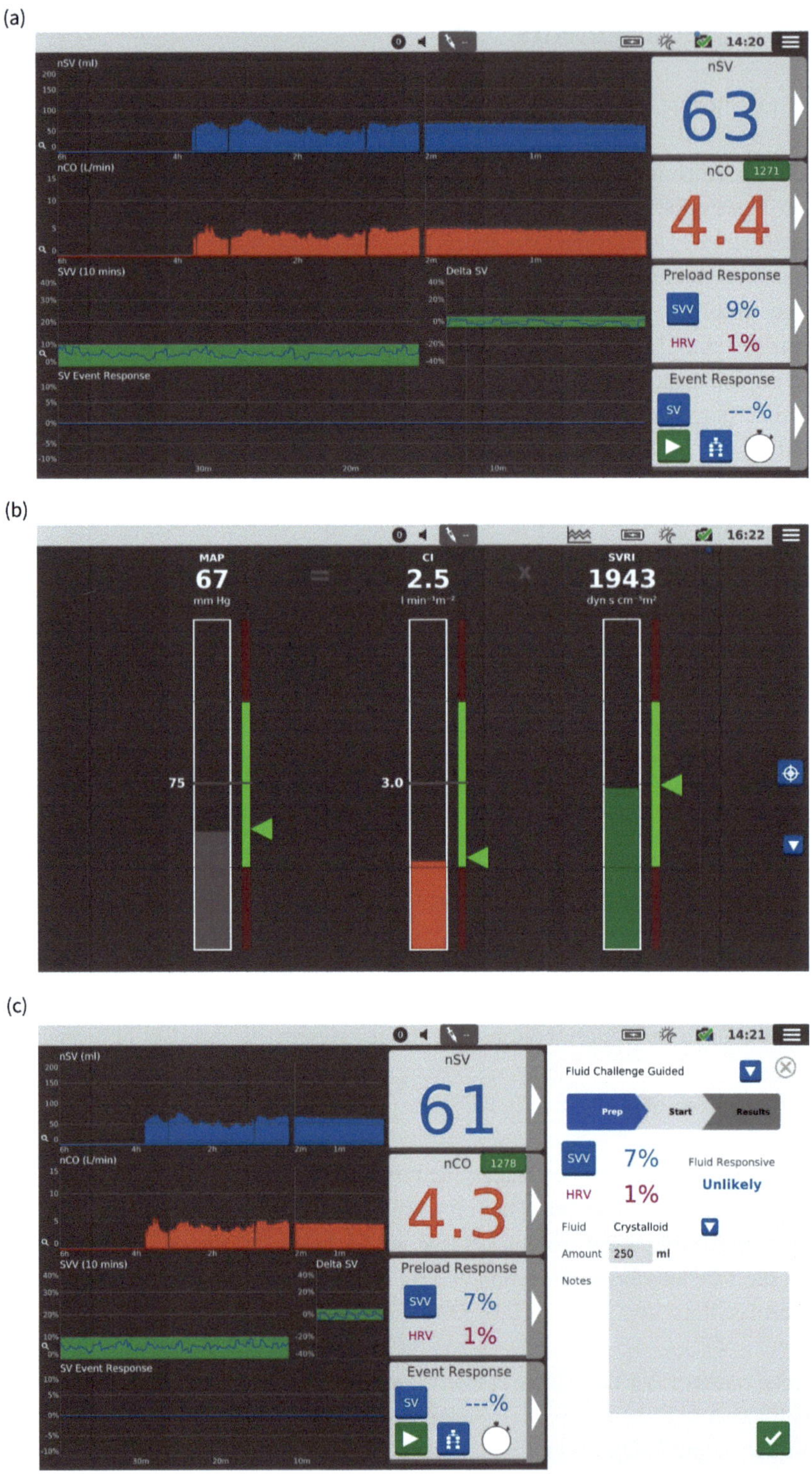

Figure 3.4.1 Indicative LIDCO® Hemodynamic Monitoring System screenshots demonstrating monitored parameters that aid delivery of anaesthesia. a. Screenshot demonstrating standard display of haemodynamic parameters. b. Alternative bar chart view of main haemodynamic values. c. The system offers algorithmic-based prediction of haemodynamic interventions through analysis of all real-time parameters.

- Stroke volume variation (SVV): a measure of the change in stroke volume across one respiratory cycle. Used to predict fluid responsiveness in mechanically ventilated patients.
- Pulse pressure variation (PPV): a measure of the change in arterial pulse pressure across one respiratory cycle. It can also be used to predict fluid responsiveness in mechanically ventilated patients.

The oesophageal Doppler: The oesophageal Doppler is a probe that is placed nasally or orally into the patient's oesophagus to the level of approximately the fifth and sixth thoracic vertebrae: the level at which the descending aorta is adjacent and parallel to the oesophagus. Using the Doppler principle, it measures the blood flow velocity in the descending aorta. This measurement is combined with the theoretical cross-sectional area of the descending aorta, defined by a nomogram when the patient's age, weight, and height are input into the monitor. The information obtained is as follows:

- Peak velocity (PV): An indicator of contractility that typically decreases with age.
- Flow time corrected (FTc): An indicator of preload.
- Stroke distance: Stroke distance is multiplied by the theoretical aortic root diameter, generated from the nomogram, to give SV.
- Minute distance: Stroke distance × HR, an estimate of cardiac output.

Thermoregulation

Temperature measurement is essential to maintain normothermia. Bladder temperature measurement using urinary catheters with temperature sensors is ideal.

In free-flap transfer, both the skin and the core bladder temperatures should be measured to ensure that the core-periphery gradient is less than 1.5 degrees, an indication of adequate tissue perfusion.

Warmed intravenous fluids, external forced air warming blankets and heat and moisture exchange filters should be used.

Multiple surgical sites

Multiple surgical sites lead to several important considerations. Anaesthetic monitoring and vascular access sites are limited and intraoperative repositioning is not uncommon. Repositioning intraoperatively poses risks to the patient; therefore, it is essential that there is a clear plan discussed in advance at the team brief. A secure airway is vital; all vascular lines should be protected and checked for length, and clear communication with a well-versed theatre team is critical to reduce the risk of complications.

Length of procedure

For lengthy operative procedures, increased attention needs to be paid to the inevitable consequences of prolonged immobility and anaesthesia-induced impaired homeostasis. Pressure areas should be padded to prevent neurovascular compression, and eyes should be protected with tapes or eye shields, if indicated. Graduated compression stockings and intermittent pneumatic calf compression devices are recommended, with consideration of preoperative low-molecular-weight heparin (LMWH) to help prevent thrombosis. A urinary catheter is essential to monitor the fluid balance and to prevent urinary retention.

3.5 **Cardiovascular considerations**

Introduction

The stress response to major surgery demands a significant increase in oxygen consumption (VO_2). In health, this is met by both an increase in cardiac output and an increase in the tissue extraction of oxygen from the blood. If the increased metabolic demands placed on the patient during major surgery and the subsequent increase in VO_2 cannot be met due to the patient's underlying physiology, then this will result in cellular and organ dysfunction.

The delivery of oxygen to tissues is described by the equation in Figure 3.5.1.

Intraoperatively, assuming haemoglobin and arterial oxygen saturations are optimized, then in order to improve the delivery of oxygen to tissues we can manipulate the cardiac output. Cardiac output is a product of stroke volume, the volume of blood ejected from the left ventricle during each systolic cardiac contraction, and the patient's heart rate. Manipulating the cardiac output is achieved using fluids, vasopressors, and/or inotropes.

Goal-directed fluid therapy

Insensible fluid and blood loss occur from both the ablative and free-flap site. Fluid resuscitation should be guided by arterial blood pressure, stroke volume variation, urine output, and arterial blood gas values.

Attention should be paid to the patient's overall fluid balance, and the fluid administered should be guided by goal-directed fluid therapy. Goal-directed fluid therapy is a patient-specific individualized approach to the administration of fluids which is guided by the patient's measurable haemodynamic parameters.

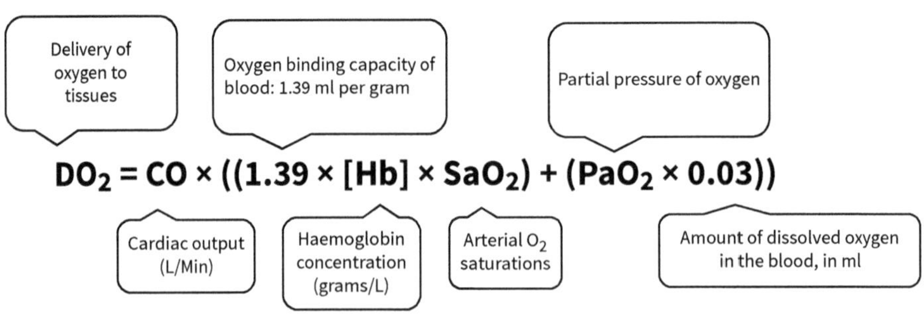

Figure 3.5.1 Equation showing delivery of oxygen (DO_2) to tissues. It is a product of cardiac output and the oxygen content of arterial blood.

It is well established that both hypovolaemia and hypervolaemia increase postoperative morbidity. Therefore, the maintenance of euvolaemia throughout the perioperative setting is desired. Isotonic crystalloid fluids should be utilized unless otherwise contraindicated. Regular electrolyte monitoring via an arterial blood gas (sampled from the patient's arterial line) will allow one to modify the choice of crystalloid fluid as appropriate. It is important to note the fluid requirements of the patient changes dependent on the operation being performed: A small ablation with a radial forearm free-flap reconstruction will require less fluid replacement than a large ablation with a composite free-flap reconstruction.

The haematocrit should be maintained at 30-35% to improve oxygen delivery to tissues and red cell velocity within the microcirculation.

Acute blood loss should be managed with the transfusion of blood products to ensure a sufficient haemoglobin concentration to allow adequate oxygen delivery to tissues (see Figure 3.5.1). Any blood transfusion should consider the patient starting haemoglobin, the intraoperative blood loss, and the patient's comorbidities.

The patient's haemoglobin and haematocrit should be monitored regularly both intra- and postoperatively. If the patient receives a large volume red blood cell transfusion, a coagulation screen should be performed and any abnormalities corrected.

Cardiovascular control

There are two main critical stages during a major head and neck cancer resection and reconstruction with free flap, whereby the anaesthetic management needs to be manipulated to achieve various goals:

1. Tumour resection
2. Flap reperfusion

Tumour resection

During the ablative phase of surgery (tumour resection), blood loss can be moderate. The principal goals of anaesthetic management during this stage are to preserve an adequate cerebral perfusion pressure and oxygen delivery while providing optimal operative conditions, i.e. minimizing bleeding by inducing hypotension to maintain a clear, dry surgical field.

Controlled hypotension (systolic blood pressure between 80 and 90 mmHg or mean arterial pressure (MAP) between 50 and 65 mmHg) can be best achieved with a combination of volatile anaesthetic and remifentanil target-controlled infusion. Additional medications that can be administered to induce hypotension include magnesium sulphate (50 mg/kg) and clonidine (1–2 μg/kg). Beta-blockers may cause relative peripheral vasoconstriction and should be used with caution.

Positioning the patient head-up improves venous return and thus helps to reduce surgical blood loss. Mean arterial pressure should be returned to the patient's normal to check for haemostasis and prior to harvesting the flap. Controlled hypotension should be avoided in patients with systemic disease compromising major organ function: in these patients, the MAP should be kept within 20% of the patient's baseline.

Flap reperfusion (vascular anastomoses).

During the microvascular anastomoses of the flap, the anaesthetic management goal is to maintain a full, hyperdynamic circulation with a high cardiac output, peripheral vasodilatation and normothermia to maintain an adequate microcirculation, and thus flap perfusion. Returning the patient to their normotension is sufficient to ensure an adequate perfusion pressure through the free-flap tissue. Composite free flaps require a higher blood pressure: a minimal MAP of 75 mmHg should be aimed for both during the anastomoses and the first 24 hours postoperatively. This is best achieved with fluid resuscitation (crystalloid fluids and/or blood products) and vasopressors, such as metaraminol.

Although historically there were concerns that vasopressors impair free-flap outcomes, there is no convincing evidence to suggest this. Conversely, there is plentiful evidence that increasing the MAP improves free-flap function.

Vasopressors (vasoactive agents)

Metaraminol is a synthetic sympathomimetic amine acting as a strong α-1 adrenergic agonist with some β-adrenergic effects, although α-agonist activity predominates, causing peripheral vasoconstriction. This in turn increases the systemic vascular resistance (SVR), increasing the patient's blood pressure. It can be used as both an intravenous infusion and given as an intravenous bolus, making it easily titratable and a good choice of vasopressor for long head and neck cases where blood pressure needs to be carefully controlled.

Noradrenaline is a synthetic and endogenous catecholamine that is a strong α-1 adrenergic agonist and moderate β1-agonist. It causes peripheral vasoconstriction, increasing SVR and subsequently the patient's blood pressure. It has some positive inotropy at higher doses. It can only be given via a central line as an intravenous infusion. Due to its potency, it can be more difficult to titrate, with resulting hypertension and reflex bradycardias. It cannot be given as an intravenous bolus and should not be ceased abruptly. Prolonged use can cause hyperglycaemia, and higher doses can result in myocardial, mesenteric, renal or peripheral (digital) ischaemia.

Dobutamine is a drug that historically has been used for free-flap surgery; it is less commonly used. It is an inotrope with a predominant and relatively selective β1-receptor effect and mild β2-receptor effect. The result is an increase in myocardial contractility and heart rate, thus augmenting cardiac output, while some vasodilation effects decrease pulmonary vascular resistance (PVR). This increase in myocardial contractility increases myocardial oxygen demands with the potential to cause cardiac ischaemia. The resulting increase in heart rate can also cause tachycardias with exacerbation of any ventricular arrythmias or ectopics. Again, this is a drug that must be given as an infusion without the ability to bolus and cannot be stopped abruptly.

Other agents such as phenylephrine (α-1 adrenergic receptor agonist with minimal to no β-adrenergic activity) and ephedrine (α-1 and β-1 adrenergic agonist) are often utilized; however, in our practice, the most commonly used vasopressors are metaraminol and noradrenaline.

3.6 Anti-coagulation and blood transfusion

Introduction

One of the most critical complications in free flap reconstruction is postoperative thrombosis that can lead to flap failure.

This can be detrimental in the patient's recovery as it may require at least one return to theatre, and further reconstructive procedures will compound the stress and the catabolic effect of surgery.

Anti-coagulation

The majority of flap failures are due to microvascular thrombosis; therefore, the administration of anti-coagulation is paramount.

Various studies have attempted to provide evidence on what is the best standard of care in the intraoperative and postoperative settings. Many surgeons administer intravenous heparin (doses range from 500 i.u. to 5,000 i.u) immediately after the anastomosis is performed, followed by various regimes of postoperative low molecular weight heparin. There is poor evidence to support this.

A recent systematic review by Dawoud et al. has concluded that the standard deep venous thrombosis (DVT) prophylaxis regime with prophylactic low molecular weight heparin (LMWH), Enoxaparin 40 mg s/c or dalteparin 5,000 units s/c (dosage of LMWH should calculated and adjusted based on the patient's weight and renal function), the day before the surgery or in the anaesthetic induction followed by a daily regime is adequate.

High doses of heparin may only disguise any technical errors of the anastomosis only to postpone the inevitable complication of thrombosis for a later stage.

It is important that any microvascular anastomosis is performed to the highest standard and the patient is anti-coagulated as per standard protocols for head and neck patients. There is no benefit, and in fact there is a higher risk of complications when administering higher doses of anti-coagulation, and hence risking bleeding diathesis and complications.

Should the patient still be in the operating theatre at the prescribed time, the dose should be administered intraoperatively after checking with the surgical team.

There is a vast amount of evidence demonstrating that additional anti-coagulation, e.g. treatment dose LMWH or unfractionated heparin infusions, over and above the standard LMWH administered for venous thromboembolism prophylaxis, increases the risk of haematoma formation without offering any benefit in preventing microvascular thrombosis and subsequent flap failure; this should therefore be avoided.

Patients with co-existing morbidities requiring regular anti-coagulation with Warfarin, or direct oral anticoagulants (DOACS) should be carefully assessed for eligibility and necessity for free flap reconstruction. Their anti-coagulation has to be carefully planned, balancing the risk of postoperative bleeding and, if appropriate, guided by a haematology specialist.

On the opposite side of the coagulation spectrum, any haemostatic agents, such as tranexamic acid, to address postoperative oozing should be strictly avoided. Local haemostatic agents such as Surgicel™ (oxidized regenerated cellulose) and Tisseel® (fibrin sealant), should be used cautiously and certainly avoided in the area of the flap pedicle and especially the anastomosis, as this may exert a thrombogenic effect and compromise the anastomosis.

Blood transfusion

Preoperative anaemia

It is not uncommon that head and neck cancer patients present with anaemia. Any preoperative anaemia, especially with haemoglobin values below 10 g/dl should be addressed as this has been proven to reflect a significant predicator for flap failure.

Postoperative haematocrit of approximately 30% should be maintained. This has been demonstrated in several studies to offer benefits from a blood viscosity and urology perspective as well as prevention of thrombosis and haemodynamic parameters.

The transfusion threshold postoperatively may vary and the individual patient's medical background context, extent of surgery, and intra- and peri-operative blood loss should be taken into consideration.

In our practice, we aim to keep the postoperative haemoglobin between 8 and 10. For patients with a significant cardiac history or cardiovascular risk factors, a blood transfusion threshold could be raised to 10 g/dl. Blood transfusion decision-making should take into consideration the individual medical background, the perioperative parameters, as well as the risk-benefits of blood product transfusion as this is not without complications, as well as local policies.

3.7 **Postoperative care**

Introduction

Major head and neck operations with microvascular free tissue transfer are highly complex surgeries in patients with often high-risk medical history. Postoperative planned elective admission to 'Level 3' (intensive care unit, ICU), or at least 'Level 2' (high dependency unit, HDU) is important for appropriate monitoring and management of cardiorespiratory function.

Goals of postoperative care

Microvascular surgery with free flap reconstruction is most often performed in patients with numerous pre-existing comorbidities. The surgery itself, often involving complex resection and subsequent reconstruction, poses additional substantial insult in their already compromised physiology. The postoperative care often requires multiorgan support.

A free flap, no matter how technically perfect the vascular anastomosis has been performed, is reliant on optimized physiology, hence diligent management of all systems is important. The main targets in the immediate postoperative care are the following:

- Airway management according to the 'Airway Plan' (Chapter 3.2).
- Normotension with a mean arterial pressure of 70–75 mmHg.

- Central venous pressure (CVP): 8–10 mmHg (if reliably measured).
- Normothermia (core temperature >36°C, with core to peripheral gradient <1.5°C).
- Haemoglobin: 8–10 g/dL.
- Haematocrit: 30–35%.
- Urine output of at least 1 ml/kg/hr.
- Head positioned 30 degrees up with tilt according to the specifics of the anastomosis (often neutral position, or head turned over to contralateral to anastomosis side to allow seamless venous outflow).
- Adequate analgesia.
- Antiemetics (as suggested in Chapter 3.3).
- Anticoagulation.
- Antibiotics according to the microbiology perioperative prophylaxis policies.
- Early commencement of nutrition.
- Flap monitoring.
- Early mobilization and physiotherapy.

Most of these targets have been endorsed and integrated into recommendations developed by the Enhanced Recovery After Surgery (ERAS) Society, as published by Dort et al.

In the following paragraphs, specific topics from above are further analysed.

Airway management

Airway management is of paramount importance in the immediate postoperative period. As described before (Chapter 3.2), head and neck major surgery is often followed by significant neck swelling. A tracheostomy, while considered to be a low-morbidity procedure, is essential for airway protection in the early postoperative phase.

Oedema of the upper airway is especially anticipated in the following scenarios:

- Resections of large oral tumours (T3 and above) and reconstruction with large flaps that tend to develop significant oedema in the first and second postoperative weeks.
- Extensive oropharyngeal resections, as they are anatomically close to the larynx and often accompanied by upper airway (arytenoid, epiglottis, upper laryngeal inlet) oedema.
- Floor of mouth and/or glossectomy resections affecting 'midline' structures may produce significant upper airway oedema or develop haematomas leading to upper airway obstruction.

For all these reasons, a surgical tracheostomy is an airway protective measure.

The technique, as described in Chapter 3.2, recommends 'rescue sutures' to add additional safety features for emergency re-insertion/re-cannulation of the tracheostomy tube, in a case of accidental displacement:

> Reconstructions with pedicled muscle flaps, large musculocutaneous free flaps with impaired lymphatic drainage at the initial stages of healing, or neck collections, increase the distance between the skin 'stoma' and the tracheal window and in the case of an emergency the absence of rescue sutures may lead to airway loss.

Tracheostomy care in the immediate postoperative period by airway trained clinical staff is important. The 'Airway Plan' as dictated by the surgeon and the anaesthetist and must be explicitly communicated with the intensive care clinical staff and documented in the patient's notes.

Weaning off the tracheostomy and decannulation is a target also endorsed by the ERAS Society protocols.

Surgical tracheostomy tubes are almost always cuffed. A trial of cuff down in the first postoperative day if the patient's clinical condition allows is recommended. This should take place with input provided by respiratory physiotherapists. It is also recommended that the tracheostomy tubes also carry a subglottic port for aspiration of secretions pooling above the level of the cuff.

The weaning process and tracheostomy decannulation is dictated by a number of criteria and parameters based on the overall recovery of the patient. Tracheostomy decannulation should not be always early and should never be rushed. It is important to be timely and methodically planned.

The basic criteria to support the decision for decannulation include:

- Absence of lower respiratory tract infection,
- Minimum amount of respiratory secretions,
- Strong cough able to expectorate secretions,
- Minimal upper airway oedema as assessed by a flexible nasendoscopy,
- Airflow bypassing of tracheostomy tube for non-fenestrated tubes, or successful capping of tracheostomy tube (for fenestrated tubes),
- Good tolerance of deflated cuff for at least 48 continuous hours.

Caution is required in extensive tongue and oropharyngeal resections with accompanying bulky flaps. When it is anticipated that the swallowing function and management of secretions will be impaired (sub-total glossectomies, total glossectomies, lateral pharyngeal/oropharyngeal resections, hypoglossal nerve compromise or sacrifice) it is recommended that the cuff remains inflated for a minimum of five days. This is to allow patients recovery from the major operation, prior to trial cuff down that may lead to aspiration and predispose to chest infections, which could be detrimental in the immediate postoperative period.

For those cases, it is imperative that the cuff pressure is regularly checked and documented to avoid overinflation and tracheal necrosis.

In patients with a known history of chronic obstructive pulmonary disease (COPD) regular carbocisteine (375 mg 4 to 6 times daily) administration should be considered, as there is the risk of mucous plugging and obstruction of the tracheostomy tube.

Postoperative analgesia

Postoperative analgesic requirements vary depending on the extent of the resection and harvest site of the free flap, but are usually moderate.

A multimodal approach to pain relief gives optimum patient comfort. Regular paracetamol, intraoperative magnesium +/− clonidine, with a long-acting opiate, such as oxycodone or morphine, administered towards the end of surgery usually provides sufficient analgesia for the initial few hours of recovery. A transdermal fentanyl patch is a good option to provide background analgesia and is best placed at the beginning of surgery. Oral morphine or oral oxycodone via the patient's nasogastric tube (NG) should be prescribed *pro re nata* (PRN). Non-steroidal anti-inflammatories (NSAIDS) are usually avoided due to the risk for bleeding.

Patient-controlled analgesia (PCA) should be reserved for patients with extensive resections or composite flaps.

The analgesic requirements for flap donor areas such as the scapula bone or the ischium in deep circumflex iliac artery bone flaps is much greater. Using local anaesthetic wound infusion catheters in these patients can help reduce opioid requirements and improve patient comfort.

Antiemetics

Following oral and oropharyngeal cancer resection and free flap reconstructions vomiting can be detrimental in outcomes risking flap dehiscence with infections and fistula formation. A combination of corticosteroids with 5-hydroxytryptamine-3 (5-HT3) receptor antagonists is proven beneficial. The ERAS Society protocols also recommend new class antiemetics such as NK1 receptor agonists.

The antiemetic regime in the postoperative period should follow the anaesthetic instructions as described in Chapter 3.3.

Postoperative antibiotic prophylaxis

Most head and neck oncology cases are classed as clean contaminated, which may risk a relatively higher rate of perioperative wound infections. Preoperative antibiotics given 1–2 hours prior to surgery (during the anaesthetic induction) and continued for 24 hours have consistently demonstrated a significant reduction in postoperative infections. There is no evidence to support that longer courses of antibiotics may be beneficial.

Head and neck patients often have pre-existing respiratory comorbidities. That, in conjunction with prolonged general anaesthesia may predispose to pulmonary atelectasis and lower respiratory tract infections. There should be an early threshold on commencing antimicrobials, upon clinical evidence of any postoperative infection, as progression to sepsis may compromise the survival of the flap and the overall recovery of the patient.

Postoperative management of infections may require input by the microbiology specialist, as often the antimicrobial agent of choice may not be the same as the regime used in the perioperative prophylaxis.

Nutrition

Approximately 35% of head and neck cancer patients usually present in a state of various degrees of malnutrition. In the most recent years, the ERAS Society, has highlighted the importance of nutritional optimization both in the preoperative and also in the postoperative period.

Malnourished head and neck patients are at risk of:

- Refeeding syndrome and electrolyte imbalance.
- Poor healing.
- Risk of postoperative complications and infections.

ERAS recommends that head and neck patients are comprehensively assessed and nutritionally supported preoperatively with specific emphasis on preoperative carbohydrate (CHO) loading.

Early commencement of nutrition even immediately postoperative is associated with better outcomes. One important component is the decision regarding the route of feeding postoperatively.

Most of the patients will be nil by mouth and fed enterically via a nasogastric tube (NG) in the postoperative period. However, when a major resection is likely to significantly affect the swallowing function, then a gastrostomy tube (peg or rig inserted) should be considered. The latter can be performed in the preoperative period or most frequently in the postoperative period and in the time window between the primary surgery and any adjuvant therapy.

Postoperative mobilization and physiotherapy

Early mobilization of patients recovering from major head and neck surgery is recommended as it is considered to be associated with fewer pulmonary complications and better outcomes.

A minimum of partial mobilization, such as sitting out on a chair can be a target for the first postoperative day and may be an important predictor of the overall recovery and hospital stay.

Pulmonary complications can be detrimental in recovery of patients following major head and neck surgery. Lower respiratory tract infections (pneumonia) may delay mobilization, prolong delayed mobilization, tracheostomy decannulation, and also have a negative impact on flap healing.

Postoperative chest physiotherapy is important to mitigate the risks of pulmonary atelectasis, also assist in the rapid recovery of the respiratory muscles and strength of expectoration, cough, and management of respiratory secretions.

Mobilization should take place with the aid of physiotherapists, as often, additional wounds in flap donor sites (fibula—lower limb, scapula—upper limb, or DCIA—core balance) may add additional difficulty and may require donor-site specific regimes.

Methods of chest physiotherapy, such as incentive spirometry (IS), intermittent positive pressure breathing (IPPB), and deep breathing exercises (DBE) have different indications and benefits depending on the patient's background and recovery needs.

Flap monitoring

For the first 3 to 5 days, monitoring the flap with explicit attention and documentation of perfusion parameters is essential. This includes:

- colour
- turgor
- capillary refill
- temperature

Most of the anastomotic problems will develop in this timeframe. The topic is best analysed in Chapter 11.

The recommended frequency of flap clinical observations is hourly for the first 2 days.

When observing a flap in head and neck reconstruction it is essential asides the flap to closely monitor the neck. Many anastomotic complications especially venous compromise will firstly manifest in the neck with fast developing swelling before a compromise is detectable in the end microcirculation of the flap.

Further reading

Ahmed-Nusrath A. Anaesthesia for head and neck cancer surgery. *BJA Educ* 2017;17(12):383–9.

Al Saied G, Almutairi HM, Alharbi Y, Almohanna M, Almutairi A. Comparison between the impact of vasopressors and goal-directed fluid therapy on the management of free flap reconstruction of head and neck and monitoring in ICU. *Cureus* 2020;12(12):e12108.

Bertelsen C, *et al.* Enhanced recovery after surgery-based perioperative protocol for head and neck free flap reconstruction. *OTO Open* 2020;4(2):2473974X20931037.

Broderick D, Kyzas P, Sanders K, Sawyerr A, Katre C, Vassiliou L. Surgical tracheostomies in COVID-19 patients: important considerations and the '5Ts' of safety. *Br J Oral Maxillofac Surg* 2020;58(5):585–9.

Broderick D, *et al.* Surgical tracheostomies in COVID-19 patients: A multidisciplinary approach and lessons learned. *Oral Oncol* 2020;106:104767.

Charters P, Ahmad I, Patel A, Russell S. Anaesthesia for head and neck surgery: United Kingdom national multidisciplinary guidelines. *J Laryngol Otol* 2016;130(Suppl. S2), S23–7.

Dawoud BES, *et al.* Does anticoagulation improve outcomes of microvascular free flap reconstruction following head and neck surgery: a systematic review and meta-analysis. *Br J Oral Maxillofac Surg* 2022;60(10):1292–302.

Dort JC, *et al.* Optimal perioperative care in major head and neck cancer surgery with free flap reconstruction: a consensus review and recommendations from the Enhanced Recovery After Surgery Society. *JAMA Otolaryngol Head Neck Surg.* 2017;143(3):292–303.

Gillan C, Goddard A. Anaesthetic considerations for major cancer resection and freeflap reconstruction in oral cancer: a review. *J Oral Maxillofac Anesth* 2023;2:18.

Jessen MK, *et al.* Goal-directed haemodynamic therapy during general anaesthesia for noncardiac surgery: a systemic review and meta-analysis. *Br J Anaesth* 2022;128(3):416e433.

Mallampati SR, *et al.* A clinical sign to predict difficult tracheal intubation: a prospective study. *Can Anaesth Soc J* 1985;32(4):429–34.

McGrath A, Bates L, Atkinson D, Moore JA. National Tracheostomy Safety Project: multidisciplinary guidelines for the management of tracheostomy and laryngectomy airway emergencies. *Anaesthesia* 2012;67:1025–41.

Myatra SN, *et al.* Identification of patients for a delayed extubation strategy versus elective tracheostomy for postoperative airway management in major oral cancer surgery: a prospective observational study in seven hundred and twenty patients. *Oral Oncol* 2021;121:105502.

Naik AN, *et al.* The use of vasopressor agents in free tissue transfer for head and neck reconstruction: current trends and review of the literature. *Front Pharmacol* 2020;11:1248.

Ormandy D, Kapoor V, Kyzas P, Vassiliou L. Tracheostomy suspension: a modified approach for securing the airway. *Br J Oral Maxillofac Surg* 2020;58:717–18.

Ormandy D, et al. Difficult airways: a 3D printing study with virtual fibreoptic endoscopy. *Br J Oral Maxillofac Surg* 2021;59:e65–e71.

Practice guidelines for perioperative blood management: an updated report by the American Society of Anesthesiologists Task Force on Perioperative Blood Management. *Anesthesiology* 2015;122:241–75.

Prout J, Jones T, Martin D (eds.) 2014. *Oxford Higher Specialty Training: Advanced Training in Anaesthesia*. Oxford: Oxford University Press.

Reiter M, Kapsreiter M, Betz C, Harreus U. Perioperative management of antithrombotic medication in head and neck reconstruction—a retrospective analysis of 137 patients. *Am J Otolaryngol Neck Med Surg* 2012;33:693–6.

Samsoon GL, Young JR. Difficult tracheal intubation: a retrospective study. *Anaesthesia* 1987;42(5):487–90.

Saugel B, et al. Cardiac output estimation using pulse wave analysis and physiology, algorithms, and technologies: a narrative review. *Br J Anaesth* 2021;126(1):67e76.

Taylor RJ, et al. Intraoperative vasopressors in head and neck free flap reconstruction. *Microsurgery* 2021;41(1):5–13.

Vincent A, Sawhney R, Ducic Y. Perioperative care of free flap patients. *Semin Plast Surg* 2019;33(1):5–12.

4
The surgical microscope

Leandros Vassilios F. Vassiliou, Panayiotis Kyzas, and Nicholas Kalavrezos

4.1 The operating microscope

Introduction

A high-quality operating microscope is integral in head and neck microvascular surgery. Surgical microscopes have evolved significantly due to advancements in optical and digital technology. Modern microscopes comprise high-precision instruments with state-of-art optics that provide stereoscopic vision with bright, co-axial illumination, adjustable magnification, and comfortable working distance.

The modern design of the clinical systems offers stability and improved ergonomics with optimum manoeuvrability, together with carrying additional appealing features such as high-resolution monitors and cameras that aid in research and education.

Fundamentals in understanding operating microscopes

Magnification: The ability to offer a view of the object at a scale larger than the actual size. The magnification offered in modern generation microscopes varies from 4 to 40 times (4×–40×). The total magnification of a microscope is calculated through a complex algorithm that takes into consideration characteristics of the focal length, the objective lens, the zoom value, the focal length of the binocular and the magnifying power of the eyepieces.

In optics, the degree of obtained magnification (V) is calculated via the following formula:

$$V = F_I/F_o \times W/16 \times V_{oc}$$

Where,

F_I is the ocular tube focal length

F_o is the objective lens focal length

W the indicated magnification on the control knob

V_{oc} the magnification provided by the eyepiece.

Stereopsis: The ability of the microscope to produce an image of three-dimensional (3D) perception. This depends on the binocular arrangement of the optical lenses and prisms, where two separate images of the object/field are combined (fused) in one.

Working distance: This is the distance from the objective lens to the point of focus. This value is fixed and is dependent on the chosen focal length of the objective lens.

Focal length: This is the distance from the focused objective length and the point of focus. This depends on the type of surgery and the magnification required, and for head and neck microvascular surgery will range from 200 mm to 375 mm.

Co-axial illumination: A feature of significant importance. The 'objective lens' is the principal optical component through which the image of the object is magnified. As the light beam travels from the light source and is directed to illuminate the target object/field if its course is at an angle to the main visual axis, the reflection will create shadows obscuring the field and reducing the quality of the image (Figure 4.1.1a). 'Co-axial illumination' refers to when the light is re-routed to the viewing axis and projected directly down through the objective lens, in order to avoid reflection and creation of shadows (Figure 4.1.1b). This is of particular importance in head and neck reconstructive microvascular surgery, where the head and neck anatomy is complex and irregular in three-dimensional (3D) configuration.

Resolution: An important component of the optical system is resolution, which measures the acuity improved by magnification. This is the ability of the system to distinguish between two separate objects.

Depth of focus: It is the area above and below (range of depth) the point of perfect focus where sharp focus is maintained. This depends on a multitude of factors, but effectively relates to the design of the optical system, the size of the objective lens aperture and the level of magnification.

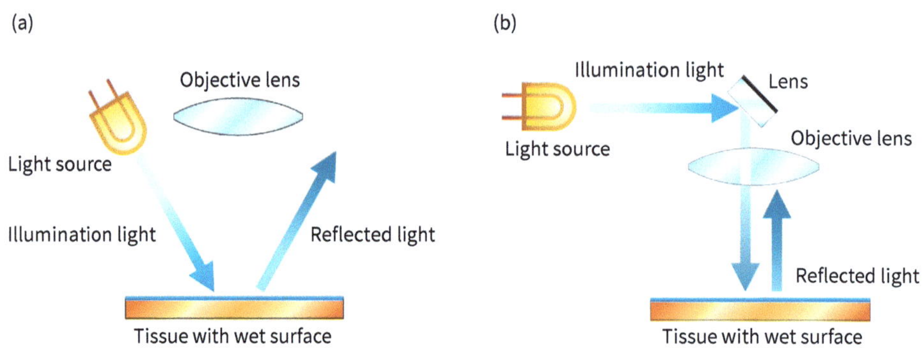

Figure 4.1.1 Co-axial illumination.
a. This figure demonstrates the light beam/rays reflected from the light source on the wet surface of the operating surgical field, at an angle, which creates shadows of the structures as viewed through the objective lens.
b. This figure demonstrates the co-axial illumination principle, where the light rays are directed through a properly angulated mirror/lens, through the objective lens following a vertical course down towards the surgical field. The angle of reflection is 180 degrees (vertical) from the surgical field and through the objective lens, eliminating any shadows of structures in the visual field.

The definition of the focal length of the objective lens is directly related to the working distance (the distance of the objective lens to the point of focus).

The 'anatomy' of an operating microscope

See Figure 4.1.2. The microscope is roughly comprised of:

a. Microscope head with the optical system
b. Light source
c. Supporting structure

Microscope head and optical system

The optical system is the main determining factor for the image quality. It is essentially binocular with optical components that include:

- The objective lens
- The magnification changer (zoom)
- The close-up lenses—eyepieces

The magnification changer comprises a series of mobile lenses designed to move closer and away from the point of focus within the viewing axis. The binocular system is effectively equivalent to two telescopes linked together.

The prism arrangement results in stereopsis, which introduces the depth of field into the surgeon's vision.

An operating microscope at 20 times magnification can achieve a resolution of 0.01 mm, whereas the human eye has an inherent resolution of up to 0.2 mm.

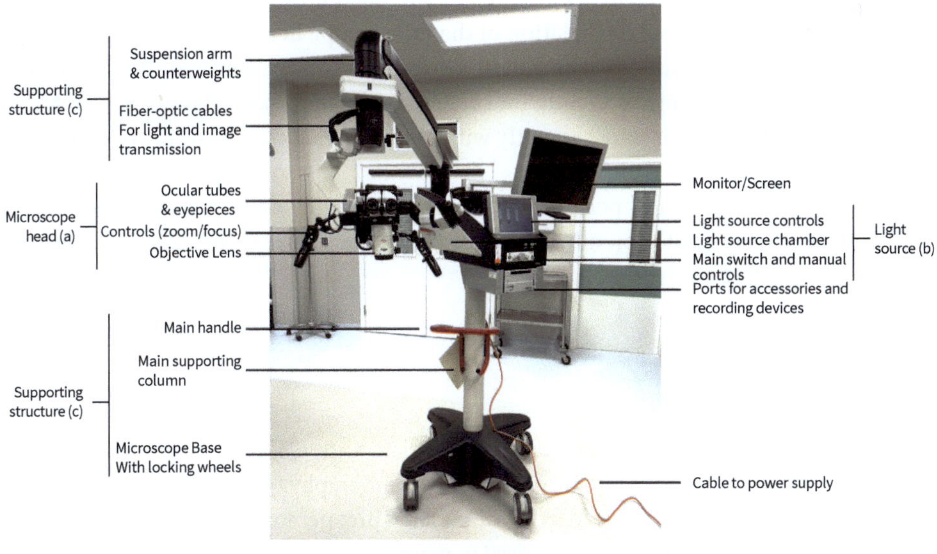

Figure 4.1.2 Indicative photograph demonstrating the critical parts of the operating microscope.

The eyepieces come in different lengths and angulations of the ocular tubes to much the surgeon's preference. Usually, they have a magnification value of 12.5× (8×–20×).

A beam splitter is incorporated in most microscopes to allow for multiple observers to multiply the produced image.

Further technological advancements mean that modern microscopes come with improved ergonomics and in compact designs. There are further developments in the technology of optics and illumination, offering augmented reality and three-dimensional visualisation as well as illumination in different wavelengths of the light spectrum, including the infra-red, ultraviolet (UV), and fluorescent. Microscopes come with a variety of adaptable imaging devices such as monitors and cameras to aid training and education.

Focus

Focusing is one of the most essential components of microvascular surgery. Three-dimensional configuration of anatomy and deep cavities makes it impossible for the whole surgical field to be visualized perfectly clear within the focal plane.

A good practice of focusing is to zoom in at the highest level of magnification and focus. Then, after this is achieved by lowering the level of magnification, the visual field should remain sharp and clear.

Modern generation microscopes have an automatic focusing device for a stereoscopic microscope that uses an infra-red beam.

Controls

The main functions of the microscope, such as the magnification control (zoom) knob, the focusing adjustment, and the position of the microscope head, come in different variations. Most regularly, handgrip controllers resemble joysticks and are attached to the microscope head with controls mainly for magnification and focus (Figure 4.1.3). Many microscopes use foot pedals, most recently wireless ones, that bear both controls for magnification and focus.

There are additional optical ports to accommodate imaging devices, such as additional liquid crystal display (LCD) monitors for assistance and cameras for capturing surgical footage of the microvascular surgeon.

Image-guided surgery

Further research allows 3D visualization to be overlaid with CT, MRI, angiography, ultrasound, infra-red fluorescence, or optical coherence tomography (OCT) images. This feature of superimposition of images derived from the patient's preoperative cross-sectional imaging is termed image 'injection' and is mainly used in neurosurgery.

Light source

The lighting sources involve LED, xenon, or halogen lamps. Illumination is transmitted from its source to the microscope via a fibre guide LED is reliable as it provides good quality

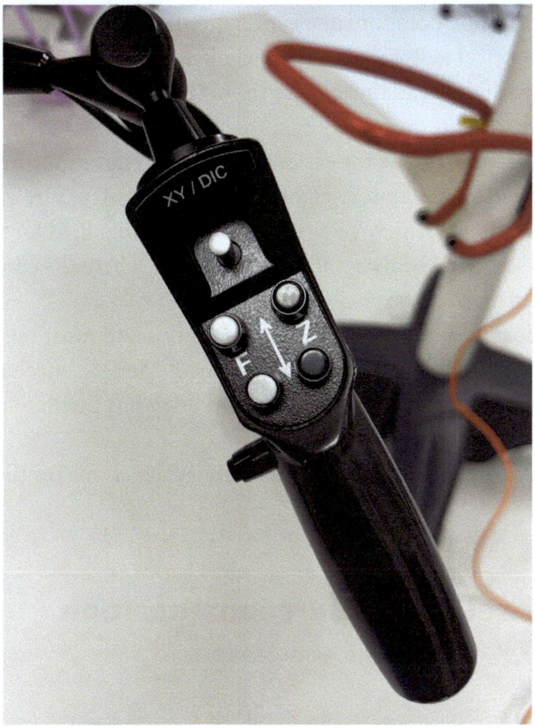

Figure 4.1.3 Demonstration of 'joystick' type hand controls, with a switch for the index fingers to move and secure the head of the microscope head, as well as the main functions of focus and zoom.

illumination within the visible wavelength, with satisfactory brightness, long life, and importantly, extremely low heat.

Modern microscopes have high-power light sources, which provide stable light intensity and are close to sunlight colour temperature. Typical light source power values are 300–600 Watts. Some models use xenon lamps (dual 300 Watt xenon) or halogen (600 Watt) lamps that can also emit on the UV and near infra-red range; however these features are less applicable in head and neck surgery.

It is important that the light source is kept away from the optical system and the operating field as it can cause significant thermal damage to tissues and the microscope optical components. Therefore, the light source is usually installed away from the microscope head(s) and the light is transmitted via fibreoptic cable through the suspension arm and supporting structure. A complex arrangement of optics is required to re-route and direct the light.

Additional modern features (BrightCare, Leica®) automatically reduce the light—and hence temperature—intensity when the working distance decreases, such as in high magnifications. Similarly, when magnification increases and hence the visual field becomes narrow, the AutoIris feature (Leica®) reduces the field (disc) of illumination to avoid unnecessary illuminating and heating of the tissues in the periphery (outside) the field of focus.

Supporting structure

The standard microscope for microvascular head and neck surgery is an 'on-caster' stand microscope. The structure needs flexibility for the microscope body to be positioned where required above the operating field, but also stability and balance.

The operating microscope components, especially the light source and the microscope body that carries the optical system, are extremely heavy, and a long suspension arm connects the light source with the head that carries the optical system.

The supporting structure sits on a heavy base that bears locking wheels. The breaks in most modern models are electromagnetic for easier control. Apart from the heavy base and main supporting column, a series of counterweights placed on the structure and suspension arm balances the microscope head, which 'hangs' over the operating field for vertical, transverse, tilt, and rotation. This structure bears a multitude of 'joints' where the components articulate via precision motorized mechanics.

Surgical microscopes should be quick and easy to move and must remain stationary and stable once the optimum position has been established. Modern mechanics offer state-of-the-art positioning, and, in most recent years, technology has further advanced to include 'auto-balance' and robotic auto-positioning features.

Modern models have the feature of position memory which makes the system more able to bookmark positions.

4.2 Microscope set-up and surgeons' position for microsurgery

Introduction

The main threat to the microvascular outcome is the surgeon's fatigue, irritation, or loss of concentration. The surgeon should be relaxed, rested, and well-hydrated.

Caffeine should be kept to what is the surgeon's 'normal'. The surgeon should avoid any physical exertion or strenuous muscle exercise the day before, as this can precipitate muscle fatigue and small muscle tremors.

It is strongly advised that the surgeon takes a break prior to the commencement of the microvascular surgery.

Operating table

It is important to request the anaesthetist to flatten the table. Often a mild head extension helps increasing the operating field in the neck and slightly moving the mandible cephalad.

The operating table must be at adequate height but as low as possible, in order to allow for maximum magnification range during the microvascular anastomoses.

In certain cases the table may be turned slightly away from the operating surgeon in order to bring lateral neck structures directly in the centre of the microvascular field.

Microscope set-up

Draping

Draping of the microscope to maintain sterility of the surgical field is of paramount importance. The material usually used is a thin, transparent, and importantly heat-resistant plastic film that encases the whole microscope. The film includes a transparent optical lens that

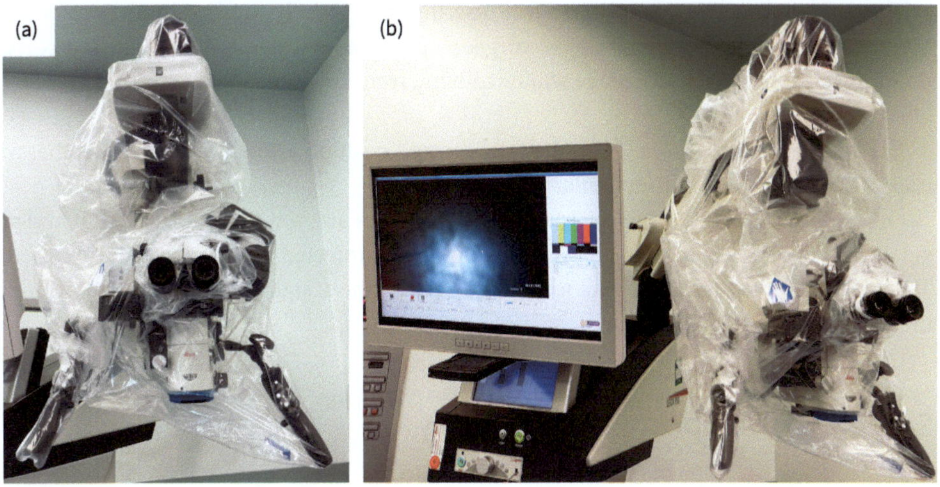

Figure 4.2.1 Microscope draping. a. demonstrating the microscope head draped with sterile film with ports for the eye and the objective lens with its respective cover. b. Whole picture of surgical microscope with the monitor on (for the scrub nurse to be able to follow the microsurgical procedure and the trainee surgeons to be able to watch the microvascular procedure).

encloses the objective lens and also the ocular housing extensions (Figure 4.2.1). There are ocular pockets for the eye pieces.

Modern microscopes have the feature of auto-draping (AutoDrape®, Zeiss®) which effectively introduces a vacuum to further adapt the film on the features and structure of the microscope.

Position of the microscope head

The microscope head should be adjusted to an optimum height that is away from the optical field to allow adequate focus. If the microscope head is too close to the neck, then the image is blurred and focus will be impossible. The tilt of the microscope's head should be approximately be between 40–60 degrees. In modern microscopes the eye pieces inclination can also be adjusted to allow optimum position.

Finally, adjustment of the interpupillary distance. This adjusts the circle of light that is projected through each eye piece to align with the pupil of each eye at the exit level. Interpupillary distance is fixed for every person, hence once you practice and achieve what is optimum interpupillary distance level you can record it for any future use and reference.

Each eye piece contains focussing adjustment that corrects for any degree of myopia or presbyopia. It depends on the surgeon's preference whether to keep the eye glasses on. However, it is preferable to eliminate any additional barriers or layers of vision when possible. Conditions such as stigmatism or hypermetropia cannot be corrected or eliminated through the microscope.

Exit pupil and optical access

It is important to comprehend the idea of the exit pupil. These are optical points that lie in a short distance from the eye piece lens. The beam of the focused light that exits the eye pieces is effectively a converging cone that reaches the narrowest point approximately 15 mm above the eye piece.

The exit pupil effectively is an optical disc that has to fully localize in alignment with the surgeon's pupil on each eye. If the surgeon's pupil on either eye is misaligned a corresponding part of the focused image will be missing from the visual field, effectively it will be blocked out.

If either eye is moved away from the fully centred position, even by a millimetre, that will lead to a partial eclipse of the circular visual field.

Optimum vision under the microscope also requires alignment of the direction and angulation of the head in relation to the direction of the projected light through the eye pieces. This is called optical access, and each eye must have its line of sight directed at the same line as the optical access of its eye piece.

Surgeons' position for microsurgery

Microvascular stools

The surgeon's stool should be chosen in accordance with the surgeon's preference. The surgeon's stool should be comfortable and allow appropriate positioning close to the operating field. Usually, the height is adjustable and the stool has wheels (rollers) to allow the surgeon to move. There are stools with pedals to allow optimum height and various back and arm supports, and so on (search for different companies that use microvascular stools).

Correct positioning of the whole body is essential for the success of microvascular surgery (Figure 4.2.2).

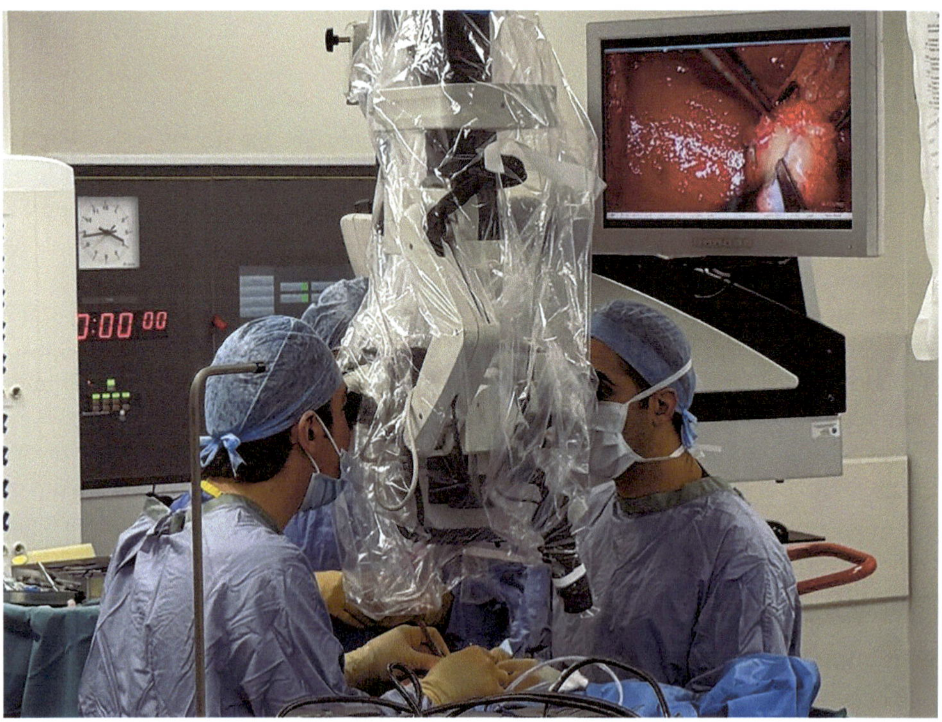

Figure 4.2.2 Microsurgeons' position performing microvascular surgery.

Surgeon's body position

In order to allow a seamless comfortable and precision movement of the fingertips it is important to sit the core body in an extremely comfortable position. Comfort is defined by the amount of muscle activity required to maintain a certain position for a duration of time.

Firstly, at a floor level, any obstacles should be removed and the table or the footstool should be adjusted at an adequate height to allow the knees to slide under the head of the table, that allows the torso of the surgeon to be as close to the operating field as possible. Any additional table-connected obstacles such as arm boards that prevent the surgeon from sliding the knees fully under the table should be removed at this point.

The position of the torso should be upright and straight without any crouching. The back should be straight and comfortable, and the shoulders relaxed at a normal height. The elbows are usually bent at 90 degrees.

The sitting position defines the ability of the surgeon to hold the upper body still. The latter is directly related to the amount of stability of the arms that affects the precision of the fingertip movement.

The neck should be in a comfortable position with the head in a relatively neutral and slightly forward tilt position, but otherwise as motionless as possible. The forearms should comfortably lie on the table with adequate support at rest.

Once the optimum position is achieved and tested it gradually becomes habit in every microvascular procedure.

Position of the hands

Microvascular surgery is all about the fingers' movements. All the other muscles of the upper limb should be relaxed, rested, and stabilized in order to allow precision and muscle movement only by the fine finger muscles.

Many surgeons would prefer to rest their elbows and to this end there are microvascular chairs with armrests. Other surgeons alternatively use gown packs or kidney dishes draped and taped on the side of the head of the table in order to rest their elbows and wrists and avoid or eliminate any tremor. Comfortable steady support of the wrists is essential to achieve steadiness of the hands.

The minimum should be adequate support of the FOREARM and WRISTS either with sterile gown packs or large surgical gauge packs. A wet large-sized gauge is recommended to be placed open on the patients face/head and/or chest and that will allow cleaning of the microvascular instruments avoiding removing the eyes off the microscope and back and forth traffic of the instruments to the scrub nurse. That saves time and unnecessary movements.

A good starting position is the 'writing position'. The forearm is gently supinated and the hand rests with its ulnar border (ring and small fingers) supported and the microvascular instrument is held between the thumb, index and middle finger (three-digit gentle grip). It is important to just GENTLY hold the instrument without applying too much force. Often novice microvascular surgeons inadvertently hold the microvascular instruments too tight due to underlying stress. This, apart from poor control of the instruments, can quickly lead to small muscle fatigue and discomfort compromising the result of the anastomosis.

Opening and closing the microvascular instruments should be achieved by FINE FINGER muscle control. Any tremor is reduced or eliminated by keeping the index finger and the thumb in contact with the middle finger which remains stable but provides a steady platform completing the tripod of fine finger surgery.

4.3 **Field division and optimum magnification**

Working under the microscope, especially in high magnification with complex structures, can initially be daunting. Structures in a three-dimensional space. Two microsurgeons are involved (one is the main operator and has the role of the assistant), and a systematic methodological approach in operating is necessary.

Eye piece focus and adjustment

The microscope hand controls adjust zoom (magnification) and focus. These are to adjust the level of magnification and to provide a perfectly sharp three-dimensional picture of the surgical field.

The focusing adjustment follows the correct set-up of the microscope head, height, tilt, and position of the eye pieces. Once the focus is correctly adjusted, then the image remains sharp regardless of the magnification level, which is called parfocal view.

Loss of parfocality is the phenomenon where the image goes out of focus every time magnification is changed.

A useful practical tip is to zoom down into the maximum magnification and adjust there the level of focus. Once this set for the respective working height where the anastomosis is going to take place then change of magnification will not defocus the image. Modern microscopes have additional aids as laser dots that meet in a complete colocalization point once the optimum focus is achieved.

Field division

The coordination of two microsurgeons in order to achieve a perfect anastomosis is of paramount importance. Each one has to stick to their role. The main operator has to act as the main operator and the assistant has to accept the role of the assistant.

The microscope field has to be broadly divided into the main operator's field and the assistant's field (Figures 4.3.1 and 4.3.2). Ideally, each instrument should not cross the imaginary line of the equator. Even during triangulation, each microsurgeon should remain in their own half of the field. This is an exercise that has to be fully explained and declared at the briefly prior to microsurgery in order to allow a seamless microvascular surgery to take place.

If in basic surgical skills crossing instruments is not allowed, then this principle becomes far more important than in microvascular surgery. As shown in figures imagine dividing the circle of the operating field into the assistant's territory and the main operator's territory and try to stay with the main microsurgical activity centred in the middle of the circle within each one's territory without crossing the imaginary line of the equator.

Optimum magnification

Modern surgical microscopes due to optical and technological advancements offer most almost three-dimensional stereotactic view, high visual clarity, and magnification levels of up to 35 times.

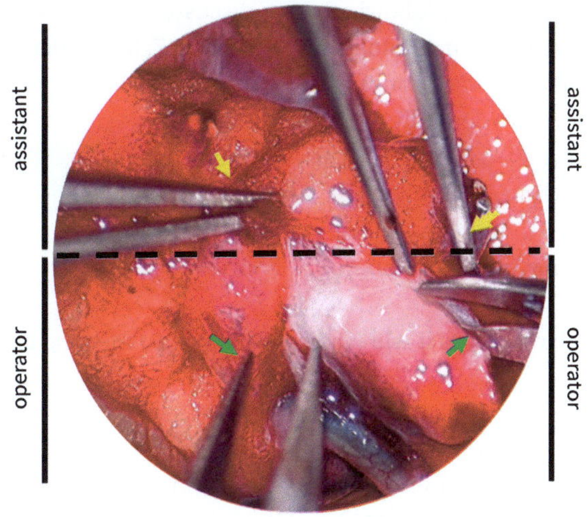

Figure 4.3.1 Appropriate division of the operative microsurgical field. Note the circular view of the operating field as sited by the operator's side. Note the imaginary line dividing the field into the assistant's half and the operator's half. Yellow arrows depict the assistant's jeweller's forceps on the assistant's operative half. Green arrows point towards the operator's jeweller's forceps (left) and the microscissors (right) for fine adventitia dissection.

Microvascular surgery, as it will be further discussed in the following chapters, entails a complex process with a multitude of different stages. For instance stages in the pedicle and vessel preparation and microsurgical suturing require different levels of recommended magnification in order to achieve the ultimate goal and also avoid pitfalls and errors.

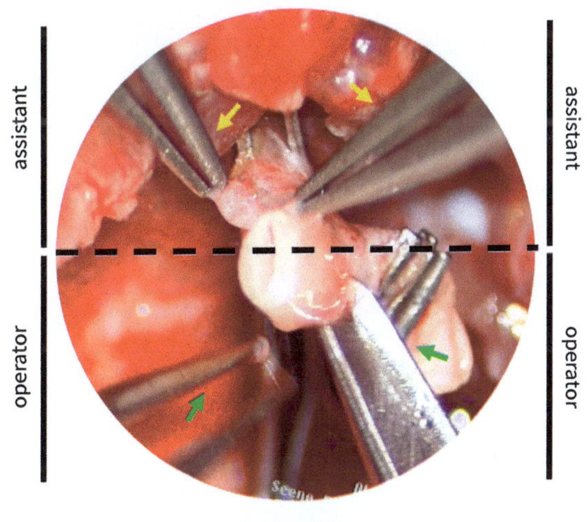

Figure 4.3.2 Appropriate division of the operative microsurgical field. This is a picture of high magnification demonstrating fine adventitia dissection. Yellow arrows point towards the assistant's jeweller's holding the adventitia using the triangulation technique. Green arrows point towards the operator's jeweller's forceps (left) and microscissors (right). Again, note the division of the operating field into two halves. Each microsurgeon keeps the instruments confined in their respective operative half of the field.

This chapter and mirroring the following topics discussed in this book (vessel preparation and microsurgical suturing in an anastomosis Chapters 6, 7, 8, 9) will provide a crude guide of which level of magnification is recommended for different stages of microvascular surgery.

Magnification levels can be broadly divided into the following:

- Low—up to 7 or 8 times magnification
- Medium—up to 15 times of magnification
- High—over 15 times of magnification

The main microvascular steps, as it will be discussed in the following chapters, comprise of the following:

1. Microvascular preparation
    1. Perivascular tissue excision—'Low' (Figure 4.3.3)
    2. Adventitia dissection—'Low/Medium' (Figure 4.3.4)
    3. Venotomy—'High'
    4. Lumen inspection and dilation—'High' (Figure 4.3.5)
    5. Fine adventitia dissection—'High' (Figure 4.3.5)
    6. Further orientation marking—'Low'
2. Microvascular anastomosis—'High' (Figure 4.3.6)
3. Pedicle check and suspension—'Low' (Figure 4.3.7)

When the microscope is first brought in and the microsurgeons (main operator and assistant) are taking positions, adjustment of the field of focus, brightness, and magnification of focus needs to take place as discussed earlier.

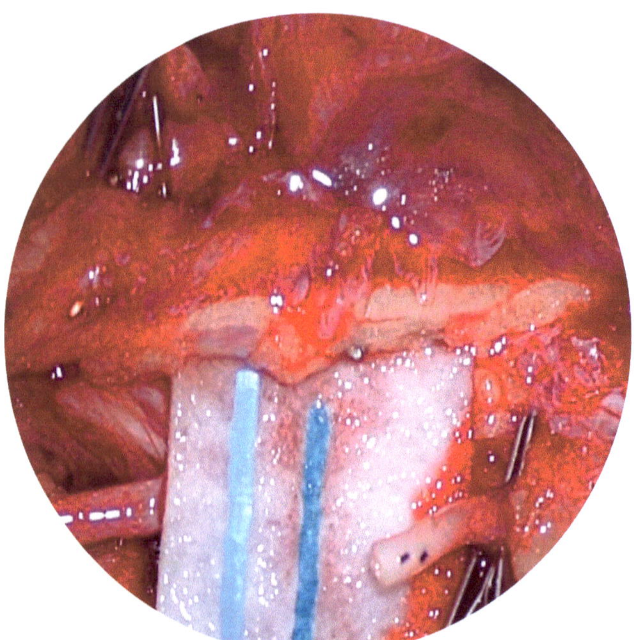

Figure 4.3.3 Optimum magnification for pedicle alignment—'Low'. Note that pedicle alignment needs a wider (lower magnification/zoom) field perspective in order to control any possible twists or kinks. The optimum magnification is kept to 'Low' (1–5× times).

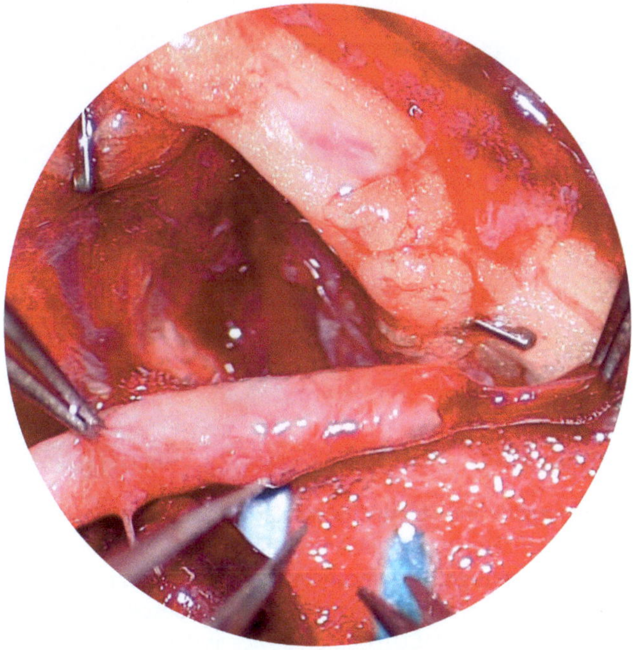

Figure 4.3.4 Optimum magnification for perivascular tissue dissection—'Medium/Low'. The picture shows low to medium magnification during an initial perivascular and crude adventitia dissection. As the microscissors may move quickly along the axis of the vessel and the tissue removed is not affect the edges of the vessels, 'Low' magnification is easier to control the vessel, set the appropriate orientation, and avoid visual fatigue of the microsurgeons.

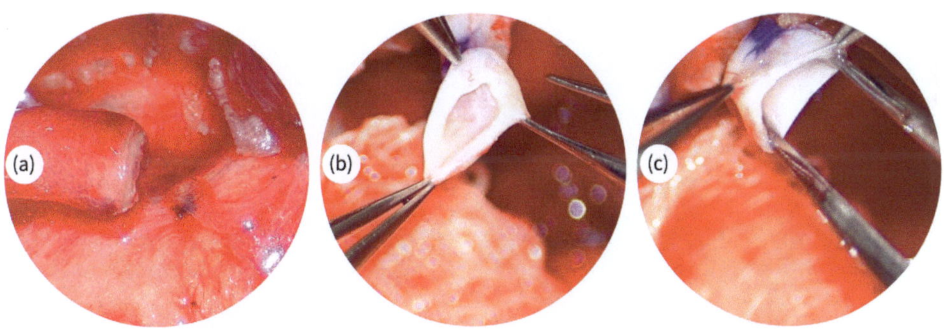

Figure 4.3.5 Optimum magnification for fine adventitia dissection 'High'. This operative step requires high magnification and sharp focus. The fine dissection prepares the vessel edges. Small 'hanging' adventitia tissue segments are to be visualized in high magnification and removed carefully, in order to achieve clean vessel edges. The next step of vessel lumen inspection requires high magnification in order to identify if any micro 'imperfections' such as small atheroma plaques, or intima tears, that may compromise the anastomosis. a. Preparation of the vessel for fine adventitia dissection. b. Using the triangulation technique, careful vessel lumen inspection is performed. c. Careful vessel lumen dilation with synchronous inspection is performed.

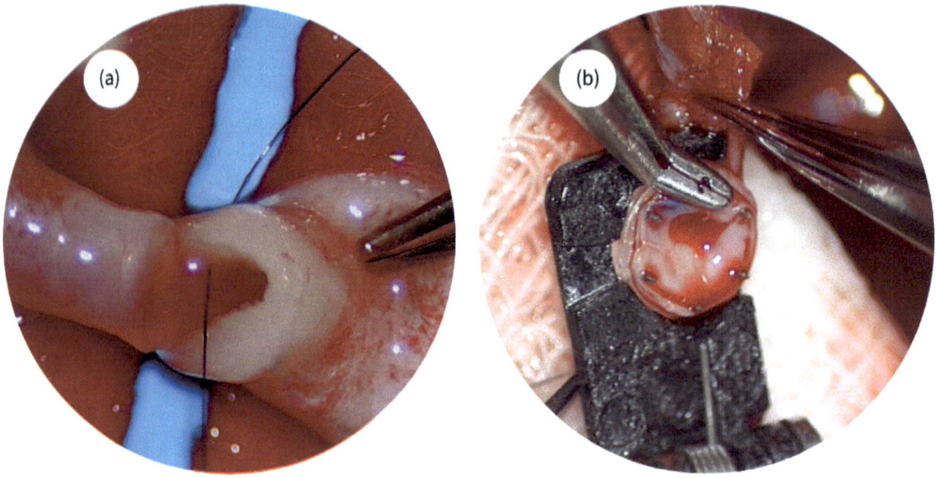

Figure 4.3.6 Optimum magnification for microvascular suture anastomosis or MACD anastomosis—'High'. a. Arterial microvascular anastomosis suturing using the back-wall-first approach. Note this needs 'High' magnification (15–25×), in order to clearly visualize the vessels' edges, inner lumen, and precisely place the sutures as described in Chapter 8. b. Venous microvascular anastomosis using a MACD (coupler) device as described in Chapter 9.4. The process needs 'High' magnification (zoom) to allow precise 'fixation' of the vessel's edges on the ring's pins with clear visualization and control of the vessel's intima and any possible interference (such as adventitia tissue segments).

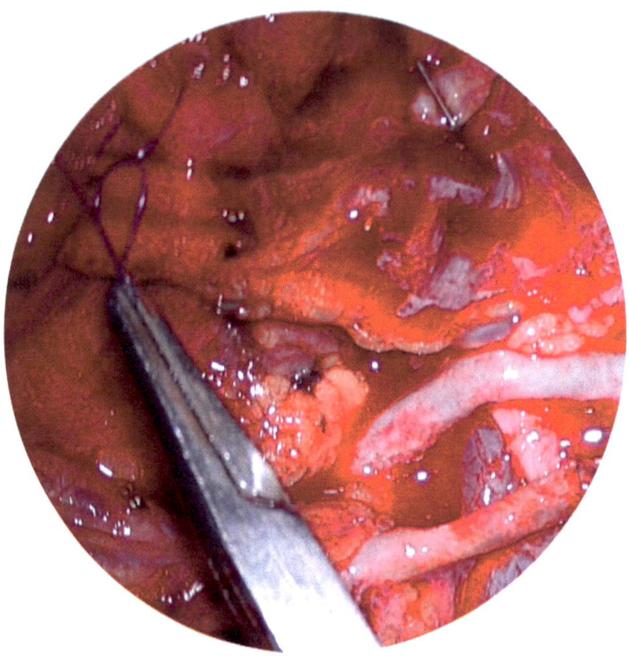

Figure 4.3.7 Optimum magnification for pedicle suspension—'Low'. Pedicle suspension as described in Chapter 10.3 requires a wide perception of the surgical field, visualization of the whole pedicle (both arterial and venous segments) course and orientation. It is important to confirm healthy blood flow (pulsatility, perfusion of vasa vasorum) and positioning of the pedicle prior to performing suturing (suspension) to neck structures.

For the initial stages of pedicle preparation, such as gross perivascular tissue excision, separation of artery from the vein, and initial pedicle orientation, only low magnification is required. For the vessel cut (arteriotomy or venotomy, dilation, and intraluminal inspection as well as adventitia fine dissection) a medium to high magnification is recommended. It will allow the operator to identify any vessel lumen and vessel edges imperfections and adjust the vessel cut and orientation accordingly.

The microsurgical operating field has to be adjusted twice: once when the donor vessel (pedicle vessels) is prepared, and once for the recipient vessel preparation. When flushing the pedicle the magnification has to be decreased to low. That will allow the operator to not only assess the pedicle pulsation and orientation, but to have a broad, wide aspect of the whole operating field. For instance, remaining in close focus (high magnification) at this stage could predispose to errors in pedicle orientation and perhaps to complications with further accomplishment of the anastomosis.

When these are completed and the main operator is satisfied, then the microvascular anastomosis (micro-suturing) will commence. This has to take place with the highest possible magnification with respect to the depth of focus.

If, for example, a vertical anastomosis is performed, then unfortunately frequent magnification changes (frequent zoom and focus adjustments) have to take place as the vessels and the working plane will be moving up and down in a vertical plane frequently. This is why a horizontal anastomosis, as described in Chapters 8 and 9, is far more preferable.

Upon completion of the anastomosis, 'zoom' (magnification) has to return to lower levels in order to allow inspection of the pedicle pulsation, behaviour, and perfusion in its entirety. The same applies for the venous anastomosis just before closure of the coupler devices or removal of the vascular clamps, the magnification is returned to low in order to allow a global inspection of the blood flow across the anastomosis and the patency across along the pedicle.

Upon completion of both anastomosis, a careful pedicle orientation configuration and course needs to take place. Of course, this must happen with the magnification level set to low in order to establish the absence of any kinks, acute angles, and twists of the pedicle. Any further steps, such as pedicle suspension or muscular gutta formation (sternocleidomastoid muscle gutta), need to be performed under low or medium magnification in order to allow a wider inspection of the regional microsurgical field and better control of all contributing factors.

The important practices that need to become a work routine for the microvascular surgeon are summarized in Box 4.3.1.

Box 4.3.1 Important reminders for when operating under the microscope

- The microvascular surgeon needs to establish a routine when operating under the microscope. Field division is important for movement, economy, efficiency, and avoidance of confusion when operating with an assistant.
- The microvascular surgeon needs to establish a routine in the practice of microvascular surgery. Each stage of the microvascular anastomosis requires a different level of magnification in order to optimize the field perspective versus focus and high level visibility for detailed work.

4.4 **Video monitoring and recording**

Introduction

Modern surgical microscopes are equipped with monitors and high-definition cameras able to record the microsurgical procedures.

Recording the procedures could be performed for medicolegal purposes but mostly is important for learning (reflective practice) and training.

This chapter provides some basic guidance on how to best record microvascular operations.

Monitor set-up

It is important that apart from the microscope that the camera and monitor are appropriately aligned and set up.

Appropriate maintenance and adjustment of the microscope's beam splitter (optical component that allows the light path to be divided and directed to multiple users such as the assistant's eyepieces or the camera) is important and if required manufacturer's service may need to be requested.

The camera is usually secured on a microscope-specific component called C-mount that comprises a special lens of appropriate focal distance to provide optimum image definition to the camera's system.

Correct alignment of the picture (real optical field as visualized by the microsurgeon and the assistant) with the image captured and projected on the monitor has three important goals:

- For the scrub nurse, the ability to observe the microsurgical operation process and proactively prepare and hand in the next instruments as they can actively participate in the overall procedure.
- If trainee microsurgeons or medical students are present in the theatre, this will allow observation of how microvascular surgery is performed for training and education purposes.
- Having the camera aligned and capturing the process of microvascular surgery allows recording for future training, education, research purposes, and also for medicolegal reasons.

Video recording

Most modern microscopes bear a medical or scientific grade charge-coupled device CCD cameras with excellent spatial resolution and acquisition speed. There is availability of high-definition (HD) or 4K equipment.

Modern microscopes come with a hard drive with a certain capacity able to store recordings from a number of operations. Ensure that appropriate coding (file name for each case) is in place with respect to patients' confidentiality. Recordings can be recognized and identified with corresponding dates of operations for future reference.

When recording microsurgery procedures, the camera has to be set up to focus at the same point as the operator's eyepieces.

Good quality videos must fulfil the following criteria:

- Optimum object centring
- Optimum brightness
- Clarity of picture
- Sharp focus

Using recordings for training and education purposes must keep in line with the respective local and national information governance (IG) policies and always guarantee the protection of the patients' confidentiality.

The recordings are usually stored in '.wmv' files that can be downloaded onto hospital-approved storing devices. Occasionally, and in older generation microscopes, the recipient hard drive has to be set to FAT32 format as most microscopes operating on Microsoft Windows environment.

Processing videos

Microvascular surgery videos are of significant importance, not only for training and educational purposes but also for reflective practice and improvement of the actual microsurgeons.

It is often the case that reviewing in detail and in-depth the steps of microvascular surgery will raise points for future improvement or reveal future pitfalls that will contribute to the microvascular surgeon's future development and further improvement.

Videos can be processed and edited in a wide range of software, such as iMovie (Apple®) for MAC operating systems. If a certain recording's format needs to be exchanged to another one in order to make the respective clip able to be processed by different software, then the recommended software called Movavi® can be recommended and utilized with a monthly or yearly subscription.

Editing of microvascular surgery videos can help isolate certain parts of the procedure that exert scientific or training interest and can also enhance the video quality.

Further reading

Acland RD. *Practice Manual for Microvascular Surgery*. St Louis, MO: C.V. Mosby Company, 1989: p. 134.

Gordon L. Advances in microsurgery. *Surg Technol Int* 1991;I:425–7.

Ma L, Fei B. Comprehensive review of surgical microscopes: technology development and medical applications. *J Biomed Opt* 2021;26(1):010901.

5
Vessel choice and preparation

Artery

Julio Acero, Danny Adam, Fernando Almeida, Leandros Vassilios F. Vassiliou, Panayiotis Kyzas, and Nicholas Kalavrezos

5.1 **Recipient artery selection**

Introduction

Successful microvascular surgery is reliant on normal flow of blood, into and out of a free flap. This requires a high-velocity, non-turbulent arterial input, and a non-obstructed venous outflow. The choice, dissection, and preparation of the recipient artery is the key first step in this circle.

There are several preoperative and intraoperative factors that aid decision-making in selecting the donor artery. Once an artery has been selected, we must have a detailed understanding of its anatomical location and its variations to ensure it is protected and dissected effectively. After we have confirmed the location of the recipient artery, we must then prepare the vessel and the surrounding tissues to set it up for a successful microvascular anastomosis.

There are several choices of recipient arteries in head and neck reconstruction due to the abundant vasculature. The 'standard' recipient arteries include the external carotid artery (ECA) and its branches, mainly the facial artery and superior thyroid artery (Figure 5.1.1). Other chapters in this textbook will cover specialist situations such as the vessel-depleted neck.

Chapter aims:

- Understand the preoperative and intraoperative factors that aid our decision-making of recipient artery selection
- Understand the detailed surgical anatomy and dissection of the standard recipient arteries for head and neck microvascular anastomosis, including the facial artery, superior thyroid artery, and ECA
- Understand the anatomy and preparation of vessels for and intraoral the anastomosis
- Understand the macro and microvascular preparation of recipient arteries for free tissue transfer

Preoperative evaluation and vessel selection

There are several preoperative factors that need to be taken into consideration. First and foremost is the patient. Any factors which may affect the quality of the patient's vessels (and

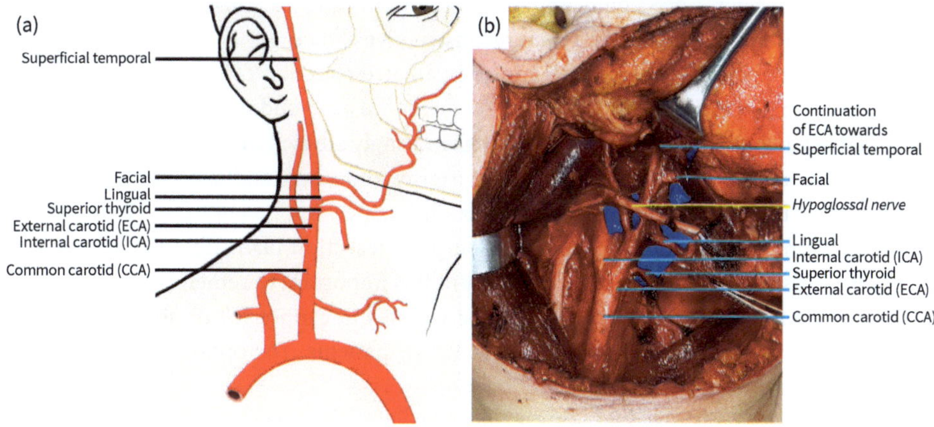

Figure 5.1.1 The standard recipient arteries of choice in head and neck microvascular reconstruction are the branches of the external carotid or the external carotid itself in selected cases. a. Schematic presentation of the external carotid system. b. External carotid artery system dissected. Note the relationship of the hypoglossal nerve to the facial and lingual arteries.

hence the success of the microvascular anastomosis) must be carefully scrutinized. Factors to consider, and not an exhaustive list) include age, history/imaging of atherosclerosis, peripheral vascular disease, coagulopathies, connective-tissue disorders, diabetes, and vasculitis. These factors must not be ignored, as they may lead to free flap failure despite a technically perfect microvascular anastomosis. It is important to consider these factors in conjunction with the patient's overall American Society of Anesthesiologists (ASA) status, underlying comorbidities and nutritional status.

Previous surgery will clearly have implications on the remaining number and quality of vessels in the head and neck. It is important for the surgeon to investigate previous interventions by utilizing medical notes and imaging. Often, however, details of previous operations, including which vessels may remain, are often lacking in operation notes. This information can not only decide if a free flap is appropriate, but also which free flap, e.g. utilizing a free flap with a longer pedicle to reach the contralateral side. If a free flap is considered, one must anticipate the altered tissue planes and scarring that make vessel harvest challenging. It would be advisable for an experienced surgeon to perform the operation in these circumstances.

In a similar manner, preoperative radiotherapy will also have significant implications on vessel selection. Radiotherapy causes tissue damage at a macro and microscopic level. It specifically leads to endothelial and leukocyte damage in blood vessels, which makes microvascular surgery challenging. It is important to assess the radiotherapy fields, and utilize this information preoperatively in the decision-making. Although previous radiotherapy is not an absolute contraindication to microvascular free tissue transfer, there is evidence to suggest that it may increase the risk of flap failure and complications. A systematic review by Mijiti (see Further reading) looked at 12,408 patients over 37 studies. This showed an increased risk of total flap failure (odds ratio [OR] = 1.80, 95% confidence interval [CI] = 1.45–2.23, $P < 0.001$) and increased postoperative complication rates (OR = 2.22, 95% CI = 1.64–2.72,

$P < 0.001$). These figures are significant and therefore need to be considered in the overall preoperative workup of a patient and their reconstructive choice.

In summary, the previously operated and/or irradiated patient is often termed the 'vessel-depleted neck' and remains a significant challenge for the head and neck surgeon. This topic is analysed in Chapter 16. Preoperative imaging is strongly advised in the form of dual-phase CT of the neck and thorax. This will visualize arteries and veins, and also alternative vessel choices such as the internal mammary. A thorough preoperative review of previous medical records, examination findings, imaging, and surgical resection plan should guide the surgeon to the possible recipient vessels that remain. It is important to remember that imaging will help guide the location and patency of the vessels but cannot tell us about the overall quality of the vessels, especially in post-radiotherapy patients. The options that remain for the vessel-depleted neck will then be as follows:

1. Ipsilateral neck
   a. Standard system (ECA, FA, STA)
   b. Alternative system (Thyrocervical trunk/transverse cervical artery, internal mammary)
   c. Vein grafts—to reach an appropriate recipient artery, however with thorough preoperative planning, correct flap choice, and appropriate recipient vessel choice, the added complexity and risk of vein grafts can almost always be avoided.
2. Contralateral neck

Finally, it is important to consider the patient's comorbidities, the complexity of surgical resection, and overall surgical time in the decision-making of recipient vessel choice. In complex cases, the surgeon should not hesitate to consider a local/pedicled flap after appropriate discussion and consent with the patient.

Intraoperative evaluation and vessel selection/preservation

Although the final decision of recipient vessel choice can only be made intraoperatively, much of the planning must be done preoperatively. The planning of the recipient artery occurs during the ablation and reconstructive elements of the surgery. During the ablation one must consider the following:

- Patient's individual anatomy: Though arterial vasculature is relatively predictable, variation in anatomy does occur and must be anticipated. Preoperative cross-sectional imaging will aid the surgeon.
- The location/size of the primary tumour and any metastasis: The surgeon must anticipate which recipient vessels may be involved or of poor quality following the resection. Nodal metastasis in level 1b, for example, may preclude the use of the facial artery.
- Location of final defect: The final defect location must be respected, as this will significantly alter the recipient vessel choice. Clearly the reconstructive choice can simplify this as a longer pedicle length will give the flexibility of recipient artery choice. It is useful to divide the location into the upper, middle and lower third of the face, and the neck as a separate entity.

- Preservation of alternative recipient vessels: until the reconstruction has been inset, the final lie of the pedicle determined, and the microvascular quality reviewed under a microscopy, one can never be certain of a recipient vessel. With this in mind, one must also have a 'plan B' in place. Therefore, it is imperative to preserve alternative recipient vessels, maintaining adequate length and handled meticulously from the beginning.
- Access: remember that the anastomosis can be made easier by better visualization and access. This begins with the neck and tumour access at the beginning of the operation. In addition, one must ensure the recipient vessels have adequate length and clearage of surrounding tissue during the ablation, thinking ahead to aid the microvascular anastomosis.

The recipient artery is of key importance when planning the reconstruction in the head and neck. Some surgeons even advocate raising the flap after the ablation is complete, to ensure the correct pedicle length is planned with the recipient artery. Given that this 'two-stage' approach can affect the length of the surgery (and therefore morbidity to the patient), it is important to weigh up the risks and benefits of this decision preoperatively. Most head and neck procedures are predictable, allowing joint operating; however, as mentioned earlier, complex cases can be anticipated preoperatively and a 'two-stage' approach may be beneficial in these cases. The choice of reconstruction may also influence the initial ablative dissection. For example, one may choose to maintain the length of the facial artery over the lower border of the mandible when planning a deep circumflex iliac artery (DCIA) flap reconstructing the maxilla. However, the same free flap in the mandible would not require such efforts.

In summary, the recipient artery is the key to adequate blood flow into and free flap. One must treat this with respect, perioperatively planning all factors which may influence the success of the microvascular anastomosis and successful free tissue transfer.

Standard recipient arteries

The remainder of this chapter will focus on the standard recipient arteries of the head and neck. These are all branches of the ECA, and include the facial artery, the superior thyroid artery, and the ECA itself. In addition, we will cover oral anastomosis utilizing the distal aspect of the facial artery.

5.2 **Facial artery**

The facial artery remains the workhorse recipient artery in head and neck reconstruction. Due to its relatively superficial course, it is easily encountered during a level 1b neck dissection. In addition, it is encountered at several different points along its long length. Therefore, with adequate planning, one can preserve as much or as little of the facial artery, considering the ablative and reconstructive principles that were discussed earlier in the chapter. The facial artery is a significant branch of the external carotid artery. Although there is anatomical variability, it often arises superior to the lingual artery. It emerges deep to the posterior belly of the digastric and stylohyoid muscle but remains superficial to the hyoglossus muscle throughout its course. It remains deep to the submandibular gland as it passes upwards and forwards towards the mandible. As it ascends, it often passes through, or just deep to the submandibular gland, giving off branches to the gland on its route. During its ascent, it also gives off a major anterior branch, the submental artery. The submental artery passes in an anterosuperomedial direction, piercing the mylohyoid muscle, to supply the submental cutaneous tissue. In addition, the facial artery gives off several smaller branches in the neck, including the tonsillar and ascending palatine branches. These can be dissected and ligated to increase the length and mobility of the facial artery prior to anastomosis. The facial artery in itself continues to loop over the submandibular gland, then passes inferiorly on the lingual side of the mandible but superficial to the submandibular gland. The facial artery then loops back superiorly over the lower border of the mandible, deep to the platysma, and anterior to the facial vein, to continue its tortuous course into the face. It gives off multiple branches, including the superior and inferior labial arteries, and passes further superior to continue as the angular artery and lateral nasal branches.

The facial artery will be encountered during the level Ib neck dissection. If a neck dissection is not clinically indicated, then an elective level Ib neck dissection could be performed for 'vessel access'. As mentioned, the decision needs to be made about how much length of the facial artery needs to be preserved during the initial dissection and ablation. The location of the primary defect and the pedicle length of the reconstruction remain in the primary determining factors. If extra length is required, this must be anticipated at the beginning of the level 1b dissection. Often, to preserve the marginal mandibular nerve, the Hayes Martin manoeuvre is performed. This is when the facial pedicle is light, dated 1 to 2 cm inferior to the lower border of the mandible. In rare cases, where recipient artery length is required or intraoral anastomosis is planned, this manoeuvre cannot be performed. One must preserve the facial artery while continuing the level 1b dissection.

Only once the final resection and neck dissection is complete, with the inset of the free flap, can one decide where to cut the facial pedicle. Though this makes the dissection more challenging, it pays dividends for future microsurgical work and the success of the free flap transfer. In routine cases, the pedicle can be located at the lower border of the mandible, preserving the marginal mandibular nerve. The submental artery is also ligated during a level 1B neck dissection. The facial artery is then re-encountered after excision of the submandibular gland, as it passes posterior to the lower belly of the gastric and stylohyoid muscles.

At this stage, it is imperative to maintain as much length as possible of the facial artery, often ligating the artery as it branches/pa$ses through the submandibular gland itself. This often gives adequate length for most mid to lower third facial defects and neck defects (depending on the reconstructive choice and its pedicle length).

At this stage, much macroscopic vessel preparation can be performed with the use of loupe magnification. The first principle is to improve visualization and access.

This is performed by dividing the posterior belly of the digastric and stylohyoid muscle, which is often more proximal than one expects to ensure optimal visualization (Figure 5.2.1). In our experience, it is important to always divide the posterior belly of the digastric and the stylohyoid muscle for the following reasons:

1. Improved access for preparation.
2. The muscles may constrict/compress the artery.
3. The natural direction of the artery is cephalad; however, when used for anastomosis the donor artery usually approaches from a caudal or anterior direction, requiring the

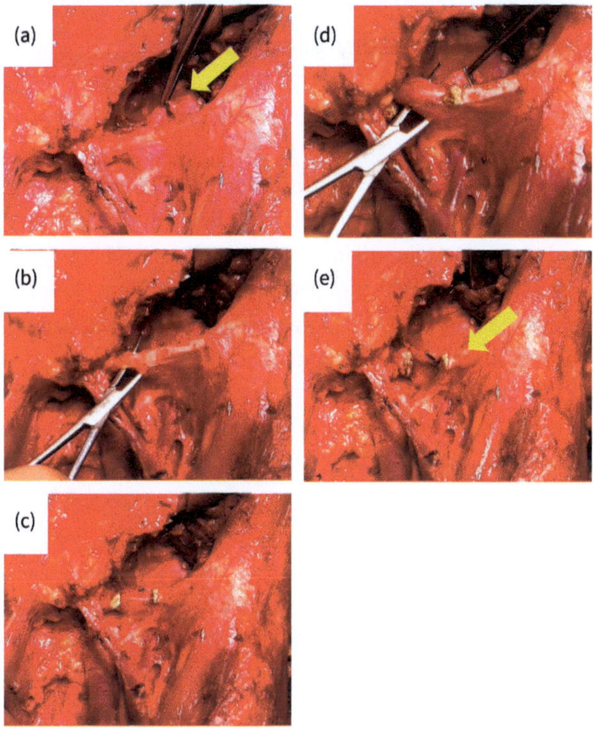

Figure 5.2.1 a. The facial artery stump (arrow) after the completion of selective neck dissection. b. An artery clip is slid under the posterior belly of the digastric prior to its division. c. The posterior belly of the digastric is divided with diathermy. d. The same process is repeated with the stylohyoid muscle. e. The stylohyoid muscle was divided, leaving the whole length of the facial artery exposed and released for preparation.

facial artery to 'bend' or change direction. Presence of strong muscle bands, such as the digastric and stylohyoid, may restrict this movement or cause kinking of the artery with possible detrimental effect on its flow.

4. The artery is wider close to its take-off from the external carotid.
5. The arterial flow is stronger close to the take-off point from the external carotid.
6. In the presence of atherosclerosis, a longer arterial stump offers more options to identify a suitable area for the arteriotomy.

It is then important to meticulously dissect the facial artery, removing any venae-comitantes, which often adhere tightly to this large artery. It is important to fully mobilize the facial artery by proximal dissection, ligating the tonsillar and ascending palatine branches which may be encountered. It is also important to carefully dissect any type of bands which may be limiting the mobility of the facial artery. How far proximally this is performed, depends on the necessary length and access required. One must ensure adequate microvascular principles, with irrigation including heparinized saline to avoid the vessel drying out, and consideration of agents to avoid vasospasm. Finally, a microvascular clamp can be applied, and the ligated end is cut with straight iris scissors. One can then release the clamp and ensure adequate flow prior to detaching the free flap.

Important tips in preparing the facial artery are summarized in Box 5.2.1.

Box 5.2.1 Tips for facial artery preparation

- The facial artery is the most commonly used recipient artery for head and neck reconstruction.
- It is highly recommended that the posterior belly of the digastric and stylohyoid muscles be fully dissected and divided. This allows the facial artery to be mobilized and prepared close to its take-off from the external carotid artery.
- Preparation of the facial artery during its proximal segment close to the take-off from the external carotid artery (ECA) offers a larger calibre vessel, better flow, and a lesser acute angle (bent) that facilitates more robust blood flow.

5.3 **Superior thyroid artery**

Introduction

The superior thyroid artery is the first branch of the external carotid artery, arising just below the greater cornu of the hyoid, though its point of origin can be relatively variable. It is the main arterial blood supply to the upper larynx, thyroid gland, and regional soft tissues. It descends inferomedially, deep to omohyoid and sternohyoid, giving off its major branch, the superior laryngeal artery, to supply the upper larynx. It continues inferiorly to give three branches:

- Infrahyoid branch: A posterior branch supplies the infrahyoid muscles behind the thyroid gland
- Thyroid branch: A medial branch supplies the superior portion of the thyroid gland
- Cricothyroid branch: A lateral branch then crosses medially to perforate the homonymous membrane and supply the cricothyroid muscle

The key structure when dissecting the superior thyroid artery is the external branch of the superior laryngeal nerve (EBSLN), which supplies the cricothyroid muscle and inferior constrictor muscle. The cricothyroid muscle has a key role in lengthening the vocal ligaments, increasing the pitch during phonation, and therefore must be preserved at all costs. The EBSLN often runs superficial to the inferior constrictors, and posteromedial to the superior thyroid artery, however, there is significant anatomic variation.

The superior thyroid artery is often visualized during the levels II–III neck dissection (Figure 5.3.1 and Figure 5.3.2). As the lymphatic tissue is dissected, the superior thyroid artery remains as the deep dissection plane. The decision to utilize the superior thyroid artery again depends on the pre- and intraoperative factors principles discussed earlier. If the lie of the pedicle suits the position of the superior thyroid artery, then this should be utilized as the first-choice recipient artery. If a level III neck dissection has not been performed, one must carry out vessel access surgery. It is simplest to perform a level III supraselective neck dissection or locate the external carotid artery in Farabeuf's triangle. This triangle is bounded by the hypoglossal nerve superiorly, the lateral wall of the thyrolingualfacial trunk and the medial wall of the internal jugular vein. Once the external carotid artery is located,

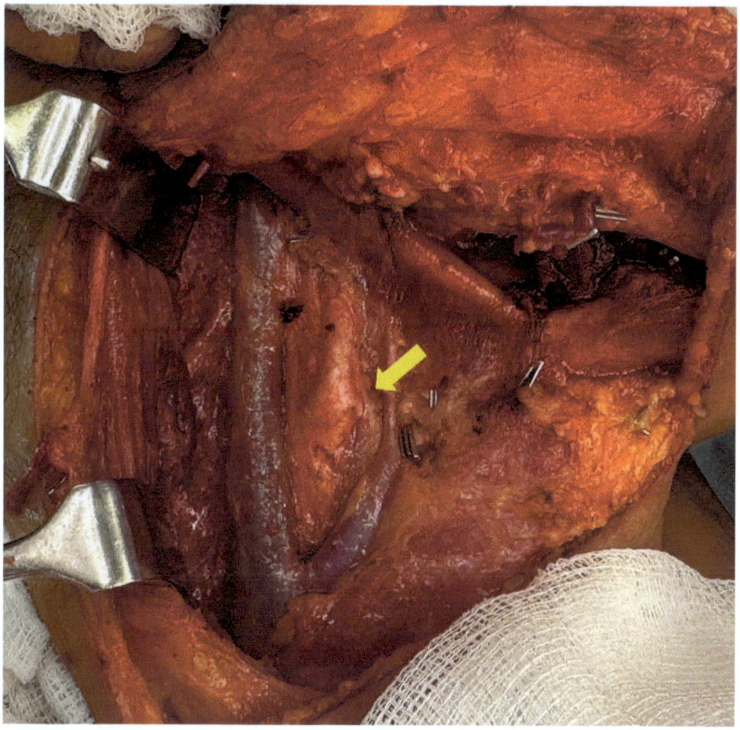

Figure 5.3.1 The take-off of the superior thyroid artery as demonstrated post-selective neck dissection (arrow).

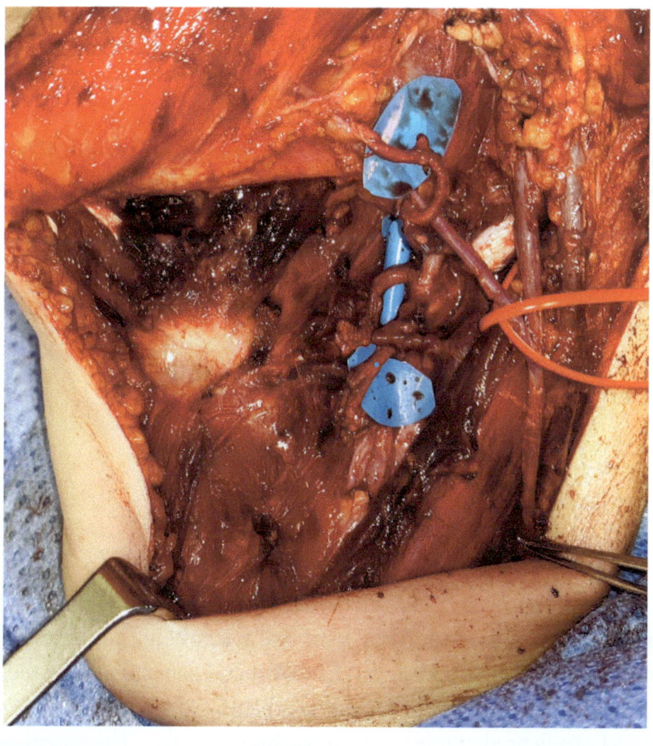

Figure 5.3.2 The superior thyroid artery (blue dot) was prepared prior to division for macrovascular anastomosis.

the superior thyroid artery can be simply dissected to the length required. As previously described, the EBSLN lies in close approximation and should be anticipated, dissected, and protected throughout. If only a small length of the superior thyroid artery, the surgeon is unlikely to encounter the EBSLN. The superior thyroid artery should then be dissected to its origin from the external carotid artery. This removes any tight bands of tissue and ensures adequate mobilization of the recipient artery, providing optimal blood flow. There are often no surrounding structures that impede visualization of the superior thyroid artery after a neck dissection, making this vessel an excellent recipient artery choice. The remaining vessel preparation is often performed under the microscope.

5.4 **External carotid artery**

Introduction

The common carotid artery arises from the brachiocephalic trunk on the right side, and directly from the arch of the aorta on the left side. It travels superiorly, deep to the sternocleidomastoid, to divide into internal and external carotid arteries between the upper border of the thyroid cartilage and hyoid bone, though there can be some variation in the bifurcation location. The internal carotid artery is often posterolateral to the external carotid artery, though there can be anomalies in its position, and this must be considered before any ligation of the external carotid artery. The internal carotid artery continues to travel superiorly in the carotid sheath, posterolateral to the external carotid artery, to enter the carotid canal in the petrous temporal bone. The bifurcation houses the carotid sinus, with extensive baroreceptors innervated by the glossopharyngeal nerve. It is important to liaise closely with the anaesthetist whenever handling, dissecting, and mobilizing the carotids in this region, as a patient with carotid sinus hypersensitivity may lead to significant decreases in heart rate, drop in blood pressure, and inevitably reduced blood supply to the brain.

The external carotid arises anteromedial to the internal carotid artery. It travels superiorly, posteriomedial to the mandible, terminating as the superficial temporal artery and maxillary artery within the parotid gland. Although its branches vary in position, there are often the following:

- Superior thyroid artery
- Ascending pharyngeal artery
- Lingual artery
- Facial artery
- Occipital artery
- Posterior auricular artery

This gives an abundant supply of blood vessel choices for the head and neck reconstructive surgeon, with the facial artery and superficial temporal artery being the workhorse for mid/lower third head defects and the superficial temporal artery being considered for the superior third of head defects (clearly depending on the defect and flap choice selected).

The external carotid artery may have several advantages and disadvantages. The advantages include its relatively predictable location and high flow rate. The potential disadvantages include the large diameter, leading to potential mismatch (almost inevitably) and the potential for atheroma formation. The carotid bifurcation leads to widening of the vessels and turbulent flow, which may be a risk factor for atheroma formation. This can not only lead to thrombus formation in the free flap, but manipulation of the area could increase the risk of stroke formation. With these potential disadvantages in mind, the external carotid artery is often not the first-choice recipient vessel for arterial anastomosis, especially close to the carotid bifurcation. However, in poor alternative recipient arteries, certain vessel-depleted cases or cases with larger donor pedicle diameter, the superior aspect of the external carotid artery may be a viable alternative option.

In most scenarios, a neck dissection will have been performed, exposing variable amounts of the external carotid arteries. If not, the external carotid artery can be found through a variety of access surgeries, many of which were mentioned earlier. Often, the decision to utilize the external carotid artery is made after the facial artery is felt to be unsuitable (Figure 5.4.1). At this point, the facial artery can be traced proximally to its origin to find the external carotid artery, often dividing the posterior belly of digastric muscle for access. The external carotid artery is then dissected and mobilized from its deeper tissues. The length of the external carotid artery can then be extended by tracing the artery superiorly, taking caution to locate and protect the hypoglossal nerve throughout. The external carotid dissection can continue

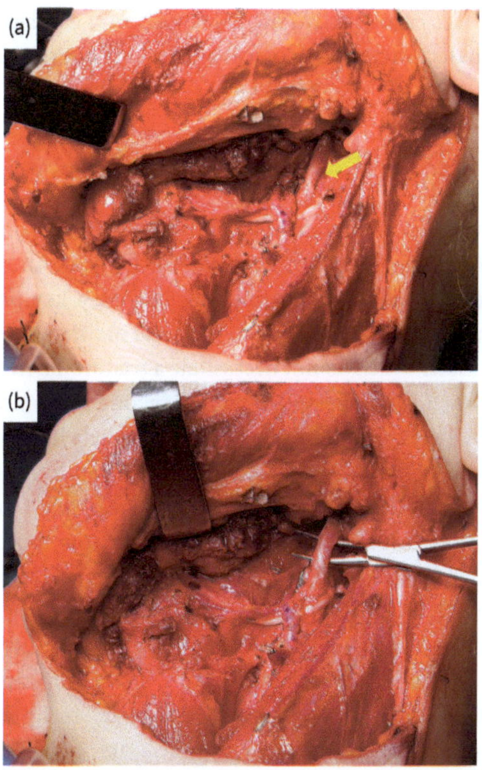

Figure 5.4.1 a. The external carotid artery in a patient who had clearance of level IB for submandibular gland adenoid cystic carcinoma, alongside selective neck dissection. The respective facial artery had poor flow and was deemed inadequate for anastomosis. b. The external carotid artery is controlled and prepared for division.

distally, ligating branches such as the posterior auricular branch to gain further length. The amount of external carotid artery dissected is often limited by the parotid gland. At this point, it is best to ligate the external carotid, then the vessel can be transposed into the neck for a suitable anastomosis position. This extra length is not always necessary if the pedicle length allows. Therefore, dissection and mobilization should be done prior to flap detachment, and the final ligation and transposition performed after flap inset and the ideal donor pedicle position is determined.

5.5 Intraoral microvascular anastomosis

Introduction

With improving outcomes in microvascular anastomosis and free tissue transfer, more challenging techniques are being developed in the pursuit of improved aesthetics and function. The intraoral microvascular anastomosis utilizes the more distal portion of the facial vessels as they are transverse to the cheek lateral to the buccinator muscle.

Intraoral anastomosis in carefully selected cases is a viable but challenging technique that can be useful for the reconstruction of maxillary defects with a short pedicle. The approach offers improved aesthetics as the neck is spared from a scar and can also be indicated for trauma and complex benign cases, such as medial femur condylar flap reconstruction in cleft patients, where a neck dissection for oncological purposes is not required.

Indications and technique

There are several indications (and therefore advantages) of an intraoral microvascular anastomosis. Aesthetics remain of upmost importance to the head and neck surgeon, and in certain benign conditions, avoiding a neck incision may be a key priority, as the intraoral microvascular anastomosis is performed via an intraoral incision only. This lends itself well to non-malignant conditions which do not necessitate a traditional neck dissection such as in benign, trauma, and aesthetic cases, for example. The second indication for intraoral anastomosis may be functional, by reducing the need for long pedicle lengths. For example, maxillary defects restored with free tissue transfer with short pedicles have always been a challenge to anastomose successfully in the neck. The intraoral facial vessels may be available and of close proximity. In addition, the free tissue transfer of flaps from more unusual sites, such as the medial femoral epicondyle flap and its naturally shorter pedicle length, can now be utilized, with the pedicle length no longer being a limiting factor.

A disadvantage of intraoral anastomosis, however, is the variability and complexity of the anatomy in this region, making the vessel location and dissection unpredictable. This can be anticipated and mitigated preoperatively as mentioned in the technique mentioned next. In addition, as the vessels are traced more distally, they become of smaller diameter and calibre. This may be advantageous for certain flaps, but it may be a disadvantage in wider pedicled donor flaps. Finally, the access and vision for both dissection and microvascular anastomosis are much more challenging; therefore, correct case selection and operator experience are of utmost importance.

A summary of the intraoral microvascular anastomosis (Figure 5.5.1) technique is written, based on the excellent review article by Zhang et al. in 2023 (see 'Further reading'):

1. Preoperative vascular assessment: The quality of the distal facial vessels must be assessed preoperatively. This is often visualized on cross-sectional angiography studies, however Doppler ultrasound is recommended to assess the quality of the vessels prior to dissection.
2. Patient positioning: the microscope is set up as any other traditional head and neck microvascular anastomosis, however the patients head should be turned 90° towards the surgeon to ensure the microscope has a direct line of vision to the anastomosis site. The use of a contrast background material propped up by swabs or neuro-patties will help keep the vessels at the correct working length throughout the procedure once the vessels have been located, dissected, and transposed to the correct position.
3. Buccal mucosa retraction: the use of a Davis mouth gag or Dingman retractor allows appropriate opening of the mouth with full exposure of the buccal mucosa throughout the procedure. This provides improved visualization and access.
4. Dissection of anastomotic vessels: an incision is made 5 mm anterior to the parotid papilla in a vertical or an oblique direction through the mucosa. Dissection then continues through the submucosa and buccinator muscle. Following this, blunt dissection then continues in the fat, to locate the facial artery which is often palpable and more predictable and its location. The facial vein is often posterior and medial to the facial

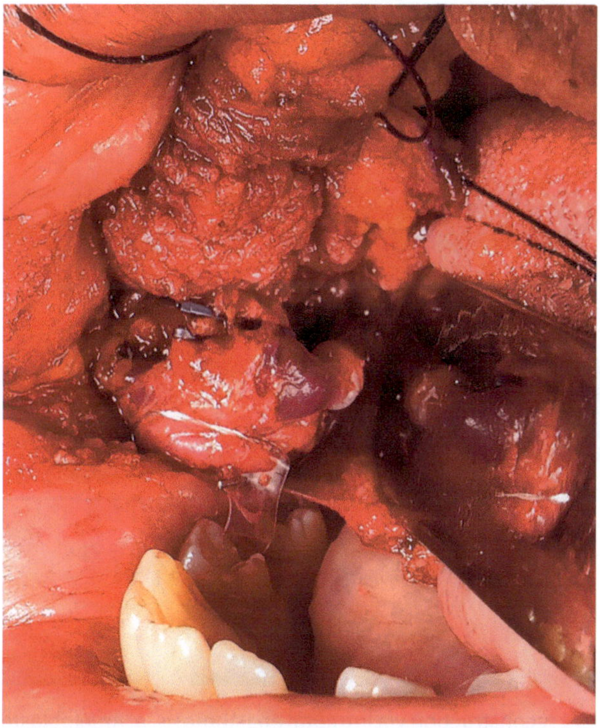

Figure 5.5.1 Intraoral anastomosis for a free flap used for maxillary reconstruction. Note the buccal mucosa incision and flap suspension to facilitate access and exposure of facial vessels.

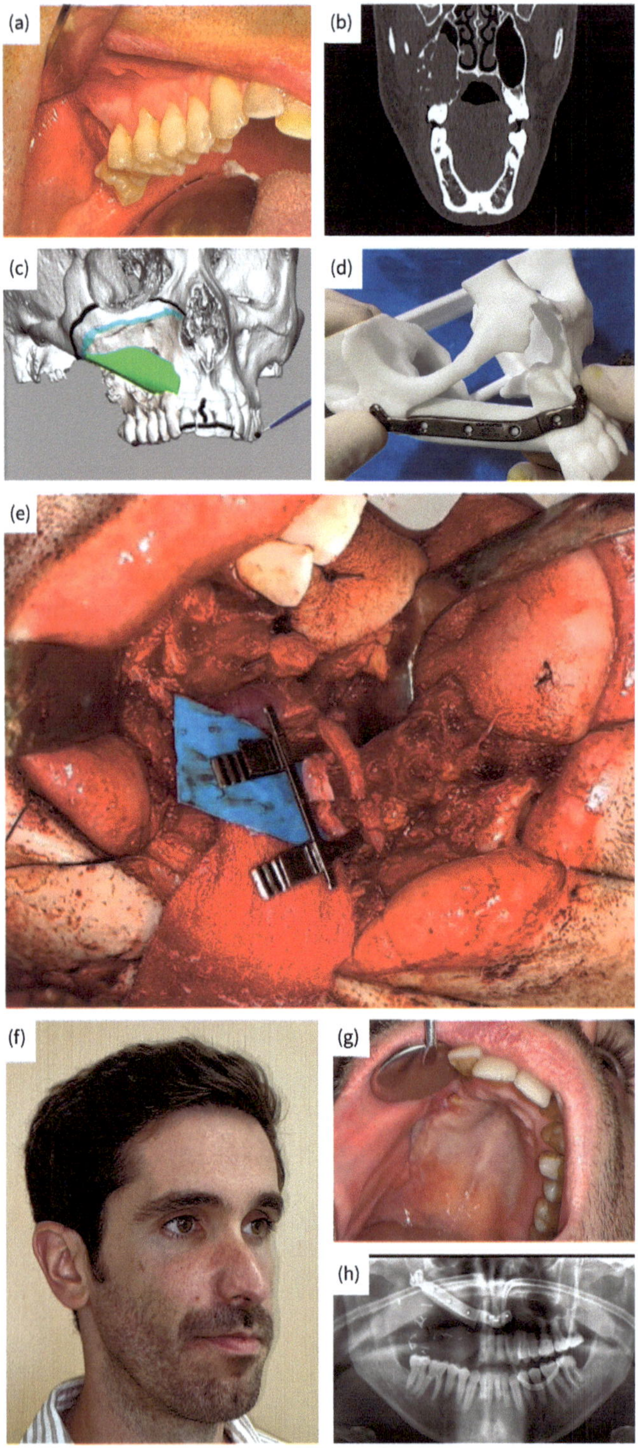

Figure 5.5.2 Maxillary reconstruction via intraoral anastomosis. a. Ameloblastoma of the right maxilla b. Axial CT. c. Virtual planning of the resection and reconstruction with a fibula flap. d. Customized plate. e. Intraoral anastomosis of the flap to the facial vessels. f. Postoperative aspect of the patient. g. Intraoral postoperative situation. h. Control orthopantomogram.
Reproduced courtesy of Professor Julio Acero, Ramon y Cajal University Hospital, Madrid, Spain

artery; however, this position becomes more variable the more superior the dissection. In difficult cases it is advised to trace and facial artery down to the mandibular inferior border and locate the facial vein in this region, as they often have a closer and more predictable relationship here. At least 4 cm of the vessels should be prepared in preparation for transposition of the vessels. During this dissection, the facial nerve may be encountered, and if so, it should be dissected and protected throughout.

5. Transposition of vessels: although there is variability in the techniques described in the literature, the most common and simple technique is to ligate the vessels as superiorly as possible and transpose these to the corner of the mouth in preparation for anastomosis. The remainder of the anastomosis technique is as described as follows for recipient artery preparation; however the surgeon must be meticulous in the assessment of the quality of the recipient vessels and its blood flow. Any doubt should prompt the surgeon to perform an extraoral incision in pursuit of adequate donor vessels.

Intraoral anastomosis offers a viable solution for complex midface microvascular reconstructions (Figure 5.5.2).

Further reading

Breik O, Praveen P, Parmar S. The vessel-depleted neck in head and neck microvascular reconstruction: extreme solutions for extreme situations. *Curr Opin Otolaryngol Head Neck Surg* 2020;28(2):129–35.

Cernea CR, Ferraz AR, Nishio S, Dutra A, Hojaij FC, Dos Santos LRM. Surgical anatomy of the external branch of the superior laryngeal nerve. *Head Neck* 1992;14(5):380–3.

Du E, Patel S, Huang B, Patel SN. Dual-phase CT angiography for presurgical planning in patients with vessel-depleted neck. *Head Neck* 2019;41(9):2929–36.

Schultze-Mosgau S, *et al.* Histomorphometric analysis of irradiated recipient vessels and transplant vessels of free flaps in patients undergoing reconstruction after ablative surgery. *Int J Oral Maxillofac Surg* 2000;29(2):112–18.

Sreedharan R, Krishna L, Shetty A. Origin of superior thyroid artery: under the surgeon's knife. *J Vasc Bras* 2018;17(4):290–5.

Zhang H-Y, Shao Z, Jia J, Liu B, Bu L-L. Analysis of intraoral microvascular anastomosis in maxillofacial defects reconstruction. *J Cranio-Maxillofacial Surg* 2023;51(1):31–43.

6
Vessel choice and preparation

Vein

Julio Acero, Danny Adam, Fernando Almeida, Leandros Vassilios F. Vassiliou, Panayiotis Kyzas, and Nicholas Kalavrezos

6.1 Recipient vein selection

Introduction

As stated in previous chapters, in the realm of head and neck reconstructive surgery, microvascular free tissue transfer is the gold standard, enabling the restoration of form and function following extensive surgical resections. Central to the success of these complex procedures is a profound understanding of the vascular anatomy in the head and neck region. In a similar manner to Chapter 5 concerned with the microsurgical details related to the arterial anastomosis, this chapter delves into the principles of venous anatomy, its variations, the critical aspects of preoperative planning, surgical dissection and preparation for successful microvascular anastomosis. Preoperatively, particular attention should be given to the patient's comorbidities, previous surgeries, the tumour site, and eventual defect. With these concepts in mind, along with appropriate preoperative imaging, the anticipated venous recipient vein(s) should be planned. This should then allow the correct selection of the appropriate flap, with a specific focus on pedicle length and calibre.

Overview of the neck venous system

The venous system in the head and neck is intricate and multifaceted, consisting of numerous veins that drain blood from the craniofacial structures into the central circulation. Smaller veins of the head and neck follow their arterial counterparts.

The primary veins of interest in microvascular free tissue transfer, and the focus of this chapter are the internal jugular vein (IJV) and the external jugular vein (EJV), along with their various tributaries.

The IJV is the principal vein of the 'deep' venous system (DVS), responsible for draining the brain, face, and neck. It originates from the jugular foramen at the base of the skull and descends within the carotid sheath alongside the internal carotid artery and the vagus nerve. The EJV and the anterior jugular vein make up the 'superficial' venous system (SVS), both deep to platysma, draining the subcutaneous tissues of the head and neck. The EJV is a superficial vein that begins at the angle of the mandible from the union of the posterior auricular

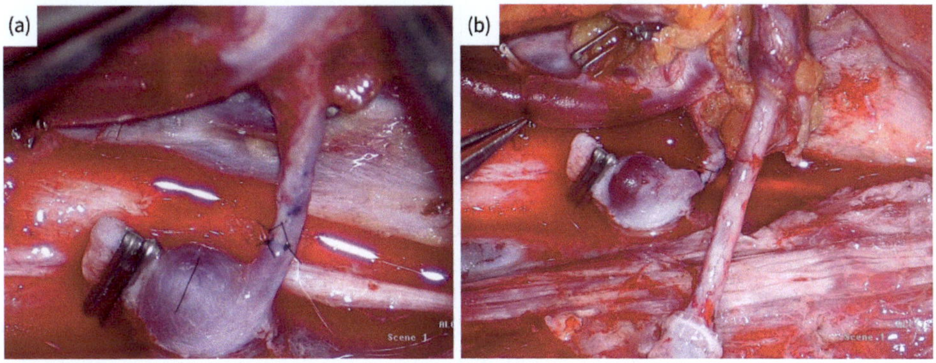

Figure 6.1.1 Importance of preservation of all veins during neck dissection—All veins matter! Neck dissection, apart from the removal of the lymph nodes for oncological purposes, must also aim to harvest vessels for reconstruction and preserve every possible vein in order to offer options for recipient vessels. a. Small radial forearm free flap vena comitans (VC) anastomosed to a small tributary draining into the common linguo-facial trunk of the internal jugular vein. b. Same operating field, zoomed out showing the cephalic vein of the flap anastomosed to the external jugular vein (EJV). This case highlights the importance of preservation of any possible vein, as it cannot always be predicted which vein will finally be the most suitable for the anastomosis(es).

vein and the retromandibular vein. It descends obliquely across the sternocleidomastoid muscle and empties into the subclavian vein.

The EJV, due to its accessibility, is often utilized as a recipient vein in microvascular anastomosis. The anterior jugular vein, which is formed by the fusion of several submandibular veins, travels inferiorly, medial to the sternocleidomastoid to enter into the EJV or subclavian vein. Due to its potential to be inconspicuously damaged during a tracheostomy procedure, it remains a high-risk anastomosis for head and neck surgery.

Anatomical variations in the venous system of the head and neck are not uncommon and can significantly impact on surgical planning and outcomes. These variations include differences in the size, course, and termination of the IJV and EJV, as well as their tributaries. Anatomical variations in venous anatomy are much more common than arterial variations and therefore must be anticipated. The specific variations will be discussed in detail later in each subchapter. An important principle in microvascular surgery is to dissect and protect all potential veins during a neck dissection or access procedures, as long as it is oncologically safe to do so (Figure 6.1.1).

Preoperative evaluation and vessel selection

Effective preoperative planning is multifaceted and involves a comprehensive assessment of the patient's medical history, including comorbidities, previous surgeries, the tumour site, and the anticipated defect. Chapter 3 delved into the detailed pre- and intraoperative analysis, and we guide the reader to this previous chapter for more detail. This section outlines the key considerations for recipient vein selection.

Patient comorbidities

The patient's comorbidities are of utmost importance when considering the reconstructive options for the patient and their eventual defect. The surgeon must firstly consider if the patient can survive the physiological burden of a free flap operation and its potential complications. Consideration should be made to alternatives, such as local or pedicled flaps, or if surgery is even the appropriate choice. These complex discussions and decisions should be made with the aid of the multidisciplinary team (MDT).

Though there is debate, there is a potential link between arterial and venous thrombotic events (see Prandoni in 'Further reading'). Due to the differences in blood pressure, flow, and the biochemical environments, the endothelial and vessel wall structure of veins differ to arteries, making veins much less susceptible to atherosclerotic disease. However, endothelial dysfunction, seen in conditions such as diabetes, obesity, and age, share pathophysiology, and must be anticipated in venous microvascular anastomosis. Several conditions may specifically increase the chances of venous complications, such as coagulopathies, vasculitides, and thrombophilias. These should always be questioned, especially in a patient with previous thrombosis or recurrent flap failures.

Previous surgery/Radiotherapy

Previous surgeries and radiotherapy in the head and neck region can significantly alter the vascular anatomy. These alterations can include changes in the position and structure of vessels, or even their absence, making subsequent microvascular anastomosis more challenging. In addition, scar tissue from surgery and radiotherapy will significantly obscure the limited venous anatomy that remains, making damage to recipient veins much more likely. It is therefore essential to utilize previous surgical documentation and up-to-date imaging to give the surgeon the best chance of success intraoperatively. As discussed in Chapter 5, radiotherapy can further damage the microvascular structures of vessels, meaning even after the challenge of finding a suitable recipient vein, it may be of poor quality.

Tumour site and defect

The location and extent of the tumour, as well as the resultant defect after resection, are critical factors in planning the reconstructive strategy. Tumours in the lower face and neck often require shorter pedicle flaps to reach suitable recipient vessels, while defects in the midface or upper face may be addressed with longer pedicle flaps. For upper face reconstruction such as orbitofrontal defects, the superficial temporal vessels or the retromandibular vein, through parotid gland dissection and facial nerve protection, are the most common options (Figure 6.1.2).

The proximity of the tumour to major vessels and the potential need for vessel sacrifice during resection must also be considered pre- and intraoperatively. The head and neck have an abundance of recipient vein options. It is therefore imperative that the surgeon has different venous options in mind once the tumour site and defect have been planned.

A potential algorithm is shown in Figure 6.1.3. It is important to note this is an extremely simplistic view, which does not take into consideration the numerous variables as discussed earlier, including the patient's previous medical history, surgical history, previous radiotherapy, defect size, and reconstructive choice. In addition, preoperative imaging should be utilized to aid

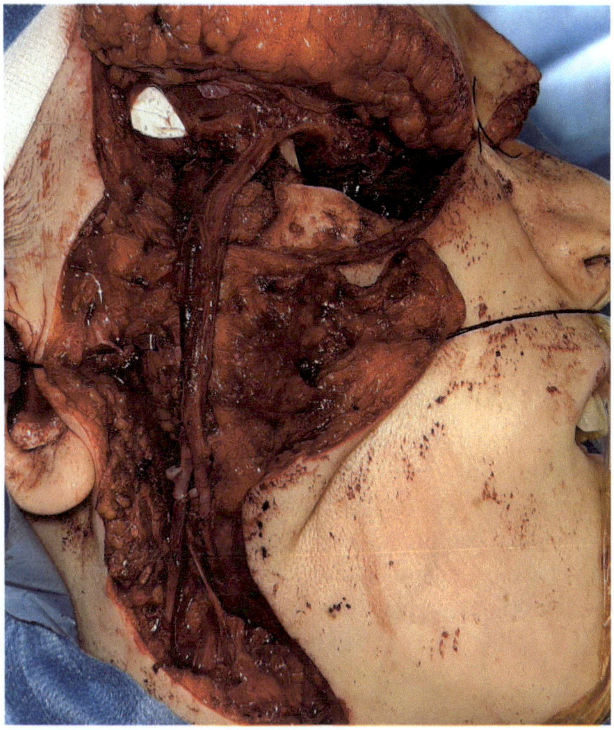

Figure 6.1.2 Repair of orbitofrontal defect with ALT flap and venous anastomosis to the exposed retromandibular vein. The latter had to be exposed following parotid gland dissection with identification and protection of the facial nerve.

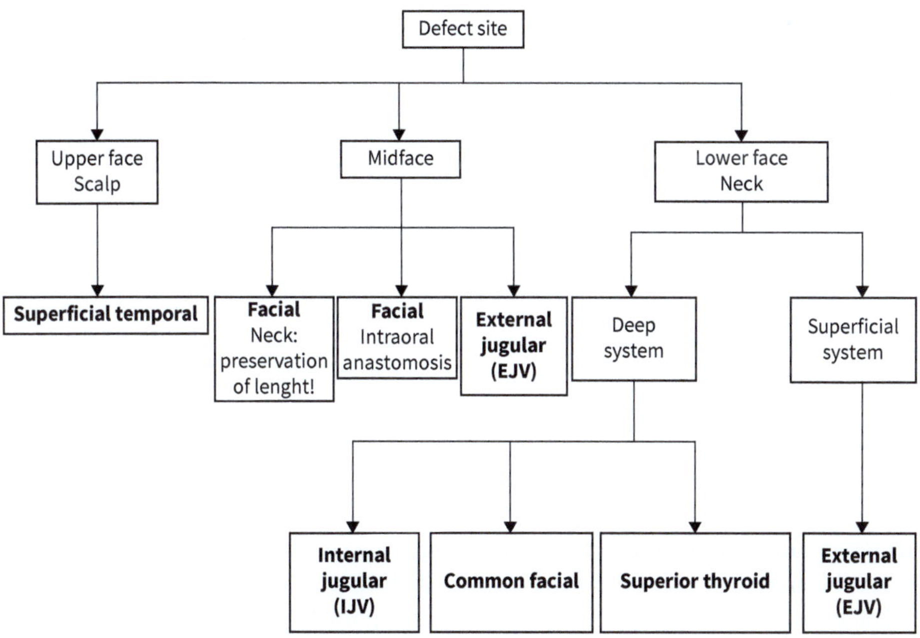

Figure 6.1.3 Algorithm for selection of microvascular recipient vein based on defect location.

Box 6.1.1 Important tips in recipient vein selection

- The anastomosis starts from the neck incision. It is important that the neck incision is performed with meticulous care in order to avoid any injury to the EJV.
- When performing a neck dissection avoid ligating and dividing veins close to the confluence with the internal jugular vein.
- Always preserve veins when possible, in order to provide alternatives for the venous anastomosis during the stage of the reconstruction and microvascular anastomosis.

Intraoperative evaluation and vessel selection

As mentioned previously, the key principle in venous recipient vessel preparation is to preserve all veins and their branches, provided it is oncologically safe to do so. This begins with the initial neck incision and continues throughout the neck dissection and resection of the tumour (Box 6.1.1). Venous dissection is less forgiving than thick-walled arteries, and hence it is important to ensure gentle tissue handling with meticulous dissection. The correct use of instruments, such as DeBakey forceps and vessel loops in the correct situations, must be in the surgeon's arsenal.

6.2 Internal jugular vein (IJV) and tributaries

Introduction

The IJV is the major venous drainage vessel of the head and neck and is a pivotal structure in head and neck surgery. Microvascular anastomosis can be performed to one of its many tributaries in an end-to-end fashion, or directly to the IJV in an end-to-side fashion.

Anatomy of the IJV

The IJV begins at the jugular foramen as the continuation of the sigmoid sinus, which fuses with the inferior petrosal sinus to form the jugular bulb, containing a valve. Superiorly, the IJV is posterior to the internal carotid artery, which enters the carotid canal anterior to the jugular foramen. The IJV lies medial to the styloid process and its associated styloid musculature. In addition, it remains medial to the posterior belly of the digastric and sternocleidomastoid throughout its course. It continues inferiorly in the carotid sheath, lateral to the common carotid artery and deep to the omohyoid muscle. It then joins the subclavian vein to form the brachiocephalic vein. Throughout its course, the IJV receives blood from multiple tributaries, each contributing to the comprehensive venous drainage of the head and neck. These tributaries tend to enter into the anteromedial aspect of the IJV, however, anatomical variability can occur, with posterior branches being reported, which can lead to unexpected and problematic bleeding (see Mumtaz and Singh in 'Further reading').

Table 6.2.1 Tributaries of the IJV and their surgical anatomy/relevance to microvascular recipient vein selection

Tributary	Surgical anatomy	Location during neck dissection	Microvascular anastomosis
Inferior petrosal sinus	Dural venous sinus draining the cavernous sinus, exits through jugular foramen.	Level: Base of skull (Irrelevant in standard neck dissection).	Not used due to deep location and small size.
Pharyngeal vein	Small veins draining pharyngeal plexus, empty into IJV near hyoid bone and thyroid cartilage.	Levels II and III, around pharyngeal constrictor muscles and carotid sheath.	Not used due to variable anatomy and calibre.
Common facial vein	Formed by union of facial and anterior retromandibular veins. Drains into IJV at the either directly or as the thyrolingualfacial trunk.	Facial vein encountered during level Ib dissection at the posterior aspect of the gland, which can then be traced proximally. Also encountered coming anteriorly over IJV during routine neck dissection. (Further detail in text).	Workhorse for head and neck surgery due to its predictable anatomy, accessibility, and adequate size for anastomosis. Preservation of length must be considered for upper and midface defects and intraoral anastomosis.
Lingual vein	Drains blood from tongue and floor of mouth. It runs parallel to the lingual artery, but superficial to the hyglossus muscle, often accompanied by the hypogossal nerve.	During level Ib dissection, the lingual vein is often located and preserved. It is closely related to the hypoglossal nerve, which must be preserved.	Not commonly used due to tortuous course alongside hypoglossal nerve and better alternatives such as common facial, IJV, and EJV.
Superior thyroid vein	Travels with the superior thyroid artery and drains blood from the superior thyroid gland and larynx, emptying into the IJV either directly, or joining the common facial vein.	During dissection of the IJV, the superior thyroid vein will be encountered on its anterior surface.	Variable size and entry into IJV, but often considered for microvascular anastomosis.
Middle thyroid vein	Drains lateral aspects of thyroid gland, travelling laterally over the common carotid artery to empty into IJV. Rarely, the thyroid vein of Kocher may exit the lateral aspect of the thyroid gland between the middle and inferior veins, draining directly into the internal jugular vein.	Levels III and IV, crossing common carotid artery, encountered in thyroid/ central compartment neck dissection.	Less commonly used due to smaller size, variable location, and fragile nature.

Although variation in the venous anatomy of the head and neck is not uncommon, for simplicity, Table 6.2.1 describes the tributaries, from superior to inferior, all of which enter the IJV anteriorly.

Though these tributaries can enter the IJV separately, it is not uncommon to find a large thyro-lingual-facial trunk centrally (Figure 6.2.1).

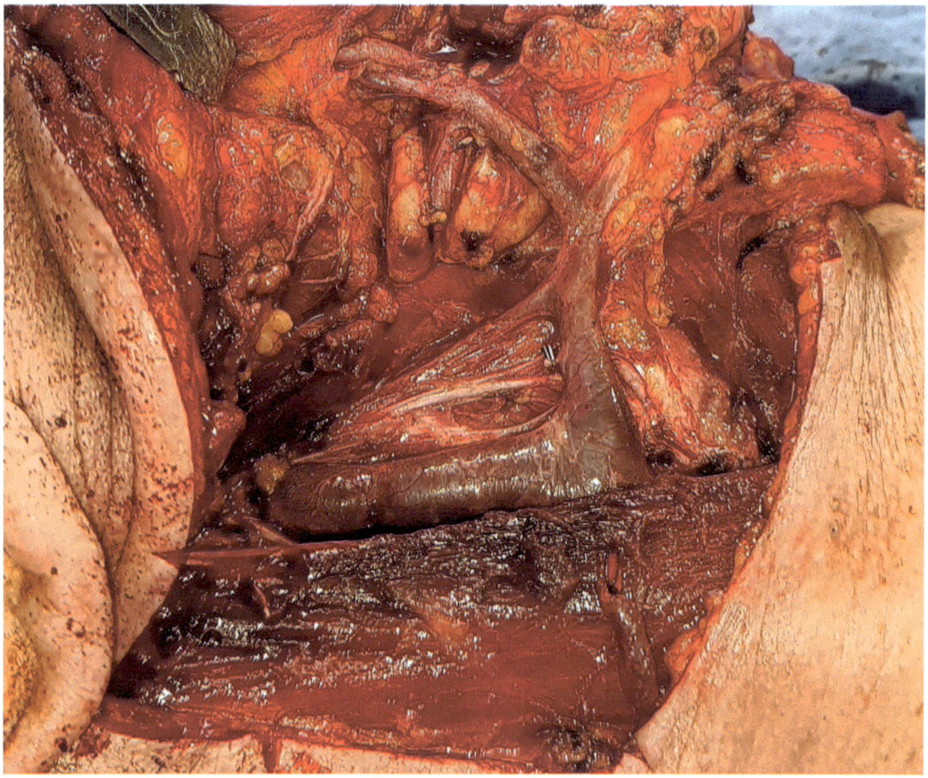

Figure 6.2.1 Thyro-linguo-facial trunk.

Common facial vein and its tributaries

The common facial vein and its tributaries will be discussed in further detail, as it remains the workhorse for microvascular anastomosis in the head and neck region. This is primarily due to the predictable anatomy, large calibre, and multiple tributaries, which often give an array of choices for the microvascular surgeon.

The common facial vein is formed by the union of the two major veins—the facial vein anteriorly, and the (anterior branch of the) retromandibular vein posteriorly, which will be discussed in turn. The facial vein is a superficial vein of the face which begins by the merger of the angular vein, and the medial canthus and the deep facial vein, draining the pterygoid plexus. It descends obliquely across the face to the lower border of the mandible, passing deep to the zygomaticus major muscle, and often crossing the lower border of the mandible posterior to anterior fibres of the masseter muscle, with studies showing a relatively consistent course (see Siwetz et al. in 'Further reading'). The facial vein remains posterior and deep to the facial artery. The reader is guided to the section on intraoral anastomosis for further details of the anatomy in this area, and the dissection of the facial vein for intraoral anastomosis. The facial vein continues underneath the lower border of the mandible, deep to the marginal mandibular nerve but superficial to the submandibular gland. Here it is often joined by superficial veins supplying the submental region. It continues along the posterolateral aspect of the submandibular gland, where it is joined by the anterior branch of the retromandibular vein to form the common facial vein. This continues superficial to the hypoglossal nerve and posterior belly of the digastric to enter into the anterior portion of the IJV.

The common facial vein and its tributaries can therefore be utilized at multiple locations during its course, depending on the defect that remains.

The second vein, the retromandibular vein (also termed the posterior facial vein), is formed within the parotid gland by the union of the superficial temporal vein and the maxillary vein, which wraps around the neck of the mandibular condyle. Within the gland, it divides into an anterior and a posterior branch. The anterior branch, as mentioned earlier, joins with the facial vein to form the common facial vein, which continues its course as described above to enter into the IJV. The posterior branch of the retromandibular vein, joins the posterior auricular vein to form the external jugular vein (EJV), which will be discussed in greater detail later in the chapter.

Anatomical variations of the internal jugular vein

An excellent review article by Mumtaz et al. in the Royal College of Surgeons Annals reviewed the anatomical variations in IJV anatomy, with a specific focus for head and neck surgeons. Common variations include duplication, fenestration, and anomalies in its course and drainage pattern. Each can present unique challenges and opportunities during microvascular anastomosis. Figure 6.2.2 and Table 6.2.2 summarizes the anatomical variables reported in the literature and the number of cases reported. In total, approximately 2% (n = 40) were found to have significant anatomical variables in the IJV. It is essential for the operating surgeon to utilize preoperative imaging, and anticipate potential anatomical variables intraoperatively, with meticulous dissection, to avoid unnecessary damage to a potential recipient vein.

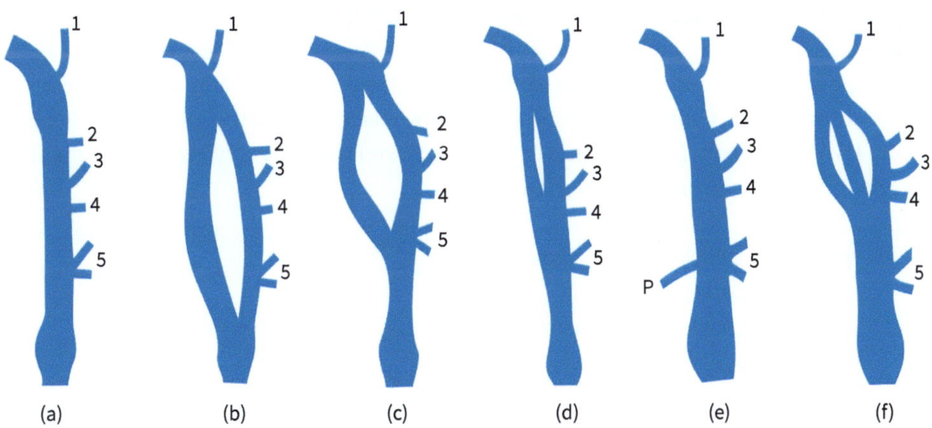

Figure 6.2.2 Anatomical variations of the internal jugular vein. a. Normal. b. Duplication. c. Bifurcation. d. Fenestration. e. Posterior tributary. f. Trifurcation. (1. inferior petrosal sinus; 2. pharyngeal vein; 3. common facial vein; 4. lingual vein; 5. thyroid veins; P. posterior tributary)

Adapted with permission from Mumtaz S, Singh M. Surgical review of the anatomical variations of the internal jugular vein: an update for head and neck surgeons. Ann R Coll Surg Engl [Internet]. 2019 Jan;101(1):2–6. Available from: https://publishing.rcseng.ac.uk/doi/10.1308/rcsann.2018.0185

Table 6.2.2 Anatomical variations of the IJV and their incidence

Anatomical variable	Description	Incidence (n = 1,197)
Duplication	Splitting of the IJV ABOVE the level of the omohyoid	14
Bifurcation	Splitting of the IJV BELOW the level of the omohyoid	4
Fenestration	A small bifurcation that reunites into a single vein creating a 'window' through which other structures may pass	16
Posterior tributary	A tributary of the IJV entering on its posterior surface	5
Trifurcation	Splitting of the IJV into three separate veins which reunite	1

Adapted with permission from Mumtaz S, Singh M. Surgical review of the anatomical variations of the internal jugular vein: an update for head and neck surgeons. Ann R Coll Surg Engl [Internet]. 2019 Jan;101(1):2–6. Available from: https://publishing.rcseng.ac.uk/doi/10.1308/rcsann.2018.0185

The duplication of the IJV (Figures 6.2.3 and 6.2.4) is a variation of particular importance for the following reasons:

- In cases of IJV duplication, there is no EJV or if it exists it will be of rudimentary size.
- All IJV tributaries will be located on the anterior trunk that lies anterior-medially to the anterior border of the sternocleidomastoid muscle and hence very easy for the unsuspected surgeon to inadvertently damage it with potential serious implications for the anastomosis (lack of recipient vein).
- The posterior trunk in usually deep and under the posterior border of the sternocleidomastoid and unsuitable for end-to-side anastomosis due to the overlying compression by the extensive sternocleidomastoid (SCM) overlap.

Although variations in the anatomy of the IJV exist, its relative location within the neck is relatively consistent. Of importance, however, is the relationship of the spinal accessory nerve to the IJV. An excellent review article by da Silva Correia et al. has reviewed the literature on its relationship, as shown in Figure 6.2.4:

- Type 1: SAN passes superficial to the IJV
- Type 2: SAN passes deep to IJV
- Type 3: SAN passes through a branched IJV (e.g. fenestration or duplication)
- Type 4: SAN splits around the IJV

From the 18 studies and 1,491 hemi-necks, type 1 had a prevalence of 79.7% (95% CI 77.6–81.7%), type 2 had a prevalence of 19.6% (95% CI 17.7–21.7%), and the type 3 had a prevalence of 0.7% (95% CI 0.0–1.4%) (da Silva Correia et al. in 'Further reading'). Of more importance was appreciating the ethnic variation in this relationship, with one study from Africa showing 85.5% of their cohort have a type 2 (deep relationship). Again, a thorough understanding of the variations of the anatomy, along with meticulous preoperative planning and dissection, should allow careful preservation of recipient veins for microvascular anastomosis.

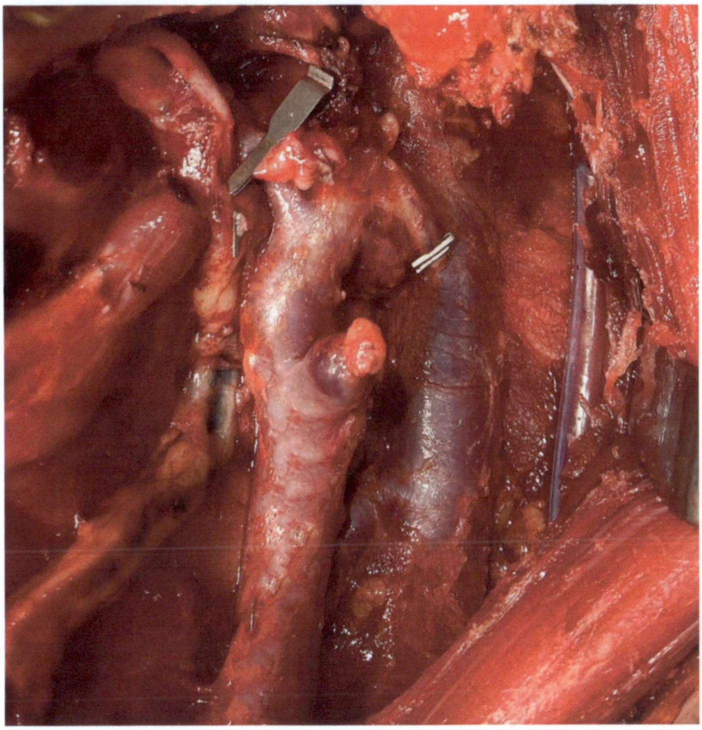

Figure 6.2.3 Internal jugular vein duplication.

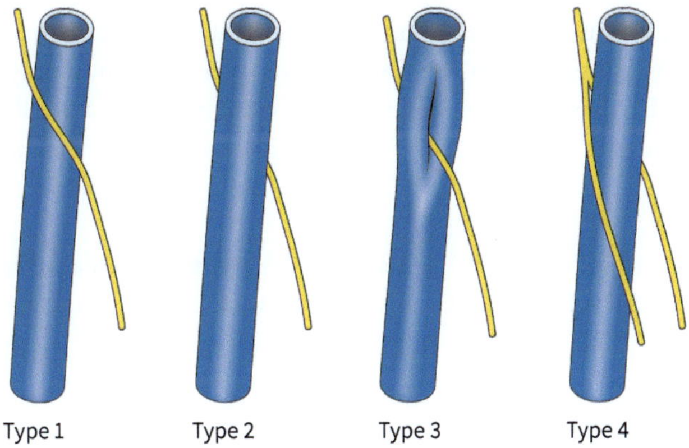

Figure 6.2.4 Schematic presentation of the four variations in the anatomical relationship of the SAN to the IJV.

Reproduced with permission from da Silva Correia AG, Alves JN, da Mota Santos SA, Guerra DR, Garção DC. Anatomical variations in the relationship between the spinal accessory nerve and internal jugular vein: a systematic review and meta-analysis. Int J Oral Maxillofac Surg [Internet]. 2023 Jan;52(1):13–18. Available from: https://linkinghub.elsevier.com/retrieve/pii/S0901502722000741

6.3 External jugular vein (EJV) and anterior jugular vein (AJV)

Introduction

The EJV is a prominent superficial vein that plays a crucial role in the venous drainage of the scalp, face, and neck.

It is an important vein for anastomosis for the following reasons:

- It is a long, straight vessel.
- It is usually of very good calibre.
- It can be chased up into the parotid (retromandibular) for extra length.
- It is easy to dissect and can be orientated variably to meet the donor vein.
- It is an excellent vessel for contralateral neck anastomosis.

The vessel must be protected at all costs at the initial stage of neck dissection as it lies superficially and can be easily damaged during the neck incision or platysma flap development (Box 6.3.1).

It is crucial hence to remember that '*The anastomosis start with the neck incision!*' and teach this to the trainee surgeons to ensure extra care during the beginning of the neck dissection.

This chapter discusses the anatomy and usual variations of the EJV.

Anatomy of the EJV

It begins at the angle of the mandible from the confluence of the posterior auricular vein and the posterior branch of the retromandibular vein. The EJV descends obliquely across the sternocleidomastoid muscle, running parallel to the greater auricular vein, deep to plastyma, within the investing layer of deep cervical fascia and terminates by emptying into the subclavian vein. The EJV has many anatomical variations in its course and tributaries, however, the potential tributaries include 100 EJVs in 50 cadavers (see Deslaugiers et al. in 'Further reading'):

1. Transverse cervical vein (88%): Joins as the EJV meets the posterior border of the sternocleidomastoid vein (SCM). Drains the skin and superficial muscles of the neck.

Box 6.3.1 Preservation and preparation of the EJV

- Remember that the anastomosis starts with the neck dissection.
- Perform the neck incision carefully to avoid inadvertent injury to the EJV.
- During the neck dissection, preserve the whole length of the EJV and only divide it once the appropriate length required for the venous anastomosis has been determined.

2. Suprascapular vein (47%): Drains the region over the scapula and joins the EJV near its termination.
3. Anterior jugular vein (46%): Joins directly into the EJV in 46% of their cadaveric dissections. This can be of major benefit for microvascular anastomosis due to its location, course, and calibre.
4. Cervical vein (13%).

Anatomical variations of the external jugular vein

A review article by Rusu et al. in 2023 (see 'Further reading') has found a plethora of anatomical variations in the superficial venous system (SVS) and the EJV. This ranged from the absence of an EJV (and other components of SVS), variation in calibre, duplication, triplication, variation in branching, and anastomosis patterns. Figure 6.3.1 shows the potential anatomical variability in the EJV taken from Dalip et al. (see 'Further reading').

The ability to classify these variabilities into clinical practice is futile due to the gross variability in individuals. In addition, cadaveric studies are limited due to challenges in the dissection of small anastomotic vessels. It is therefore of more importance for the microvascular surgeon to maintain the key principles of this chapter; thorough preoperative planning and meticulous dissection of all key veins and their branches, provided it is oncologically safe to do so. An excellent article by Honda et al. shows the potential for contrast-enhanced CT in preoperative planning and individualizing treatment (see Honda et al. in 'Further reading').

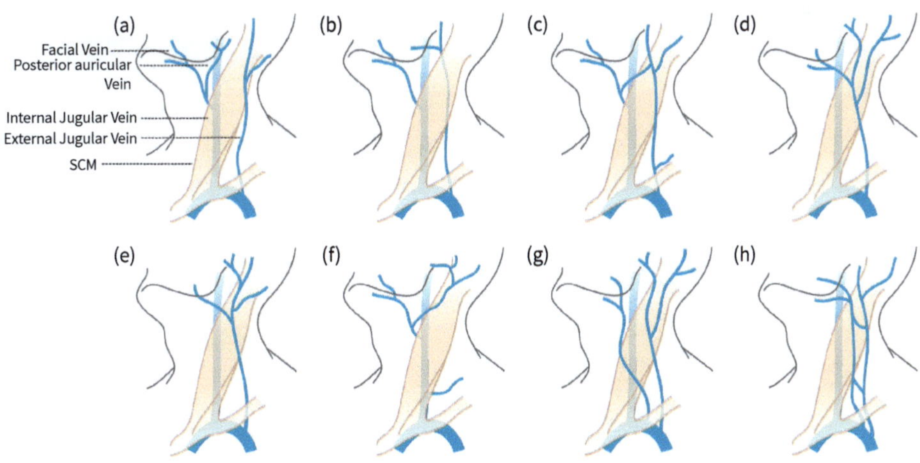

Figure 6.3.1 Anatomical variations of the external jugular vein (EJV).

Adapted from Dalip D, Iwanaga J, Loukas M, Oskouian RJ, Tubbs RS. Review of the Variations of the Superficial Veins of the Neck. Cureus [Internet]. 2018 Jun 18, under the Creative Commons Attribution License CC-BY 3.0. Available from: https://www.cureus.com/articles/13083-review-of-the-variations-of-the-superficial-veins-of-the-neck.

Anterior jugular vein/anterior branch of the external jugular vein

The anterior jugular vein (AJV), is a smaller tributary that runs parallel to the main EJV. It originates from superficial veins in the submandibular and submental regions and descends along the anterior aspect of the neck. There are typically two key branches that run in parallel, a medial AJV (MAJV), that runs medially over the sternohyoid, and a more laterally based lateral AJV (LAJV), which courses along the medial aspect of the SCM. The MAJV and LAJV typically unite inferiorly, running deep to the SCM to enter into subclavian, interior jugular vein (IJV), or EJV. Similar to the EJV, there is significant anatomical variation in terms of absence, duplication, branching and anastomosis (see Honda et al. in 'Further reading').

The clinical case in Figure 6.3.2 shows a dominant anterior jugular vein, which was a continuation of the retromandibular vein, with multiple tributaries, with the IJV lacking any branches. Again, this shows the variability in the SVS, reinforcing the need for the microvascular surgeon to be meticulous in the awareness and dissection of all veins in the head and neck. In Figure 6.3.3 a more rare and complex combined duplication with dominant AJV is shown.

The AJV can serve as an alternative recipient vessel in microvascular free tissue transfer, particularly when the main EJV or IJV are not suitable due to size mismatch, previous surgery, or anatomical variations. Its superficial location and typical course make it a potential option in certain reconstructive scenarios. As the AJV runs medially in the neck, there is a significant risk of damage to the vessel during the tracheostomy procedure. This can sometimes be damaged unknowingly, making the vessel appear large and of suitable calibre. It is therefore essential that the microvascular surgeon is aware of this from the very start of the tracheostomy procedure, and all efforts are made to preserve this vessel. If there is any doubt about damage to the AJV during the tracheostomy procedure, this vessel should not be used for microvascular anastomosis.

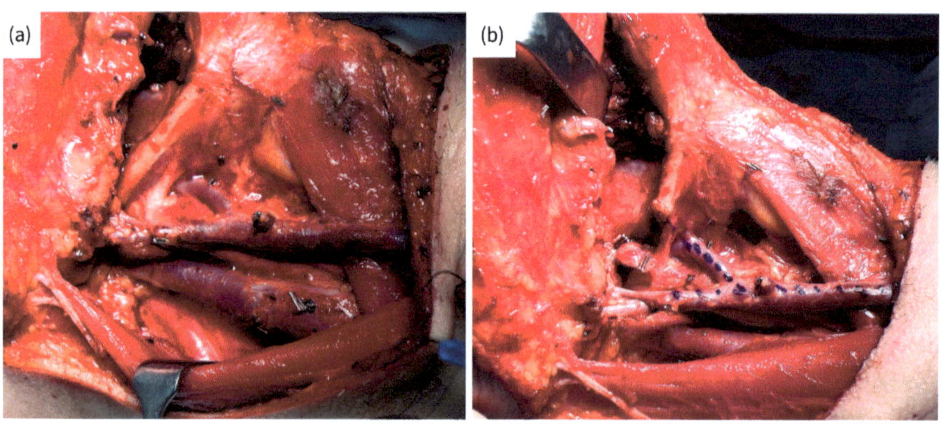

Figure 6.3.2 Dominant anterior jugular vein (AJV). a. The AJV is the continuation of the retromandibular vein, with all the tributaries, with the IJV lacking any branches. Note the position of the AJV superficial to the omohyoid muscle. b. The AJV marked to maintain orientation and prior to division of the recipient vein.

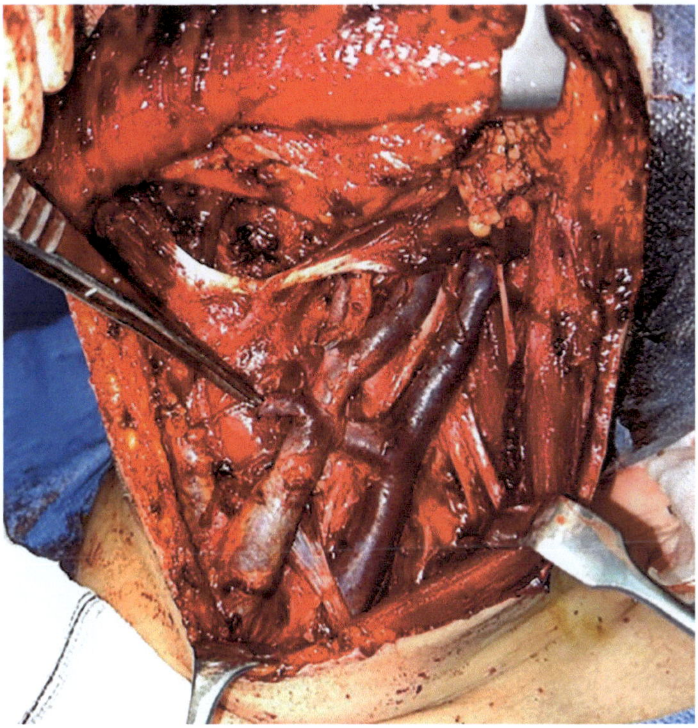

Figure 6.3.3 Rare variation of combined dominant anterior jugular vein and IJV duplication. Note the anterior trunk, which corresponds to a hypertrophic AJV and lies above the omohyoid muscle and the IJV. Note the wide interconnecting vein in the middle that bridges the two systems. Again, and as discussed in the subchapter on IJV, duplication of the posterior trunk is depleted of tributaries (aside the 'bridging' vein with the IJV) and lies deep in the neck under the posterior border of the sternocleidomastoid muscle.

6.4 **Preparation for end-to-end anastomosis**

Once the ablation has been completed and meticulous haemostasis must be achieved, the attention should turn to preparation of the remaining recipient vessels for microvascular anastomosis and receipt of the free flap reconstruction. Prior to performing the microvascular anastomosis, the veins must be prepared for an end-to-end (ETE) or end-to-side (ETS) anastomosis. This decision often depends on several factors, namely the available anatomy, lie of the recipient and donor vessels, and the surgeon's preferred technique. A meta-analysis by Ahmadi et al. in 2017 (see 'Further reading') compared ETE vs. ETS and found no statistically significant difference in outcome between the two techniques (see Ahmadi et al. in 'Further reading'). Therefore, the decision to use one technique over another should depend on the available anatomy, optimal configuration, and minimizing vessel mismatch.

ETE venous anastomosis is a cornerstone of microvascular reconstructive surgery in the head and neck region. Success in these procedures relies heavily on meticulous vein selection and preparation. This section provides a guide to the preparation of veins for ETE anastomosis, covering both macrovascular and microvascular principles.

Proposed sequence

The following is a suggested comprehensive sequence, which ensure economy of time and movement, with minimal vessel handling to prepare the recipient vein for microvascular anastomosis. This mirrors the steps for the preparation of the artery as discussed in Chapter 7:

1. Recipient vein
   i. Macrovascular preparation (performed prior to flap detachment)
      a. Identification, dissection, and mobilization of an appropriate recipient vein
      b. Orientation and marking of the vein
      c. Clamping of the vein
   ii. Microvascular preparation
      a. Perivascular tissue excision
      b. Adventitia dissection
      c. Venotomy
      d. Lumen inspection and dilation
      e. Fine adventitia dissection
      f. Further orientation marking
2. Donor vein preparation follows the same sequence (further discussion in Chapters 7 and 9)

Macrovascular preparation

Identification of recipient vein in the head and neck and with full dissection and mobilization

Identifying a suitable recipient vein is the initial step and is crucial for the success of the anastomosis. Selection criteria include anatomical location, vein size, and flow characteristics. It is important to maintain as many potential recipient options as possible, as the ideal recipient vein cannot be confirmed until transfer of the free flap and donor vessels is complete. There may be failures in anastomotic attempts, or valves which may not permit the use of a tributary.

We support the concept that a single venous anastomosis is sufficient as the feasibility of the flap, because the use of a single vein significantly increases the speed of blood flow through the microanastomosis, obtaining lower rates of venous thrombosis (see Dediol et al. and Dornseifer et al. in 'Further reading'). However, in the literature this appears controversial and others support the anastomosis of two veins rather than one, when the opportunity arises (see Christianto et al. in 'Further reading'). For this reason, we come back to the key principles of this chapter:

1. Preoperative planning: Meticulous interpretation of preoperative imaging and clinical examination will ensure optimal planning and selection of recipient veins.
2. Maintain all veins and tributaries, provided it is oncologically safe to do so: This begins at the start of the neck dissection, from the initial incision to the completion of the resection. All veins should be maintained with maximal length of tributaries where

possible. It is important to bear in mind that veins may principally have adequate length, but maybe unsuitable microscopically due to valve position. Therefore, by maintaining maximal length to the microscope, one can ensure the best chance for a successful anastomosis.

The detailed anatomy of the venous systems has been discussed earlier in the chapter. The workhorse for ETE anastomosis includes the common facial vein (and its tributaries) from the deep venous system, and the external jugular vein from the superficial venous system. If both systems are available with a good calibre match and pedicle orientation, the question lies on which system to use. A recent meta-analysis suggested a reduced rate of venous thrombosis in the internal jugular vein (IJV) system rather than the external jugular vein (EJV) system (RR 0.55) (see Yin et al. in 'Further reading'). This, however, has not been the experience of the authors, with the EJV often having an excellent calibre match and pedicle orientation, with no difference in thrombosis rate. In fact, the EJV is the author's preferred venous anastomotic vein when the option permits.

Gross preparation ensures that the vein is adequately exposed, mobilized, and oriented, ready for fine microscopic dissection. It is essential to fully dissect and mobilize the recipient veins, prior to detaching the free flap and transfer to the head and neck. Mobilization involves the careful dissection of the vein from surrounding tissues to allow for tension-free anastomosis. In addition, it allows the safe clamping of the vessel during the anastomosis. The combination of blunt and sharp dissection will ensure complete dissection and mobilization while preserving the vasa vasorum to avoid ischaemia to the vein wall. The use of surgical loupes is essential to enhance the visualization and precision, ensuring small side branches are ligated safely and not torn. Incomplete mobilization can lead to tension at the anastomosis site, potentially causing failure due to twisting or excessive strain on the anastomosis.

Orientation and marking

Once the veins have been fully dissected, the vessel should be marked in a similar manner to marking the pedicle prior to detachment (please see Chapter 7 for further details). After meticulous haemostasis, the vein should be dried and placed in its passive and relaxed position. At this point, the vein is simply marked with methylene blue at regular intervals on its superior surface. It is of critical importance to appreciate that the dots from the pedicle MAY NOT necessarily line up dots on the recipient vessels. The dots simply give an indication of the relaxed, natural orientation of the vessel, aiding the microvascular surgeon prior to microvascular anastomosis.

Clamping of the veins

Once the macrovacular preparation of the recipient vein is complete, with meticulous haemostasis, full mobilization, and marking of the recipient vein, the clamping of the vein may be performed before or during the microscope work, depending on the size of the recipient vein. It is the author's preference to place a surgical drain behind the sternocleidomastoid prior to any microscope work. This can be applied under suction during the microvascular work, which keeps the field dry and avoids suction near the pedicle and anastomosis.

The artery is typically anastomosed first to reduce the ischaemic time. The attention then turns to the venous anastomosis and preparation of the vein for ETE anastomosis. Clamping the veins is essential to provide a bloodless field and minimize trauma during microvascular preparation and anastomosis. During the microvascular procedure, veins will be clamped at various points. However, it is best to keep the veins unclamped as much as is practically possible. This approach prevents blood stagnation and the accumulation of metabolic byproducts. If the opportunity allows, for example, with two veins available on the free flap (e.g. a cephalic and VC in a radial forearm free flap), it is best to keep on vein open while the other is being prepared and during the anastomosis.

Various clamps exist on the market, and are discussed in detail in Chapter 1. They aim to exert minimal pressure on the veins, occluding the blood while minimizing endothelial damage. These range from microvascular clamps, to bulldogs and Satinsky clamps, depending the size of vessel to be clamped. The vein in gently manipulated into position, at this point the appropriate clamp can be placed as proximal as possible to ensure it does not disrupt the field of microvascular work and allows full mobilization of the vessel during the anastomosis. For an ETE anastomosis, a 3V clamp is appropriate for smaller veins, with bulldog clamps being utilized for larger veins. Once the vein has been clamped, the position the vessel has been ligated can be cut with straight microvascular or iris scissors perpendicular to the vessel. The vein can then be ligated with heparinized saline, moving onto the crude perivascular dissection under the microscope. As mentioned, in small recipient veins, this entire stage can be performed under the microscope.

Microvascular preparation

Perivascular tissue excision

It is the author's preference to detach the flap and perform the recipient and donor microvascular work together. This improves the overall economy of movement with all microscope work being performed in one sitting. Removing perivascular tissue is the first step in refining the vein for anastomosis. A basic understanding of the venous anatomy is critical to a successful anastomosis. The anatomy of a vein is similar to an artery, but it has several key differences due to the reduced blood pressure:

- Tunica adventitia: Also termed *tunica externa.* This outermost layer is made up of connective tissue, which mainly consists of loosely arranged collagen fibres and much fewer elastic fibres when compared to an artery. This provides structural support and protection to the vein, but the loose arrangement of collagen and the relative lack of elastic fibres acquires flexibility to the vein, allowing it to accommodate varying volumes of blood. Similar to an artery, adventitia of larger veins contain the vasa vasorum (small blood vessels that supply the walls of larger veins) and nerves (nervi vasorum). The vasa vasorum supplies nutrients to the outer layers of the vein wall, while the nerve fibres help regulate vascular tone, though this role is much less pronounced than arteries. Smaller veins will lack any significant vasa vasorum, with diffusion becoming the primary source of nourishment. Physiologically, the adventitia has an important role in growth, repair, and immune surveillance.
- Tunica media: In comparison to its arterial counterpart, this layer is much thinner, with fewer smooth muscle and elastic fibres. The smooth muscle is less organized, and there is a higher proportion of collagen fibres relative to arteries. The reduced number of elastic

fibres in the tunica media of veins results in less elasticity. Veins are more distensible and can expand to accommodate varying blood volumes, functioning as capacitance vessels.
- Tunica intima: This layer is again, relatively thinner than its arterial counterpart. It includes an endothelial cell layer and a thin subendothelial layer. Veins lack a well-defined internal elastic lamina. The tunica intima in veins provides a smooth surface for blood flow. Maintaining the integrity of the tunica intima is crucial to prevent thrombosis and ensure smooth blood flow through the anastomosis. Gentle handling and suturing techniques are critical to avoid damaging the intima and media layers, which can instigate a catastrophic thrombotic event. This is even more important in veins, due to slower flow, allowing more time for platelets to aggregate. The thinner structure and absence of an internal elastic lamina reflect the lower pressure conditions in veins. This is of critical importance, allowing both suturing and microvascular anastomotic devices to be utilized, given the thin, pliable nature of the vein. Finally, the endothelium in veins often contains valves, which must be avoided for a successful microvascular anastomosis.

With this anatomical and physiological understanding, the adventitia can be dissected. This initially begins with gross dissection of the loose perivascular tissues, followed by finer dissection of the more adherent adventitia. A key principle of microvascular surgery is to only dissect what is necessary for a safe and successful anastomosis, no more and no less.

The first step, if not already performed before the microscope is introduced, is to clamp the vessel. An appropriate clamp is chosen based on the size of the recipient vein for the ETE anastomosis, usually a 3V for smaller or a bulldog for larger tributaries. It is placed proximally, away from the anastomosis site to avoid interruption the technical aspect of suturing or placement of a microvascular anastomotic device (MAD). The vessel is then irrigated with heparinized saline to remove any stagnant blood which may initiate a thrombus.

Adventitia dissection

Dissection of the adventitia in a vein should be handled gently and with intelligence. The vein should only be handled from its adventitia. Unlike the arterial adventitia, the plane of dissection is often more challenging to find, and due to its thinner wall, damage to the vein can easily be accomplished. Removal of the loose perivascular tissue can be achieved by gently picking this layer up with a pair of jeweller's forceps and using curved microscopic scissors to gently cut away this fluffy layer. This sharp dissection technique is generally preferred to blunt dissection that tears the adventitia using two sets of jeweller's forceps (see Lohman et al. in 'Further reading').

Initial adventitia dissection is performed using the 'triangulation technique'. Here, the assistant uses two straight jeweller's forceps and the surgeon uses a single straight jeweller's forceps to gently grasp the adventitia only, forming a triangle at equal distances apart. This allows the surgeon to precisely remove the more adherent adventitia around the proposed anastomosis site, using straight microscope scissors. The scissors are used in parallel to the vessel wall to ensure the pointed tips do not damage the vein itself. Remember, only the minimum necessary adventitia should be removed that may affect the bites of the suture of the placement of a MAD. Underpreparing can lead to loose fragments, which are extremely thrombogenic and may get caught intraluminally during suture placement. Overpreparing can remove the important physiological role that the adventitia plays, again leading to anastomotic failure. Leaving a small amount of adventitia a small distance from the anastomosis site can be useful to allow minimal trauma to the wall of the vein during placement of sutures or the MAD. Bear in mind that the final adventitial prep will come later, after venotomy and inspection of the lumen.

Venotomy

The next critical stage for a successful ETE anastomosis is a venotomy of the recipient vessel. This ensures a minimally traumatized, clean-cut edge, with all layers of the vein intact for suture or MAD placement. Prior to selecting the venotomy site, it is essential to ensure that no valves are present which may interfere with the flow of the anastomosis. It is also ideal to leave enough of a stump to ensure adequate mobilization during the anastomosis.

Once the position of the anastomosis has been selected, the adventitia is gently grasped with straight jeweller's forceps. The assistant can also grasp the adventitia near the vessel end, with minimal pressure. The aim is to place the recipient vein under gentle tension to allow a single clean cut. With the vein stabilized, straight iris scissors are used to make a single perfect cut perpendicular to the vein. Placing the vein well into the scissors, rather than cutting with the tips increases the probability of cutting the vein in one single cut. Ensure the scissors are sharp, to avoid tearing or chewing through the vessel, which will damage the most critical point of the recipient vein. If there is a calibre mismatch, an angled cut can be considered to try and correct this vessel mismatch, however it comes with its own inherent risks.

Lumen inspection and dilation

Once the venotomy has been performed, the vein is irrigated with heparinised saline to ensure any loose tissue and remaining blood are removed, in addition to checking the lumen patency. With gentle handling of the adventitia, the lumen is inspected to ensure the health of the vein and also ensuring there are no valves near the anastomosis site which my hinder the flow.

The next stage is to dilate the vein if required. There are several reasons to consider gentle mechanical dilation of the vessel prior to suturing or MAD placement. Firstly, dilation often allows better visualization, which can help identify any narrowing, spasms, or pre-existing thrombi in the vein that could compromise the anastomosis. Addressing these issues beforehand can prevent complications. Dilation helps in assessing the true diameter of the vein, which is crucial for size matching with the donor vein prior to the anastomosis. Proper size matching minimizes the risk of complications such as turbulence, which can lead to thrombosis. Dilating a vein can also make it easier to handle during the suturing process. The increased diameter can provide more space for placing sutures accurately, therefore reducing the risk of intimal damage or catching the back wall with suture placement.

Dilation is performed using vessel dilators (instrument shown in Chapter 1). The surgeon should gently grip the adventitia close to the anastomosis site. This allows more control of the dilation process and reduces the risk of kinking or endothelial damage. Under excellent visualization under the microscope, the dilators are inserted into the lumen. Using a combination of tactile and visual feedback, the pressure is released on the dilators to apply gentle pressure on the vein for 1–2 seconds. The dilators are then turned 90 degrees, and a further 1–2 seconds of pressure can be applied. The vein should only be dilated a maximum of 50% greater in its diameter to avoid catastrophic damage to the venous endothelium.

Box 6.4.1 Sequence of vein preparation (end-to-end)

A. Macrovascular preparation (performed prior to flap detachment)
   i. Identification, dissection, and mobilization of an appropriate recipient vein
   ii. Orientation and marking of the vein
   iii. Clamping of the vein
B. Microvascular preparation
   i. Perivascular tissue excision
   ii. Adventitia dissection
   iii. Venotomy
   iv. Lumen inspection and dilation
   v. Final adventitia dissection
   vi. Further orientation and marking

Fine adventitia dissection

Once the correct vein position has been achieved, with the lumen inspected and adequately dilated, the final fine adventitia dissection should be performed. This should be performed using the triangulation techniques described earlier. If the earlier dissection has been performed with a perfect venotomy cut, little to no dissection may be required at this stage. Remember, the aim is to ensure no adventitia is introduced during the anastomosis, while keep as much adventitia present to provide its physiological benefits.

Further pedicle marking

At this stage, although the pedicle has been marked earlier, due to the anatomy, passive lie of the vein and position of the venotomy, the orientation for suture or MAD placement may be difficult to see under the microscope. It can be beneficial therefore to place one further dot near to the anastomosis site at the 12 o'clock position. This is often performed with a surgical marking pen onto a dried vein, to ensure any dye does not flow into and compromise the anastomosis field.

This is a suggested protocol that is methodical, comprehensive, and efficient. The microvascular surgeon should develop their own order to achieve these goals. Once the recipient vein has been prepared, the same protocol is suggested for preparation of the donor vein.

The steps for vein preparation discussed in this chapter are summarized in Box 6.4.1.

6.5 **Preparation for end-to-side anastomosis**

Introduction

End-to-Side anastomosis is a technique where the free end of the donor (pedicle) vein is anastomosed on the side of the recipient vein (almost always the internal jugular vein, IJV) through a hole (venotomy) that the microsurgeon creates in it (Figure 6.5.1).

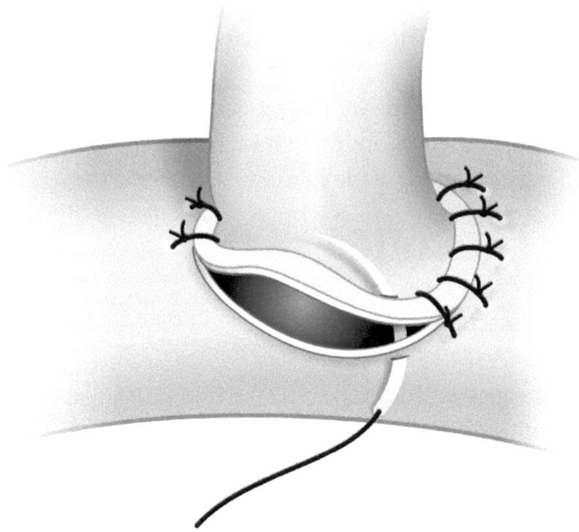

Figure 6.5.1 Schematic illustration of an end-to-side anastomosis in the IJV.

As mentioned earlier, there is no difference in outcomes between an end-to-end (ETE) and an end-to-side (ETS) anastomosis (Ahmadi et al. in 'Further reading'). The decision to use the ETS technique depends on the available anatomy, optimal configuration, and minimizing vessel mismatch. Due to the variability in the anatomy of the veins, but the relatively consistent anatomy of the IJV, this technique is of critical importance to the head and neck microvascular surgeon. The following is a suggested protocol for ETS anastomosis preparation:

1. Donor vein preparation
   a. Same protocol as ETE recipient vein preparation, with some key adaptations
2. Recipient vein (IJV) preparation
   a. Macrovascular preparation
   - Dissection, mobilization of IJV, and selection of venotomy site
   - Clamping of IJV
   b. Microvascular preparation
   - Adventitia dissection
   - Venotomy and flushing
   - Lumen inspection and final adventitia dissection

Donor vein preparation

For ETS anastomosis, preparation of the donor vein is performed first, then the clamp is released while preparation of the IJV is performed for the ETS anastomosis. This ensures minimal clamping of both the donor vein and the IJV. The aim of the ETS preparation is to have the donor vein entering the recipient vein (IJV) at a maximum 30–70 degree angle at the correct position on the IJV in a three-dimensional plane.

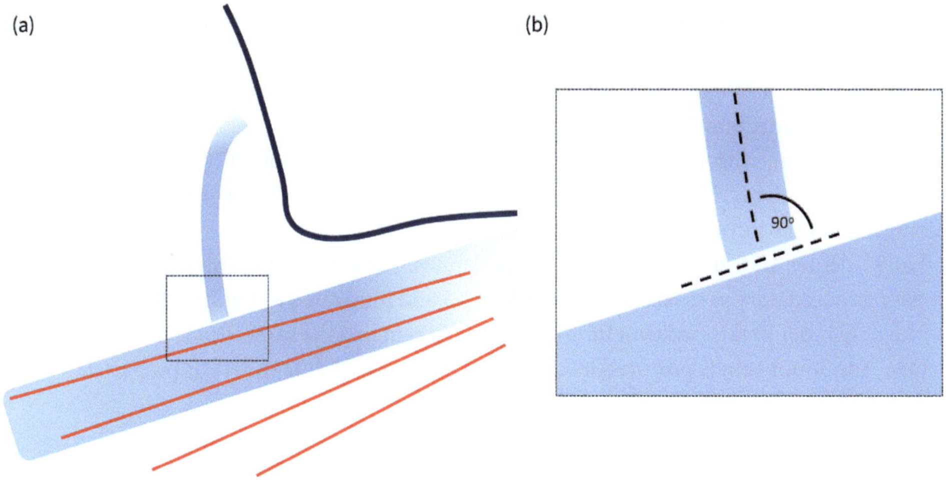

Figure 6.5.2 Straight donor vein venotomy, depending on the entry angle into IJV. a. The orientation and the length of the venous pedicle favour a direct 90-degree entry to the IJV (end-to-side anastomosis). b. Anastomosis site magnified to demonstrate the straight venotomy, tangent to the axis of the donor vein.

When the donor vein is prepared, the protocol for ETS is performed. The venotomy can be performed, either at a tangent plane (90 degrees to the vessel axis straight clean cut) to the axis of the vessel (Figure 6.5.2), or a bevelled cut is performed (Figure 6.5.3), in a similar way to when an angled cut is performed to increase the vessel diameter is a mismatch case.

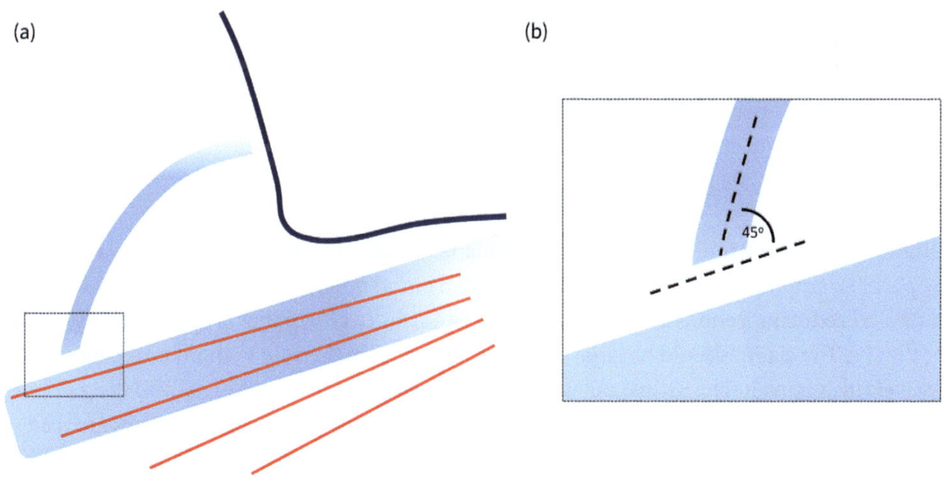

Figure 6.5.3 Bevelled donor vein venotomy. a. The orientation and the length of the venous pedicle, forming a gentle curve, favour an angled entry to the IJV (end-to-side anastomosis). b. Anastomosis site magnified to demonstrate the bevelled, almost 45-degree venotomy of the donor vein. A 90-degree angle of anastomosis in a configuration like this could predispose to kinking of the venous anastomosis, resulting in flow obstruction and thrombosis. It is always important to check the need for pedicle suspension as discussed in Chapter 10.3.

Angled venotomy (Figure 6.5.3) on donor vein depends on the intended orientation of the pedicle and how the operator designs the final configuration of the venous connection. Occasionally an abrupt 90° connection may predispose to kinking of the anastomosis hence an angulated connection maybe preferred

The angulation, with the peak inferiorly, will reduce any abrupt 90° degree turns in the vein as it enters the ETS anastomosis, maintaining roughly a 30–70-degree entry and optimizing blood flow through the anastomosis.

For 90-degree ETS anastomoses and if the flap vein is at risk of kinking then pedicle suspension is mandatory as discussed in Chapter 10.3 and illustrated in Figure 10.3.2.

The remainder of this protocol for the donor vein remains the same.

Once the donor vein is prepared its clamp can be released while the IJV is prepared.

Recipient vein preparation

Dissection, mobilization of IJV, selection of venotomy site

The entire 360 degrees around the IJV needs to be meticulously dissected and mobilized to allow the placement of the clamp. This should be performed superiorly and inferiorly the planned ETS entry point to allow clamp placement.

With the donor vein already prepared, the position for the venotomy and its entry point in the recipient vein should be determined. The tributaries of the IJV all enter along an imaginary line, from superior to inferior on its anteromedial surface. The donor vein should therefore enter into the IJV along this imaginary line.

The operator needs to 'visualize' the intended configuration of the veins after the completion of the anastomosis and try to recapitulate this image from his imagination to reality.

Ensuring the length of the donor vein is passive, but under enough tension to avoid kinking of the vessel with head and neck movement, the optimum angulation of how the donor vein enters the IJV needs to be carefully determined.

When the position is selected, a small dot can be placed in the approximate position using a surgical marker pen onto the dried IJV. Once the position has been determined, the surgeon can move on to clamping of the IJV.

Clamping of IJV

Although there are a multitude of clamps available, a Satinsky clamp (see Chapter 1) allows the partial clamping of the IJV, allowing controlled blood flow, preventing distal vein thrombosis, and reducing venous congestion. Choose a Satinsky clamp that is appropriately sized for the IJV. The clamp should be large enough to encompass the vein without crushing or excessively distorting it. The Satinsky clamp will be placed proximally and distally to the marked site of the ETS entry point. The Satinsky clamp is then partially opened, so the jaws are ready to engage the vessel without excessive force. Position the clamp so that one jaw is placed behind the IJV and the other jaw is in front, encircling the vessel. The clamp should be oriented such that it will partially occlude the IJV longitudinally, leaving the opposite side of the vein free from occlusion. Gently close the clamp to partially occlude the IJV. The clamp's design allows for partial occlusion, meaning that blood flow is maintained through the unclamped portion of the vein, reducing the risk of distal congestion and allowing venous return. Be cautious not to apply excessive pressure, which could cause vessel damage or complete occlusion. It is then essential to ensure the clamp is securely in place and stable. The clamp should not slip or rotate, as this could cause unintentional vessel damage or disrupt the remainder of the anastomosis. When the clamp is secured, it can occasionally be beneficial to place a sterile tonsil swab below the anteromedial aspect of the IJV. This procedure helps rotate the medial aspect of the IJV away from the patient. This often gives better visualization of the venotomy site and subsequent suturing.

Microvascular preparation

Adventitia dissection

Adventitia dissection is performed in a similar manner to that described earlier, with removal of the loose perivascular tissue, followed by the more adherent adventitia. Again, this should only be prepared over the area required for venotomy and subsequent suture placement. Achieving the correct balance of adventitia removal, to maintaining as much as possible for its physiological role, is of critical importance to a successful anastomosis. It is advisable to remove the adventitia for twice the diameter as the entry donor vein. This should achieve the correct balance.

Venotomy and flushing

With the IJV clamped, the next critical stage is to perform the venotomy as the planned entry site of the donor vein. There are several techniques to perform this:

Incision with micro scissors (this is the preferred technique by the authors): This is performed by gently grasping the adventitia at the point the venotomy will be performed with straight jeweller's forceps. Using straight microvascular scissors, two cuts 180 degrees to each other are made, at 45 degrees to the vessel wall in a 'V' shaped pattern. The aim should be to make the diameter approximately 50% larger than the donor vein diameter. It is key to perform this in two clean cuts to achieve straight edges on the venotomy. Using sharp micro scissors is essential. This is the preferred method by the authors, as the microscissors allow excellent control over the venotomy size and shape. Some surgeons prefer to place an 8-0 suture into the venotomy site and use this to lift the vein wall prior to performing the cuts in the method described.

Straight No.11 blade: The No. 11 blade, which has a sharp, pointed tip, is used to make a small puncture or nick in the vein at the desired venotomy site. The incision is often started by gently stabbing the vessel with the point of the blade. The blade is then carefully drawn along the length of the vessel to extend the venotomy. This is usually done in a single, smooth motion to ensure a clean cut. The sharpness of the No. 11 blade allows for a clean, sharp incision, which can be ideal for anastomosis. There is however a risk of making the incision too long or deep, which can complicate the anastomosis or cause excessive bleeding.

30 G needle: A 30-gauge (30 G) needle is used to puncture the vein at the chosen site. The puncture is usually made at the edge of where the venotomy will be. The initial puncture can be gently extended by carefully dilating the vein with fine forceps or by inserting micro scissors into the puncture and cutting to create the desired venotomy. The fine needle causes minimal trauma to the vessel wall, reducing the risk of complications such as thrombosis. The small puncture size allows for careful control over the venotomy size and can be gradually extended as needed. This can be of benefit it smaller donor vein diameters where precise control is needed. The disadvantages however are that the puncture itself is small, so the incision often needs to be manually extended using additional tools like microscissors, which can be time-consuming.

Punch biopsy tool: A punch biopsy tool is used to create a round or oval hole in the IJV. The tool is pressed against the vein at the desired venotomy site, and a circular or oval section of the vessel wall is removed in one motion. A paper by Chung et al. explains this technique in detail, suggesting a more efficient venotomy of consistent size and a uniformly circular edge (Chung et al. in 'Further reading').

Whichever technique is chosen, it is essential to aim for the correct size venotomy, with minimal trauma to the surrounding tissue, with clean cut edges, with the venotomy being at least 60% larger than the diameter of the donor vein. Once the venotomy has been performed, the IJV is copious flushed with heparinized saline to avoid any stagnant blood and clot formation. The size of the venotomy should be checked against the donor vein, and any last dilation can be performed at this point.

Lumen check and final adventitia dissection

In a similar manner to described earlier in the chapter, the lumen of the venotomy is checked for its overall health for ETS anastomosis. Any final adventitia should be removed; however, if the pre-venotomy adventitia is dissected correctly, and the venotomy performed with perfect technique, no further adventitia dissection should be required.

At this point, the donor and recipient veins are perfectly prepared for the suturing process. The donor vein should be clamped appropriately, proximally to allow mobilization, and no interference with the suturing process. The donor vein should be irrigated thoroughly with heparinized saline after clamp placement to remove any stagnant blood. The vessels are now fully prepared for an ETS anastomosis.

The key steps in preparing the IJV for ETS anastomosis are summarized in Box 6.5.1.

Box 6.5.1 Sequence of recipient vein preparation (end-to-side)

A. Microvascular preparation
   - i. Dissection, mobilization of IJV, and selection of venotomy site
   - ii. Clamping of IJV

B. Microvascular preparation
   - i. Adventitia dissection
   - ii. Venotomy and flushing
   - iii. Lumen inspection and final adventitia dissection

Further reading

Ahmadi I, Herle P, Miller G, Hunter-Smith D, Leong J, Rozen W. End-to-end versus end-to-side microvascular anastomosis: a meta-analysis of free flap outcomes. *J Reconstr Microsurg* 2017;33(06):402–11.

Christianto S, Lau A, Li KY, Yang WF, Su YX. One versus two venous anastomoses in microsurgical head and neck reconstruction: a cumulative meta-analysis. *Int J Oral Maxillofac Surg* 2018;47(5):585–94.

Chung J-H, *et al.* Use of a biopsy punch for end-to-side anastomosis in free-tissue transfer. *J Plast Surg Hand Surg* 2020;54(4):215–19.

da Silva Correia AG, Alves JN, da Mota Santos SA, Guerra DR, Garção DC. Anatomical variations in the relationship between the spinal accessory nerve and internal jugular vein: a systematic review and meta-analysis. *Int J Oral Maxillofac Surg* 2023;52(1):13–18.

Dalip D, Iwanaga J, Loukas M, Oskouian RJ, Tubbs RS. Review of the variations of the superficial veins of the neck. *Cureus* 2018;10(6):e2826.

Dediol E, Uglesic V, Knezevic P, Milenovic A. Single versus double venous microvascular anastomoses. *Plast Reconstr Surg* 2011;127(6):2513.

Deslaugiers B, *et al.* Contribution to the study of the tributaries and the termination of the external jugular vein. *Surg Radiol Anat* 1994;16(2):173–7.

Dornseifer U, *et al.* Less is more? Impact of single venous anastomosis on the intrinsic transit time of free flaps. *J Reconstr Microsurg* 2017;33(2):137–42.

Hedayat F, Lauder JJ, Kyzas P, Vassiliou LV. Internal jugular vein duplication: clinical significance for head and neck cancer ablative and reconstructive surgery. *J Surg Case Rep* 2021;2021(7):rjab300.

Honda K, Omori K, Kishimoto Y. Anatomical variations in the superficial venous system of the neck: an image-based study using contrast-enhanced computed tomography. *Surg Radiol Anat* 2024;46(5):669–77.

Lohman R, Siemionow M, Lister G. Advantages of sharp adventitial dissection for microvascular anastomoses. *Ann Plast Surg* 1998;40(6):577–85.

Mumtaz S, Singh M. Surgical review of the anatomical variations of the internal jugular vein: an update for head and neck surgeons. *Ann R Coll Surg Engl* 2019;101(1):2–6.

Prandoni P. Is there a link between venous and arterial thrombosis? A reappraisal. *Intern Emerg Med* 2020;15(1):33–6.

Rusu MC, Tudose RC, Vrapciu AD, Toader C, Popescu ŞA. Anatomical variations of the external jugular vein: a pictorial and critical review. *Medicina (B Aires)* 2023;59(3):622.

Singh R. Variations of venous drainage of the thyroid gland and their surgical implications: a narrative review. *J Vasc Bras* 2023;22:e20220163.

Siwetz M, *et al.* The course and variation of the facial vein in the face—known and unknown facts: an anatomical study. *Medicina (B Aires)* 2023;59(8):1479.

Yin S-C, *et al.* Comparison of internal jugular vein system anastomosis and external jugular vein system anastomosis in free flaps for head and neck reconstruction: a meta-analysis. *J Oral Maxillofac Surg* 2020;78(1):142–52.

7
Pedicle orientation and vessel preparation

Leandros Vassilios F. Vassiliou, Panayiotis Kyzas, and Nicholas Kalavrezos

7.1 Pedicle orientation and marking prior to detaching the flap

Introduction

Small changes in the laminal blood flow can cause turbulence and trigger the coagulation cascade. A twist of the vascular pedicle can be catastrophic, and this is often one of the main reasons of technical failure identified during flap-salvage exploratory procedures. The vein is more susceptible to twisting due to its thin-walled structure. Subsequent flow changes can quickly lead to thrombosis.

The artery isn't immune to pedicle twisting; this can cause vasospasm and/or increased resistance through the contorted segment, turbulent or reduced arterial flow, and eventually arterial thrombosis.

Pedicle management is absolutely crucial for the survival of the reconstruction. Most flap failures, when the problem is not due to technical anastomotic pitfalls, are attributed to pedicle positioning issues, such as torsion (twist) in the neck or withing the tunnel, or acute angles (kinking).

Pedicle management starts before the operation by careful **pedicle exit planning.** At the time of the operation, pedicle management requires **pedicle marking** on the donor site prior to flap detachment, meticulous **tunnel creation** in the recipient site, careful gentle **pedicle passage** through the tunnel and precise **pedicle orientation** prior to the anastomosis. The microvascular surgeon must plan the position and orientation of the vascular pedicle in such a way that avoids any possibility of flow disturbances in any of the vessels.

This subchapter elaborates on the four out of five principal steps of the aforementioned pedicle management:

- Pedicle exit planning
- Pedicle marking
- Tunnel creation
- Pedicle passage through the tunnel
- Pedicle orientation.

The last step, 'pedicle orientation', is also the first step in preparation of the microvascular anastomosis and is described further in Chapter 8.

Pedicle exit planning

Although this topic has been discussed in Chapter 2, the decision as to where the pedicle will emerge after the flap inset directly correlates with its orientation.

For example, having a long pedicle from a composite flap with different components (i.e. chimeric scapula) emerging posteriorly (at the angle), while aiming to use the facial artery as the donor artery, dictates that the pedicle should loop in a rather acute and risky fashion.

Similarly, when a fibula free flap is used to reconstruct defects that reach high at the ramus of the mandible, one should avoid having the vascular pedicle emerging from that area, as the angle will be too acute and the risk of thrombosis high.

We next outline a few 'generic' examples of preferred pedicle exit (emergence) to facilitate a safer orientation. The list is not exhaustive, but the principles remain the same. One should consider **the pedicle length and its expected course of travel to the recipient vessels (i.e. loop or not), in the most favourable configuration:**

1. Chimeric scapula tip—latissimus dorsi for mandibular reconstruction (harvested from the contralateral side): Pedicle emerges anteriorly.
2. Composite deep circumflex iliac artery (DCIA) for mandibular reconstruction (harvested from the ipsilateral side): Pedicle emerges posteriorly (at the angle).
3. Composite DCIA for mandibular reconstruction (harvested from the contralateral side): Pedicle emerges anteriorly—beware of the length constraints!
4. Composite fibula free flap for hemimandible reconstruction up to the sigmoid notch (harvested from the ipsilateral side): pedicle emerges anteriorly.
5. RFFF for hemi-glossectomy (harvested from either side): pedicle emerges posteriorly and forms a large U-shape loop. In case of anterior emergence, the neck pedicle loop will be gentler, **BUT** the angle of the pedicle when it meets the intraoral flap is far too acute; we recommend avoiding it.

Pedicle marking prior to flap detachment

This can be achieved by respecting the passive, natural and 'relaxed' position of any blood vessel at its donor side. As such, it is imperative that the flap and vascular pedicle is left to settle in this passive position in the donor area prior to detaching. The surgeon aims to replicate this orientation by recording the position of the vascular pedicle.

A simple, cost-efficient, and quick way of ensuring pedicle orientation is marking the surface of the pedicle with methylene blue dye immediately (see Ardehali et al. in 'Further reading') prior to detaching the flap (Figure 7.1.1). This should be done after meticulous haemostasis in a very dry surgical field. Small, well-defined dots are placed along the course of the pedicle with emphasis on marking both the artery and the vein in a clear and easily identifiable fashion. The marking (dots) indicates *the superior aspect of the pedicle in its donor side*; this doesn't necessarily mean that the dots will appear upwards in the neck (see next).

This simple and quick technique provides an accurate reference point of the appropriate and twist-proof spatial orientation of the pedicle.

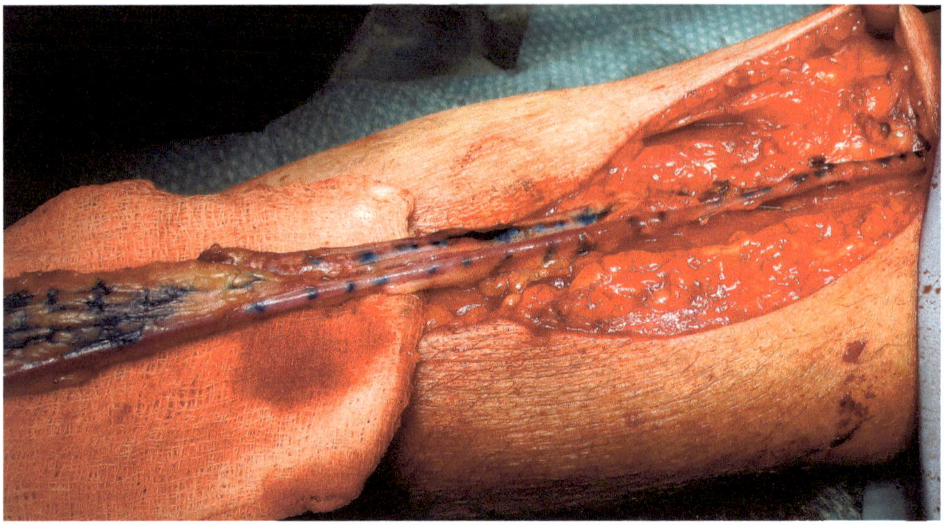

Figure 7.1.1 The length of the pedicle is dotted with methylene blue dye prior to detachment. This reduces the risk of twisting the pedicle during flap inset.

Special care is given when the flap has two or more venous systems or, crucially, when these venous drainage systems join to form a common drainage tributary (Figure 7.1.2). The orientation of these might be different at different levels of the pedicle at the donor side; this should be carefully addressed and recorded to ensure no twist in the recipient side.

Once marking is done, the expected flap and pedicle orientation ***on the recipient side*** is noted. A soft tissue flap used to reconstruct a floor of the mouth defect will have a different pedicle orientation than when the same flap is used to reconstruct a posterior maxillectomy defect or a buccal mucosa defect. The marking dots might appear up, down, medial, or lateral,

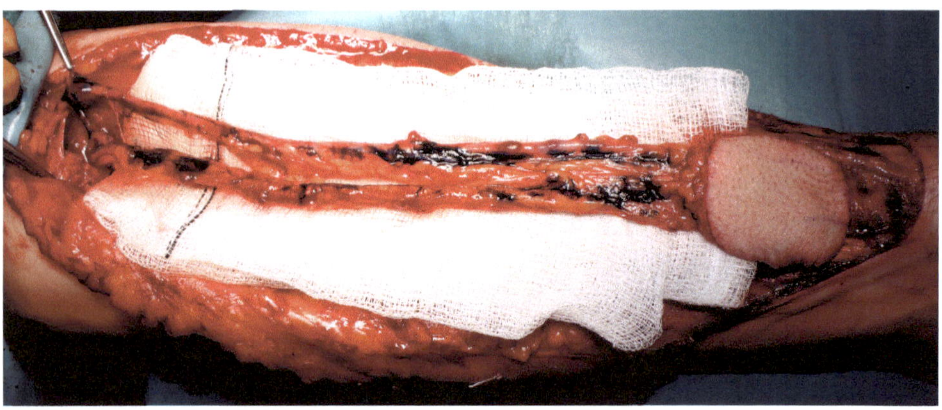

Figure 7.1.2 Special care is given when two or more venous drainage systems join together to form common tributaries. In these cases, the orientation might change; this needs to be recorded carefully. The case illustrates a radial forearm free flap vascular pedicle; the cephalic vein joins with the conjoint venae-comitantes (VC) tributary to form a common drainage pathway.

and these combinations depend on the defect and the side of the neck that is used for the microvascular anastomosis. These are easy to predict and confirm intraoperatively, but they require careful preoperative planning and intraoperative confirmation prior to flap detachment. Similar to the flap design, the pedicle orientation must be rehearsed in the surgeons' planning sessions.

The methylene blue dye should be allowed to fully dry prior to manipulating the flap or detaching the vascular pedicle. Otherwise, the dye might spread, dilute with blood, and tissue fluids and stain the pedicle in a messy, unrecognizable fashion. This can be counterproductive. Should this occur, the vascular pedicle is washed with copious amounts of heparinized saline, and the marking/orientation process starts again.

The importance of pedicle orientation is even more obvious in composite and chimeric flaps. The volume and the weight of the flap can act as a twisting factor and the different components can act as lever points for twist. This is common when one harvests chimeric flaps from the scapular system. The soft tissue component might be based on the thoracodorsal vessel as a myocutaneous latissimus dorsi flap or as a thoracodorsal artery perforator (TDAP); the bone component can be based on the angular branch (scapula tip). Often, when bone length is needed, both scapula vascular pedicles need to be utilized (circumflex scapular and angular branch). In this case, there are several potential twisting points, and this can be exacerbated if a bone osteotomy is performed. Therefore, additional orientation techniques can be utilized in these cases. The methylene blue marking is meticulously done; it can be extremely difficult as the surgical field is blood-stained due to the oozing from the bone and muscle cut-ends. The surgeon can use anchoring points at the pedicle bifurcation areas to ensure appropriate orientation. This can be done with a perpendicular piece of background material that is sutured at the adipose tissue of the pedicle in those points. The background material is removed after the flap is inset in the recipient side.

Tunnel creation

The vast majority, if not all, of head and neck reconstructive cases involve a tunnel through which the flap pedicle transits into the neck, for the donor vessels to meet the recipient ones.

Geometry

For oral and facial reconstructive procedures, one crucial aspect of the tunnel is the rigid bony mandible.

Most tunnels have conceptually four walls. For example, a tunnel for the reconstruction of a unilateral floor of the mouth and ventral tongue defect has the following four walls:

Anterior: Lingual aspect of mandible symphysis
Medial: Tongue intrinsic and extrinsic musculature (hyoglossus, genioglossus)
Lateral: Lingual aspect of the mandible body
Posterior: Posterolateral floor of the mouth

Intraoral reconstructions (tongue, floor of mouth, inner cheek, and palate) most often require the flap pedicle to pass medially to the mandible (**inner mandible side**), whereas in extraoral (face) defects, the pedicle can pass laterally to the mandible (**outer mandible side**).

Length

Tunnels vary in length (floor of mouth, tongue, mandibular reconstructions require relatively short tunnels, whereas maxillary and upper face defects result in long tunnels), and tissue laxity (floor of mouth, tongue, maxillary reconstructions involve a bony tunnel wall due to the mandible).

Specifications

In order to facilitate good flap blood flow, the tunnel must be:

- Spacious
- Straight

Space

The tunnel needs to allow passive passage of the pedicle with no constriction. The tunnel needs to have space not for the pedicle to pass passively and freely when not perfused and deflated, but also when the flap is anastomosed and fully running, allowing for vessel expansion and degree of reperfusion injury and surgical oedema.

A minimum of four finger spaces is the standard requirement. For maxillary, palatal, and midface defects this may require additional to the ablation cuts, mucosal incisions, and relieving incisions through muscle layers to create space.

Straight configuration

A good tunnel is the tunnel that allows the pedicle to pass through in a completely straight and passive course with no bends, no curves, no complex course.

Any of the above may cause kinking of the pedicle with impact on the blood flow and may risk turbulence, compression, or constriction and ultimately ischaemia (arterial failure), or congestion (venous failure)

The surgeon must visualize the configuration of the tunnel and remove any obstacle that stands in the course of the flap pedicle.

A typical example is the mylohyoid muscle. This muscle sits as a sling between the inner mandible and the hyoid bone and extends posteriorly till its free edge at the posterior molar area. An anterior floor of mouth or tongue T1/T2 resection may not require resection of the mylohyoid, and a conservative surgeon may choose to preserve this muscle. Coming to reconstruction next, when the flap is inset in the anterior floor of mouth, the pedicle may form a loop posteriorly, curving over the posterior free edge of the mylohyoid prior and exiting with anterior direction prior to forming a second loop for it vessels to reach the facial (recipient) artery (Figure 7.1.3a). This configuration may risk substandard flow and flap ischaemia or congestion. This highlights the importance of the tunnel configuration being 'straight' as it is far more preferable that the mylohyoid muscle is divided during the tunnel formation to

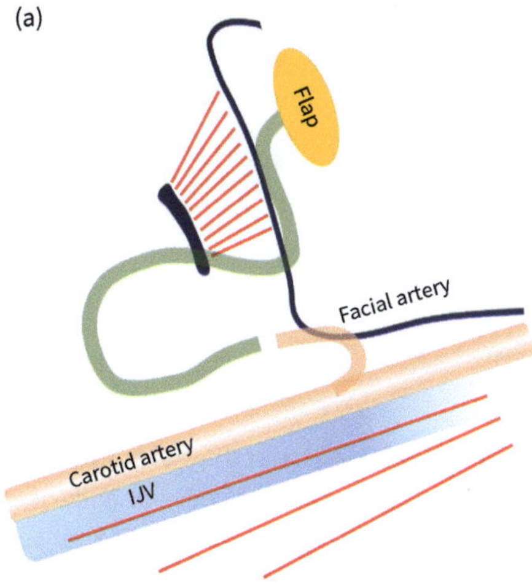

Figure 7.1.3 Division of the mylohyoid muscle to facilitate an unhindered pedicle course. a. Schematic presentation showing a free flap (yellow) reconstructing an anterior floor of mouth defect, in the presence of intact mylohyoid muscle (top red stripes). The flap pedicle (green) has to bend around the bend of the mylohyoid free edge (posteriorly) and again form a lazy 'S' curve prior to reaching the free stump of the recipient facial artery (pale orange). This acute bend around the mylohyoid can predispose to reasons for flap failure. b. Division of the mylohyoid muscle allows the pedicle (green) to pass directly caudally through the tunnel into the neck in a straight configuration, maximizing optimum flow with no acute bends, kinks, or areas of constriction or turbulence.

avoid this scenario (Figure 7.1.3b). Division of the mylohyoid allows the pedicle to directly drop into the neck with so 'S' bends, no kinking, no complicated course.

Tunnel and passing the flap through

When passing the flap through the tunnel and prior to the inset, it is important that the flap is passed from the neck and through the tunnel to the defect site, as opposed to placing the flap in the defect and pulling the pedicle through the tunnel!

This manoeuvre is crucial, as pulling the pedicle through the tunnel will cause twisting or stretching with a detrimental effect on the anastomosis and the survival of the flap.

The suggested technique is to pass from the defect and through the tunnel into the neck a long pair of forceps (Spencer-Wells, or Fraser-Kelly) and grasp a point of the flap (muscle or subcutaneous fat) with its tips. Once the flap is held by the forceps, it is pushed gently through the tunnel towards the defect with the forceps holding hand extremely lightly pulling it. During the passage of the flap through the tunnel, the pedicle needs to be constantly visualized, and extra care needs to be taken to avoid twisting or stretching the pedicle (Figure 7.1.4).

It is important to emphasize here that the passage of the flap through the tunnel is facilitated mainly by PUSHING it gently through, rather than PULLING it. The latter may

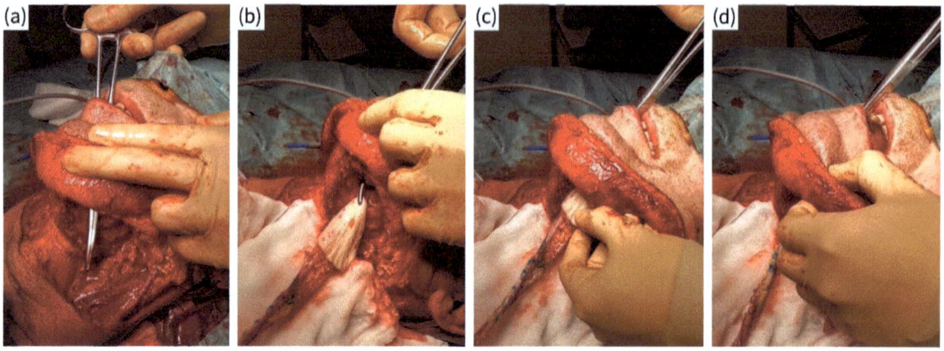

Figure 7.1.4 Technique of passing the flap through the tunnel. a. Anterior floor of mouth defect about to be reconstructed with an RFFF. Note the ipsilateral mylohyoid and anterior belly of digastric muscles have been divided to allow unhindered flap and pedicle passage. A Spenser-Wells forceps is passed through the defect and tunnels into the neck and held with the surgeon's right hand. b. The flap is laid on a heparinized saline-soaked gauge with the pedicle orientation markings clearly visible. The area of the flap that will reconstruct the medial part of the defect is grasped with the tips of the Spencer-Wells forceps to facilitate transition through the tunnel. c. The surgeon's left hand is gently guiding the flap through the tunnel while attention is kept on the pedicle markings. The process continues slowly and carefully with focus not to twist the pedicle as the flap moves towards the defect. d. Passing the flap through the defect is mainly performed by pushing the flap with the left hand through the tunnel and less by pulling it with the forceps-holding hand. The opposite can damage the flap's microcirculation or even avulse the skin paddle.

introduce shear forces between the skin and the underlying microvascular supply bed, or even worse, in heavy-handed surgeons, complete avulsion of the skin paddle, especially in composite or perforator-based flaps.

The manoeuvre must be executed slowly, gently, with extreme caution and care and only after confirmation that the tunnel is of adequate width to allow the bulk of the flap to traverse through it.

Attention must be given to the dotted points on the pedicle (Figure 7.1.1). The dotted surface (side) of the pedicle must remain unchanged and any for any suspicion of twisting the flap is better removed and the manoeuvre repeated, until it is established that the pedicle withing the tunnel rests comfortably without pressure, twisting, stretching, or kinking.

If for any reason the surgeon has even the most minute doubt, or suspicion that the pedicle encountered a twist or stretch during the passage through the tunnel, it is imperative that the process is repeated again until the surgeon is fully satisfied with the 'feeling' of the pedicle through the tunnel, its passivity, and the lack of any torsion as evident by the pedicle markings.

It is far better to repeat this step as many times as required in order to secure a safe pedicle, than rushing through this crucial stage of the operation, only to compromise completely the final result afterwards.

Important highlights of this subchapter are summarized in Box 7.1.1.

Box 7.1.1 Important recommendations regarding pedicle marking, orientation, and passage through the tunnel

- It is important to mark with methanol blue the course of the pedicle prior to detachment of the flap.
- For the anterior floor of the mouth, ventral, and alveolar defects, it is important during the creation of the tunnel to divide the mylohyoid muscle in order to avoid acute pedicle bends and kinking.
- The flap has to pass from the neck towards the defect through a very careful and meticulous technique. The markings along the pedicle help avoid any twisting in the tunnel.
- Passage of the pedicle through the tunnel is crucial for the survival of the flap. Complex flap failures often relate to mistakes at this stage of the operation (see Chapters 13.3 and 14.3).

7.2 **Adventitia dissection and arteriotomy**

Introduction

Vessel preparation and, specifically for this chapter, artery preparation is of uttermost importance for a successful anastomosis.

The microsurgeon needs to develop in their practice a standardized, reproducible, and efficient sequence in preparing both arteries (recipient and donor) for the anastomosis.

As the flap pedicle artery is given as *de facto* we propose the preparation starts with the recipient artery first, as any potential problems (atherosclerosis, poor vessel flow, etc.) can be identified early prompting additional preparation or even selection of an alternative vessel without causing anxiety for the ischaemia time.

Proposed sequence

In our experience, the following sequence is practical, logical, and ensures economy of time and as minimal vessel handling as possible:

1. Recipient artery (flow/pressure check performed prior to committing to vessel preparation):
   a. Perivascular tissue excision and ligation of side branches
   b. Adventitia dissection
   c. Arteriotomy and dilation
   d. Lumen inspection (flow/pressure check can be confirmed at this point)
   e. Fine adventitia dissection
   f. Orientation marking
2. Donor artery:
   a. Vessel separation: artery from veins
   b. Adventitia dissection

c. Arteriotomy and dilation
d. Lumen inspection
e. Fine adventitia dissection
f. Orientation marking

In this chapter, a more detailed description follows on the technical aspects of the aforementioned steps.

It is important for the operator to remember that each of these steps needs to be performed in a 'balanced' and controlled manner.

Vessel overpreparation can be worse than underpreparation

Blood vessel structure

The arterial wall structure can be divided into three discrete layers starting from outside:

- Adventitia (tunica adventitia, tunica externa)
- Media (tunica media)
- Intima (tunica intima, tunica interna)

The adventitia is known to be the external layer of blood vessels. This outermost layer of the vessel wall is also referred to as *tunica adventitia* or *tunica externa*. Its main histological composition is of collagen (type I) and lasting fibres. Within this connective tissue there are nerves (nervi vasorum) that control the smooth muscle tone and carry sympathetic fibres as well as a well-developed network of blood vessels (vasa vasorum) that nourish the main vessel. This outer perivascular tissue is connected with the surrounding connective tissue stroma and is often surrounded and invested by adipose tissue.

From a histological and cytological point of view the adventitia is important biological functional layer of the vessel as it significantly controls retrieval, integration, storage, and release of key molecular regulators. Cellular types consist of fibrous immunomodulatory cells, stem cells, endothelial cells, pericytes, and adrenergic nerves.

The media is the predominant layer of the arterial vascular wall. It consists mainly of smooth muscle and elastic fibres and actively regulates the blood flow and pressure through the vessel by vasoconstriction or vasodilation, respectively, causing narrowing or widening of the vessel diameter. Technically perfect approximation of the arterial media layers is key for a successful anastomosis. Fine—gentle and atraumatic—handling of the vessel aims to avoid stimulation of vasospasm that may threaten the result of the anastomosis.

The intima is composed of endothelial membrane and subendothelial connective tissue. This layer is highly active metabolically and plays important role in controlling blood flow, and coagulation as well as regulating the media and causing changes in the vessel diameter. Safeguarding the integrity of this layer is crucial for a successful anastomosis as any microsurgical trauma, tear, or surface imperfection during suturing may trigger the coagulation cascade, leading to thrombosis and failure.

Many arteries of the calibre often used for anastomosis have an internal elastic membrane that connects the intima to the underlying media. This layer can often become fibrotic or calcified in patients with previous radiotherapy or atherosclerosis. Extra care must be given in such cases as described before, as the intima is prone to separation (dissection) from the underlying media layer (see Chapter 7.3).

Recipient artery

The recipient artery of choice must have been identified during the neck dissection and vessel harvest stage of the operation and an artery flow check (perfusion check) must have been performed. This is to minimize the chance of any surprises and the need to look for and prepare another artery, while flap ischaemia time is clocking.

The following are a list of minimum requirements performed prior to 'microscope time':

- Elimination of anatomical constrictions and mobilization of the vessel. This refers to any overlapping muscle or connective tissue fibres that pose risk of compression of the anastomosis. For the facial artery, the posterior belly of the digastric and the stylohyoid muscle need to be divided to free up the vessel from any constrictions.
- Separation of the recipient artery from accompanying vessels (Figure 7.2.1).
- Ligation of side branches.
- Flow/pressure check. This is described next.

Recipient artery flow/pressure check

No flap can perfuse and survive, unless the blood flow from the donor vessel is satisfactory and constant. This needs to be ascertained prior to detaching the free flap from the donor side.

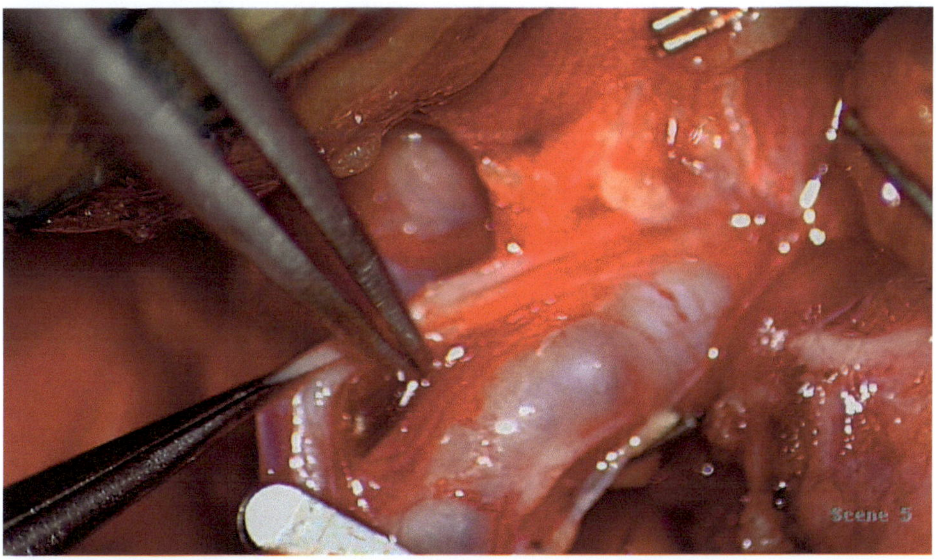

Figure 7.2.1 Preparation of the recipient artery. The microscope photograph demonstrates the gentle separation of collateral blood vessels that follow the main facial artery trunk. It is recommended that these vessels be ligated with two Liga clips at the base, a reasonable 1 cm of clean vessel (artery) is the goal to allow seamless handling for anastomosis.

Before committing to vessel preparation the blood flow has to be assessed. Once the recipient vessel is dissected out, a 3A microvascular clamp is placed proximally and the vessel is cut. The clamp is released, and the flow is checked (Figure 7.2.2); if the flow is satisfactory, the mean arterial pressure at that point is recorded. If the flow is not adequate (as it often happens due to vasospasm as a result of the dissection manipulations), then the anaesthetic team is asked to increase the blood pressure and papaverine is applied (see earlier). This usually resolves the issue within 5–10 minutes, and the flow is rechecked. If at that point, the flow remains unsatisfactory, an alternative donor vessel needs to be sought.

We need to emphasize here that the mean arterial pressure (MAP) at which there was satisfactory donor arterial flow, MUST be the minimum MAP prior to releasing the clamp to restore flap perfusion after completion of the arterial suturing. It is our practice to inform the anaesthetist 5 minutes before completion of suturing (usually 2–3 last stitches) so that there is adequate time to restore the MAP at the desired level.

Composite flaps are dependent on the blood pressure more so than soft tissue only flaps. In our practice, we have noticed that soft tissue flaps perfuse adequately with a MAP around 70 mmHg, whereas composite flaps require MAP closer to 80 mmHg. This of course varies in individual patients.

The vessel most commonly used in head and neck (H&N) microsurgery is the facial artery (see Chapter 5). This artery is favourably located close to the ablation side, allowing for the pedicles of most flaps to reach it. It has a calibre (2.5–3 mm) that is an almost perfect match

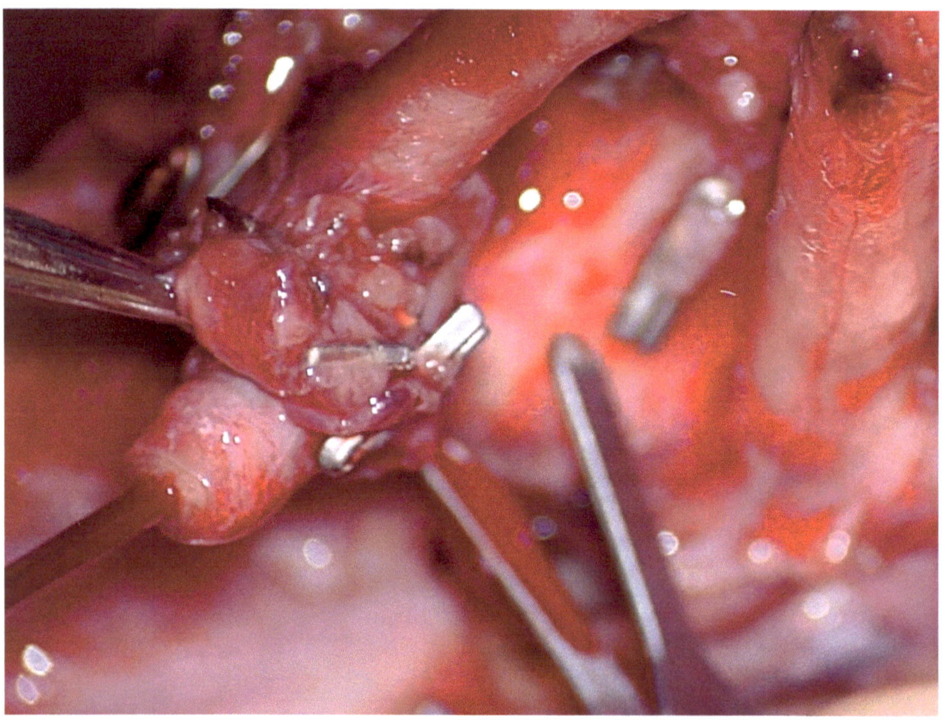

Figure 7.2.2 Transient release of the microvascular clamp (3A) demonstrates a good jet of blood flow, indicative of good perfusion power for the free flap.

to the diameter of most recipient flap arteries. Most importantly, its diameter varies, from its origin on the external carotid artery towards its upward course to the face. This allows the microsurgeon to choose which part of the artery will use, in order to achieve the closest possible match. We often use the first 2 cm of the vessel at its origin on the external carotid. At that point, the facial artery runs deep to the posterior belly of the digastric muscle; this has to be divided to allow good access, and to avoid untoward pressure to the arterial anastomosis side.

The superior thyroid artery and the external carotid artery are also good candidates for donor vessels, but these options are reserved for cases when the facial artery cannot be used (e.g. when it has to be resected very close to the external carotid as part of the ablative procedure).

If all these have not been performed prior to microscope time, then they can be achieved using magnification loupes only, as these do not require magnification and in fact attempting to perform those under the microscope risks prolonging time in the expense of flap ischaemia.

Adventitia dissection

Adventitia dissection refers mainly to the removal of all the perivascular loose connective tissue that surrounds the main vascular stem.

Stripping the adventitia from the donor and recipient arteries serves two purposes.

- First and foremost, when adventitia tissue is impinged at the suture lines, it acts as a thrombogenic factor. It allows an easier, cleaner, and more meticulous suturing during the anastomosis and makes life easier during this stressful task.
- Secondly, it protects the anastomosis in several ways: It avoids the anastomosis catching in surrounding structures (liga clips) or twisting on its own weight.

Histological studies on the effects of microvascular surgery and adventitia preparation on the actual vessel wall have demonstrated that what is termed as 'adventitia dissection' does not effectively remove the whole adventitia, but the vast majority of loose connective tissue that may impede the anastomosis.

Technique

In the process of adventitia dissection, the rule is that the MV surgeon should strip and prepare only what's needed; nothing more and nothing less.

Vessel overpreparation can have worse implications than underpreparation.

Some surgeons peel the adventitia away bluntly, whereas others trim the adventitia sharply with scissors.

There is substantial evidence that sharp dissection reduces the risk of arterial thrombosis (see Lohman et al. in 'Further reading'); this is what we practice and recommend.

Moreover, as the adventitia tissue is composed of connective tissue that contains fibrous bands and septations, pulling this around the vessel may introduce areas of fibrous band ring-like constrictions that run circumferentially and may 'strangulate' the artery later on (Figure 7.2.3).

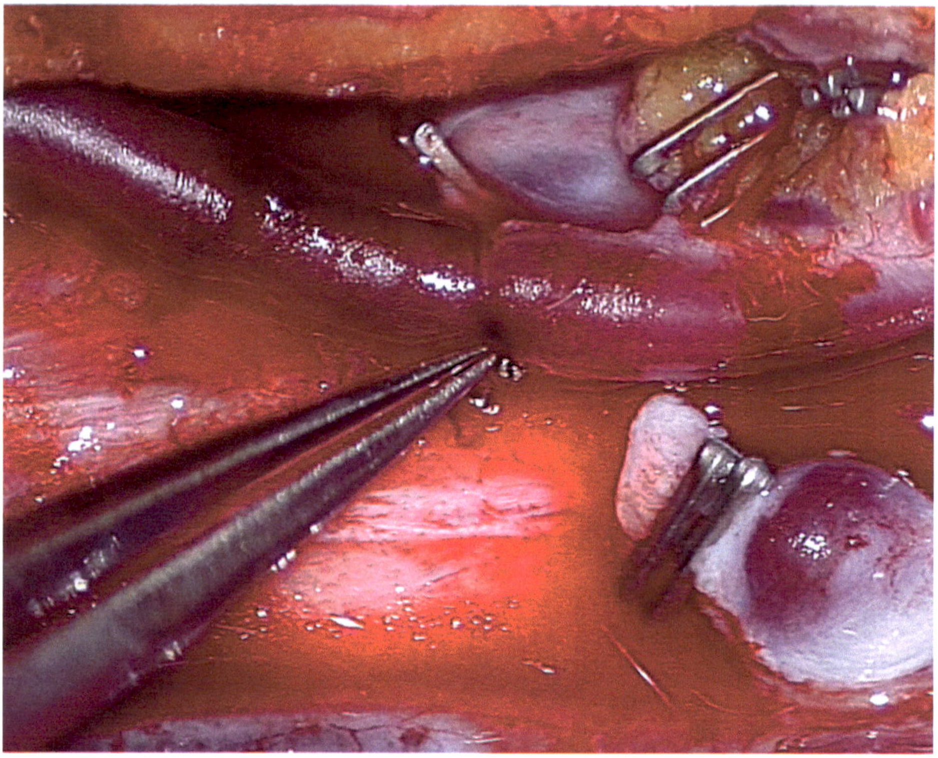

Figure 7.2.3 Post-artery anastomosis constriction band. The figure demonstrates the flap artery post anastomosis. The artery is running, however, during the adventitia prep, instead of sharp dissection, pulling of tissue was performed. That resulted in the pulling of tight constricting bands that may affect the intraluminal blood flow. The recommended technique for adventitia preparation is sharp dissection.

The adventitia layer can be crudely separated into i. loose perivascular connective tissue, and ii. more adherent adventitia layer.

a. Perivascular loose tissue excision and ligation of side branches
b. Finer adventitia dissection

Perivascular loose tissue excision

The suture line and the last couple of millimetres of the arterial ends must be clean of adventitia; we are very particular and meticulous about it.

In vessels with quite rich perivascular and adventitia tissue it is appropriate to pull the adventitia gently alongside the long axis of the vessel and start trimming it by sharp dissection (Figure 7.2.4). The adventitia looks woolly and fluffy and there is always a degree of transparency, and this is not comprised of solid tissue. Further final dissection can proceed using the triangulation technique.

Sharp dissection is fairly easy to do, provided the surgeon and assistant understand the principle of 'triangulation' and can coordinate their moves.

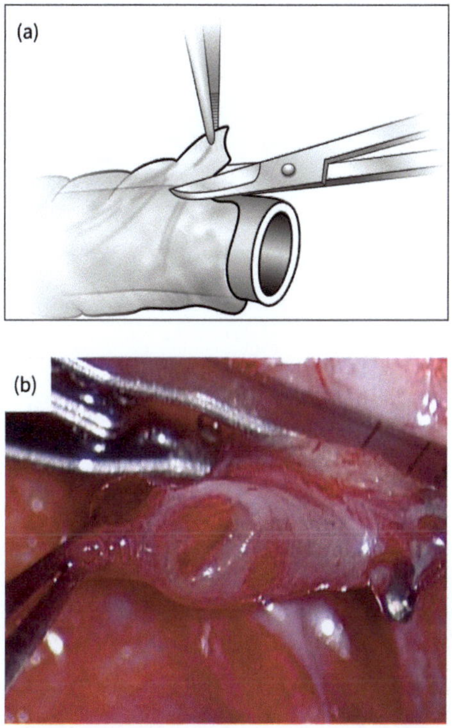

Figure 7.2.4 a. Schematic illustration of crude perivascular removal. b. Microscope photograph that demonstrates the loose perivascular tissue removal. This could be a quick step, especially with the triangulation technique prior to fine adventitia dissection, dilation, and final trimming of the adventitia as described in this chapter.

The assistant picks and tents up the adventitia from two points while the surgeon completes the triangle with the jeweller's forceps held in one hand, while sharp dissecting with curved micro scissors with the other hand. With a combination of dissecting and a gentle push, the artery is slowly rolled over (Figure 7.2.5) and cleaned in a 360-degree way for the desired length, the same way as unfolding a paper roll.

In addition, having a bit of adventitia not far off the anastomosis, allows the assistant to support and turn the vessel during suturing, without manipulating the arterial muscular wall.

Underprepared adventitia

Microleaks, especially when the arterial clamp is released, can initiate external microthrombi on the suture line, which in turn can propagate, resulting in arterial thrombosis with catastrophic consequences.

Overprepared adventitia

At the same time, we discourage overpreparing and overstripping adventitia from a large proportion of the vessels. This is due to the fact that the adventitia is a very important layer of the arterial wall, with well-established functions that must not be disturbed.

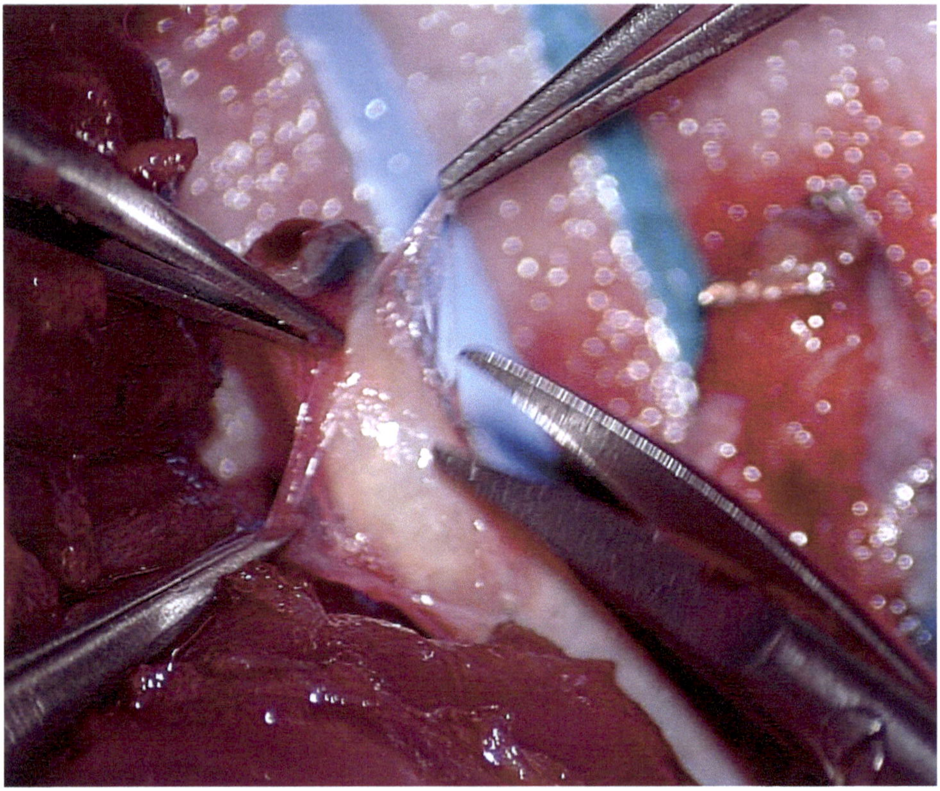

Figure 7.2.5 Fine adventitia dissection using the triangulation and rolling technique.

Arteriotomy

Following dissection of the adventitia as described earlier, it is time for the arteriotomy.

This is a crucial step as it will define the arterial vessel edge that will be available for the anastomosis. That sets the platform for the vascular anastomosis.

The aim is that the vessel ends are clean, the vascular wall layers are all intact, the vessel lumen under the microscope perfect, and that there is enough vascular length stump to manipulate and mobilize the vessel as required during suturing.

Prior to the arteriotomy, a careful inspection of the vessel end takes place, and the most optimum site is selected.

Avoid making the arteriotomy close to ligaclips or side branches, and leave as much as length as possible for the vascular clamp and for adequate mobilization.

Once the site of the arteriotomy has been selected the main operator stabilizes the recipient artery, holding it with the jeweller's forceps by gripping the adventitia only, a few millimetres close to the arteriotomy site. In order to full stabilize the vessel, the assistant holds the vascular ends (Figure 7.2.6a).

As these may have minimum adventitia due to preparation, it is not going to cause harm if the assistant holds the vessel end with a full thickness grip. The vascular end that the assistant

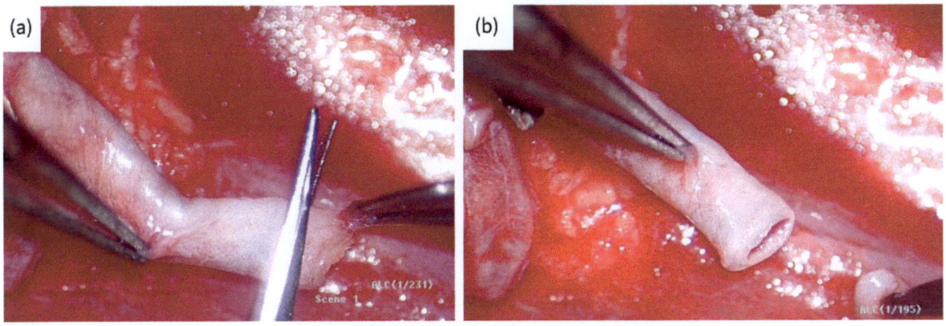

Figure 7.2.6 Arteriotomy. a. Note the stabilization of the artery between the two forceps. The edge of the vessel is held by the assistant in a direction that allows the main operator to perform a straight cut perpendicular to the axis of the vessel. The instruction has to be sharp, the cut has to be straight, clean, and direct. b. The artery post-arteriotomy. Note the clean cut demonstrating an even vessel edge wall.

holds is going to be discarded regardless. It is crucial that the vessel is adequately mobilized in order to avoid the arteriotomy cut slipping away its target.

Once the vessel is stabilized the operator makes the cut using sub iris scissors. It is important that the scissors are sharpened, otherwise if their jaws accidentally (chew) the vessel end that may damage the vascular walls with a detrimental effect for the anastomosis.

It is important that the arteriotomy is achieved with one single, clean, decisive cut (Figure 7.2.6b). The cut has to be completely perpendicular to the vascular axis, unless calibre mismatch indicates a bevelled incision.

A bevelled incision may lead to formation of a kink in the anastomosis changing the orientation of the arterial flow.

The arteriotomy has to achieve a full thickness vessel wall cut that transects evenly all the layers. Once the arteriotomy is performed the arterial lumen is irrigated and an inspection is performed.

The key points of optimum arteriotomy are summarized in Box 7.2.1.

As described in Chapter 7.4 dilation further takes place and a more careful inspection of the intima is performed prior to orientation and commencement of the anastomosis.

The whole sequence of adventitia dissection and arteriotomy as described in this subchapter is demonstrated in Figure 7.2.7. and summarized in Box 7.2.2.

Box. 7.2.1 Key parameters for optimum arteriotomy

- Choice of site—not close to ligaclips or side branches
- Leave length for vascular clamp
- Stabilization of the vessel
- Firm grip of the vessel end
- Sharp, straight iris scissors that will not ‘chew’ the vessel end
- Perpendicular to the vessel axis
- One single clean decisive cut
- Full thickness cut—all layers transected evenly
- Lumen inspection dilation

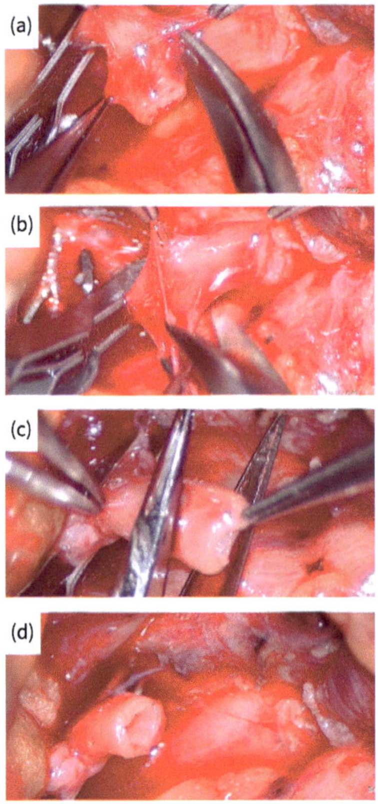

Figure 7.2.7 The representation of the whole sequence (key steps) in the adventitia section and arteriotomy. a. Triangulation technique for adventitia dissection. b. Further adventitia dissection releases a good length of clean vessel for preparation for anastomosis. c. Note the stabilization of the vessel. The assistant holds the vessel edge, and the main operator performs a clean perpendicular to the muscle axis. d. The artery post-arteriotomy shows a clean vessel edge.

Box 7.2.2 Proposed sequence for recipient artery preparation

1. Recipient artery (flow/pressure check performed prior to committing to vessel preparation):
   a. Perivascular tissue excision and ligation of side branches
   b. Adventitia dissection
   c. Arteriotomy and dilation
   d. Lumen inspection and flow/pressure check
   e. Final adventitia dissection
   f. Orientation and marking
2. Donor artery:
   a. Vessel separation: Artery from veins
   b. Adventitia dissection
   c. Arteriotomy and dilation
   d. Lumen inspection
   e. Fine adventitia dissection
   f. Orientation marking

7.3 Control of atheroma/intima condition

Introduction

Microvascular surgery for patients with head and neck cancer poses significant surgical challenges not found in other patients requiring free tissue transfer. The high incidence of smoking and alcohol abuse in this patients' population, alongside old age, diabetes, and peripheral vascular disease, results in poor vessel quality. The clear, pristine vessel lumen, without atheromatic plagues that is often found in young healthy patients (i.e. female patients undergoing post-mastectomy reconstruction) is a rarity in the head and neck (H&N) cancer population. Surgeons often have to deal with vessels full of atheromatic plagues often in an unpredictable cobblestone fashion.

The potential catastrophic effect of atheromas in microcirculation is well known. This becomes even more pronounced if the atheromatic plague is disturbed, broken or manipulated in a careless/reckless way.

Key considerations in patients with vascular disease

We have therefore adopted a trail of thinking and a technique to minimize the deleterious effect of atheromatic plaques in arterial microvascular anastomosis.

Flap selection

We pay special attention to known or potential peripheral vascular disease when we decide what flap to utilize for reconstruction. Old age, diabetes, and hypertension guide our planning thought process centrally (closer to the heart) and away from the periphery. We would, for example, opt for a scapula free flap instead of a fibula, irrespective of three-vessel run off, purely because of vessel quality.

Recipient vessel

The facial artery is the vessel of choice in most instances. We have noticed that the closer one gets to the external carotid artery (ECA), the cleaner the lumen; the atheromatic plaques are less frequent. We therefore focus our vessel dissection and preparation to the 2 cm of facial artery as it originates from the ECA. That avoids extensive vessel manipulation, saves time in not dissecting the torturous intra-gland part of the vessel and results in a wider vessel calibre and easier suturing.

Despite these precautions, there is always a chance that some atheroma might still be present (Figure 7.3.1). In that case, it is crucial not to dilate the vessel extensively, and certainly avoid dilating directly on the atheromatic plaque. Minimizing handling is key to avoiding plaque disturbance and microemboli.

Care should also be taken when positioning/repositioning the vascular micro clamp. A pair of sharp, straight scissors is essential to ensure a clear final cut at the mouth of the vessel.

Donor (flap) vessel

It is paramount to check for vessel quality during flap harvesting. If the quality of the vessel is doubtful, and atheromatic plagues are obvious throughout the course, it might be prudent

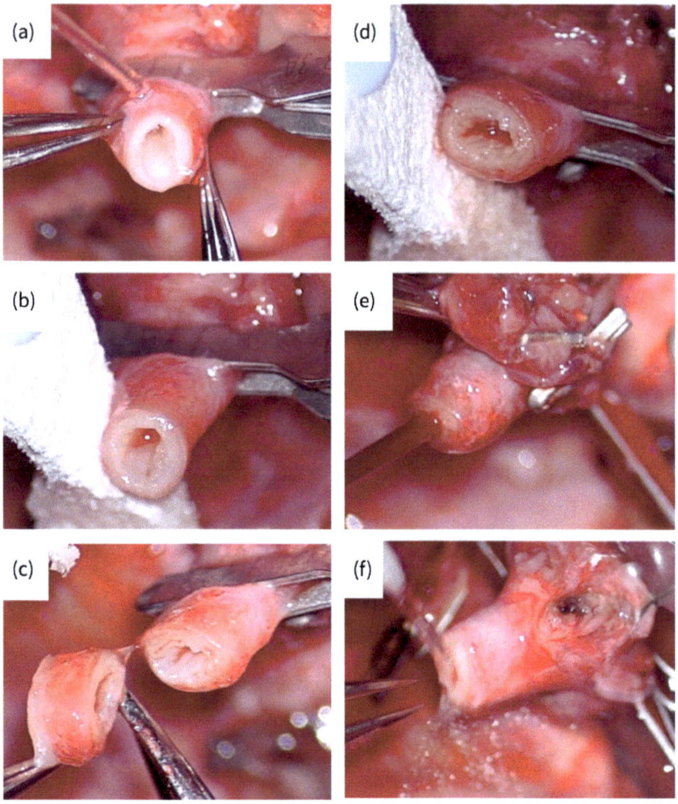

Figure 7.3.1 Vessel with atherosclerotic disease. a. The vessel after the arteriotomy. Careful inspection of the lumen demonstrates an intraluminal plaque (fluffy structure). b. Careful use of an arrow demonstrates the presence of atheromatous plaque the vessel edge. c. Further proximal arteriotomy onto an area of the vessel without any atheromas at the vessel edge. Note the fibrotic appearance of the intima, which is one of the very common features in atherosclerotic disease. d. Inspection of the lumen after the careful use of an arrow shows the absence of atheromatous plaques. e. Transient release of the vascular clamp confirms good power of blood flow, a sign of suitability for flap perfusion. f. The vessel is washed, and the preparation starts for the anastomosis.

to abandon the flap and consider alternatives. Appropriate pre-op planning often avoids this untoward situation. During vessel preparation of the recipient artery under the microscope, the same principles as those of the donor vessel apply. If pedicle length is ensured, the surgeon should persist in identifying an artery part of adequate length that is free of atheromatic plaques for the anastomosis. Gentle loop and reduced pedicle manipulation are important.

Suturing

Suturing of atherosclerotic vessels is difficult as it risks disrupting the plaque. This risk can be reduced when the needle passes from the lumen outwards; the opposite can be catastrophic. This increases the technical difficulty of the case and often requires vessel repositioning by the assistant. Minimizing the number of sutures is also important. The rule is that the less you handle atheromas the least the chance of problems.

Box 7.3.1 Preparation of atherosclerotic vessels

- It is preferable to avoid the presence of atheromas at the site of the anastomosis. In globally atherosclerotic vessels if there is no other option then minimal handling is required.
- In atherosclerotic vessels, avoid dilation as this may break the atheroma and also may predispose to intima dissection.
- Atherosclerotic vessels need extremely gentle handling and suturing from inside the lumen out in order to 'splint' the intima to the underlying wall rather than separating the vessel wall layers.

Microsurgical technique in atherosclerotic vessels

In addition to the potential problems from atheromas, there is a second intraluminal arterial threat that surgeons must be aware. This refers to the intima separation/dissection (Figure 7.3.1) of the donor artery and requires particular attention. Free-floating or torn intima is extremely thrombogenic and is a well-recognized cause of arterial thrombosis and failure. It results either from indigenous vessel weakness (i.e. due to age) or (more frequently) due to manipulation, use of blunt scissors and in atherosclerotic vessels passage of the needle in an out-in fashion and applies shear forces to the delicate intima.

It is imperative to ensure instruments are well maintained and vessel handling is gentle.

Should intima separation/dissection occur, one should cut the recipient artery back, close to its origin from the ECA. However, this doesn't always solve the issue and the surgeons must deal with the problem during suturing.

The technique modification is simple to comprehend but technically difficult to achieve: The suture must pass from the lumen outwards (intima-to-adventitia) aiming to 'pin' and secure the intima to the underlying media layer, avoiding tears. This might require a slightly bigger suture bite (in width) than normal, and it needs to be balanced out appropriately on the recipient vessel.

Suture numbers must follow the atheroma guidance—as few as possible. Any tears or loose intima within the lumen must not be accepted; in this case, the anastomosis must be revised if possible. If this isn't achievable (i.e. due to remaining vessel length), then an alternative donor vessel must be sought.

Important highlights in the preparation of atherosclerotic vessels are summarized in Box 7.3.1.

7.4 **Dilation and flushing**

Introduction

Dilating the artery is a very important step in the context of vessel preparation but is also fraught with danger. It helps consolidating the vessel wall layers and redefining the vessel edge rendering it easier for microvascular suturing and causes some degree of transient smooth muscle paralysis preventing early post-anastomotic vasospasm.

It has to be done with care and elegance, in the appropriate timing, and should not be repeated constantly. The aim is to help the artery return to its original shape and lumen diameter; this would inevitably have been reduced due to vasospasm occurring during vessel preparation.

Technique

Dilation is done with a vessel dilator (see Chapter 1.4). The vessel is immobilized held by its adventitia, with the operator's left hand holding jeweller's forceps and the instrument is inserted into the arterial lumen so that the tips are fully inside the vessel.

Insertion must be in a direction parallel to the vessel axis (Figure 7.4.1). Although the dilator's tips are blunt, care must be given to avoid injuring the extremely delicate intima with the dilator tips during the insertion.

Once in the dilator is then allowed to spring out, controlling the expanding force with a combination of observation and tactile sensation. This requires fine fingertip control of the instrument. It is very important to keep in mind that uncontrolled release of the dilator tips can overstretch the vessel. Overdilation or overstretching can tear thin-walled vessels or

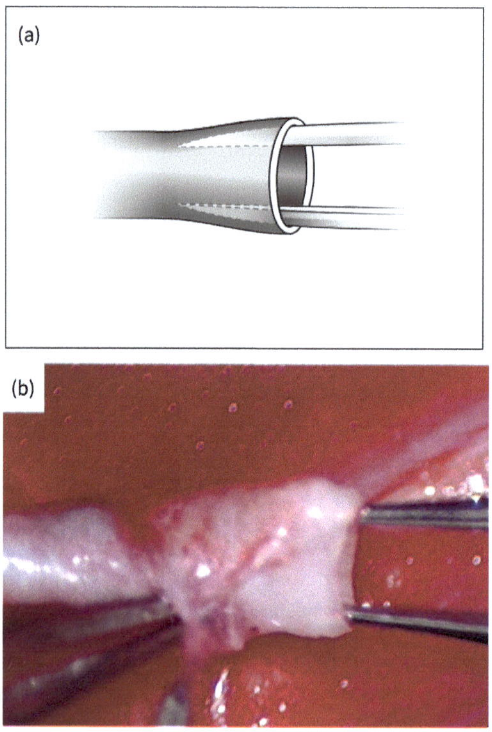

Figure 7.4.1 a. Schematic representation of insertion of the dilator tips inside the vessel lumen and careful release (opening) of the dilator tips to stretch the vessel wall. b. Microscope photograph showing the assistant immobilizing the vessel and the tips of the dilator inserted into the vascular lumen.

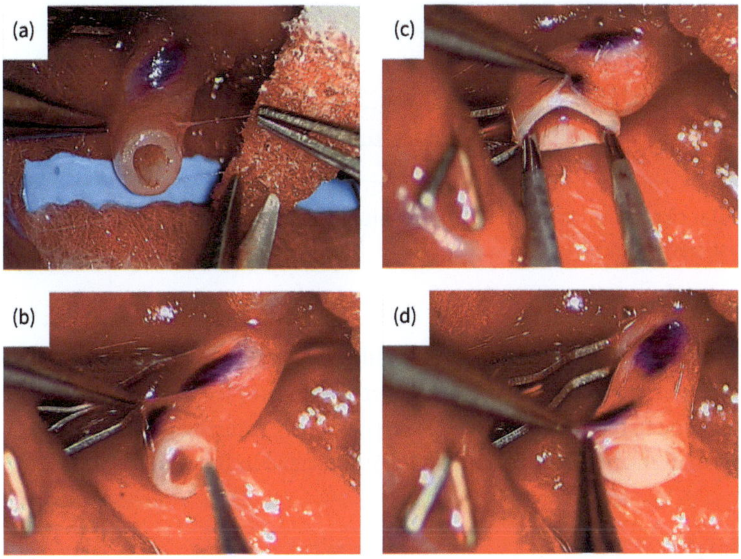

Figure 7.4.2 Artery dilation following arteriotomy and lumen inspection. a. The artery immediately after the arteriotomy. Note the clean vascular edges. An arrow tip has been used to drain the vessel to allow inspection of the intima condition. b. The vessel is prepared for dilation after blood flow check. c. Dilation of the vessel. Note the reconfiguration of the vessel wall and the increase in the dimension of the vascular lumen. d. Following final dilation, fine adventitia trimming is performed as the last step prior to microvascular suturing.

cause intima dissection in atherosclerotic vessels with detrimental effects on the outcome of the anastomosis.

The dilator stays open, stretching the vessel's lumen for 1–2 seconds and then carefully closed and slid out. This is repeated one or two times until a visible change in the vessel's edge morphology is evident.

Dilation is done in two directions, horizontally and vertically (180 degrees apart), so that the round shape of the arterial lumen is restored.

For the recipient artery, this is close to the end of the vessel preparation; however, most often following dilation, some fine adventitia trimming for perfection might be required (Figure 7.4.2). Once performed the artery is washed, dried with an arrow, and left to rest until suturing begins.

For the donor vessel, dilation is done just before the thorough and copious flushing of the flap with heparinized saline. This allows easy insertion of a cannula inside the artery to facilitate washout/flushing (Figure 7.4.3). Following that, the microsurgeon proceeds with the final preparation of the recipient vessel edge and considers a final dilation prior to commence suturing.

Vessels with atheromatic plaques pose a risk during dilation (see Chapter 7.4); touching and/or manipulating the plaque might lead to breakdown or microemboli. For that reason, we strongly recommend avoiding dilation at the part of the lumen that has atheromas, and minimal/gentle dilation for the rest of the vessel lumen. The ideal scenario would be to identify a segment of the vessels without plaques (see earlier—atheromas), but we appreciated that this is not always possible.

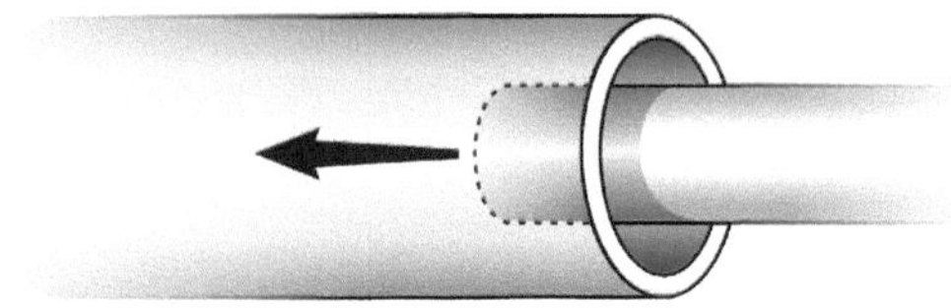

Figure 7.4.3 Flushing of the pedicle artery with heparinized saline in order to clear the flap microvascular circulation from any stagnant blood that can precipitate microemboli and compromise perfusion.

Lastly, in the case of intima separation, dilation must be done in a gentle way and in all areas of the vessel where the intima has started to separate (see Chapter 7.4). This gentle touch allows the intima to rest on the muscular layer, making suturing it and securing it easier.

Key information about vessel dilation is summarized in Box 7.4.1.

Papaverine

Papaverine is an opium alkaloid antispasmodic drug, used primarily in the treatment of visceral spasm and vasospasm (especially those involving the intestines, heart, or brain), and occasionally in the treatment of erectile dysfunction. Like other antispasmodic drugs (i.e. verapamil) it has been used in microsurgery for decades. Its pharmacological effects cause vasodilation, which in turn allows perfusion of the flap, especially at the critical time of ischaemia reversion. We advocate the use of papaverine during the following steps of free flap microsurgery:

1. After completion of free flap and pedicle dissection, and while the flap is allowed to rest and re-perfuse, still attached to its blood supply. This causes hyperdynamic flap circulation, 'supercharging' the flap, prior to detaching it, and ischaemia clock is set. We normally let the flap rest for 20–30 min prior to detach; in some cases (i.e. deep circumflex iliac artery (DCIA) flaps) this time is even longer.
2. Prior to begin donor artery preparation, so that we can safely check the arterial flow of the donor vessel.

Box 7.4.1 Important tips for vessel dilation

- Correct dilation is key for a successful anastomosis. Never underestimate the importance of appropriate vessel dilation. The vessel dilation has to be performed in all directions of the vessel lumen in order to equally expand the vessel walls.
- An artery prior to dilation is usually crumpled and deformed. After successful dilation the arterial walls open up and thin up and the artery has the appropriate form for anastomosis.
- The dilation relaxes the smooth muscle and eliminates post-anastomotic spasm that could predispose to obstruction and thrombosis.

3. Prior to tightening the last suture on the arterial anastomosis (see Chapter 8), we flush the arterial lumen with papaverine. This helps identifying any potential anastomotic leak points, but crucially, it allows the blood flow to carry papaverine into the flap microcirculation, and to cause vasodilation even to the smallest arteries of the flap, hence helping perfusion. We found this to be of extreme importance in composite flaps and in cases of flap exploration and salvage.

It is important to note that, like any other medication, the use of papaverine has to be cautious and not exaggerated. Papaverine (or any other medication) will not save a flap that has unresolved technical issues (i.e. anastomosis suturing, pedicle orientation, etc.). There are also publications suggesting that excessive use of papaverine can cause dryness to the vessels or even cause a chemical burn; it has, therefore, to be used with due care.

Pedicle flushing with heparinized saline

Flushing the vascular pedicle with heparinized saline is one of the most important steps of free-flap microsurgery.

Other agents have been used in the literature, such as urokinase in the past or agratroban (thrombin inhibitor) for specific patients with heparin-induced thrombocytopenia (HIT).

Blood clots, microemboli, and free radicals due to ischaemia are major threats to the microcirculation of the flap. Mechanical washout, aided by the thrombolytic medicinal effect of heparin, helps to clear the microcirculation of the flap from these unwanted elements. The use of heparinized saline in vascular surgery goes back many decades, with an abundance of literature to support its use (see Further Reading). However, there are salient points that need to be looked at when it comes to microsurgery, mainly due to the size of the vessels used.

Following completion of the preparation and dilation of the recipient vessel, a cannula is carefully inserted into the lumen of the donor (flap) artery (Figure 7.4.4). For most flaps, a pink (20 gauge) cannula is the size of choice; however, pedicles with narrow arteries (i.e. lateral arm flap, DCIA flap) might require a smaller blue (22 gauge) cannula. After insertion, the microsurgeon gently holds the artery with his fingers, while the assistant is supporting the vein.

Mimicking the normal blood pressure rhythm, the microsurgeon is then flushing the flap. Significant resistance at this point indicates pedicle twist or compression of the pedicle in the tunnel.

A total volume of 20–40 ml of heparinized saline are usually enough for soft tissue flaps; we advocate the use of 60–80 ml for composite flaps.

The microsurgical team is satisfied when the flushing pressure is low and uninterrupted, when no arterial leaks are seen on the pedicle (if there are any, now is the time to ligate these side branches) and when clear heparinized saline comes through the flap vein.

At that point, the orientation of the pedicle is reconfirmed, another marking dot is placed close to the edge of the artery and micro suturing can commence.

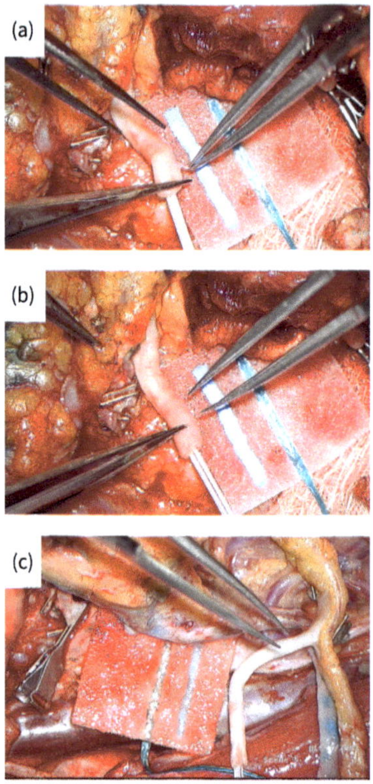

Figure 7.4.4 Flushing of the pedicle. a. The edge of the artery is carefully held by jeweller's forceps and the tip of the cannula is gently inserted. b. The vessel is held by the jeweller's, and the tip of the cannula is slowly advanced. It is important at this stage to try and maintain the artery straight in order to allow atraumatic insertion of the cannula inside the lumen. c. The flushing of the pedicle has started, and clear saline flows out from the draining veins.

7.5 **Separation of artery from vein(s) (flap pedicle)**

Introduction

This part of vessel preparation depends on the type of flap, the length of the pedicle and the recipient vessels. This step (Figure 7.5.1) is performed with sharp dissection and the triangulation technique as described next.

The length of separation of the artery from the veins depends on the distance between the recipient artery and the recipient vein.

Technique

The general principle is that dissection should be minimal BUT to the extent that allows passive and secure orientation of the venous and the arterial component of the pedicle.

Pedicle vessel separation is important, and the extent of it is dictated by the location and the distance apart between the recipient artery and the recipient vein. For example, if the

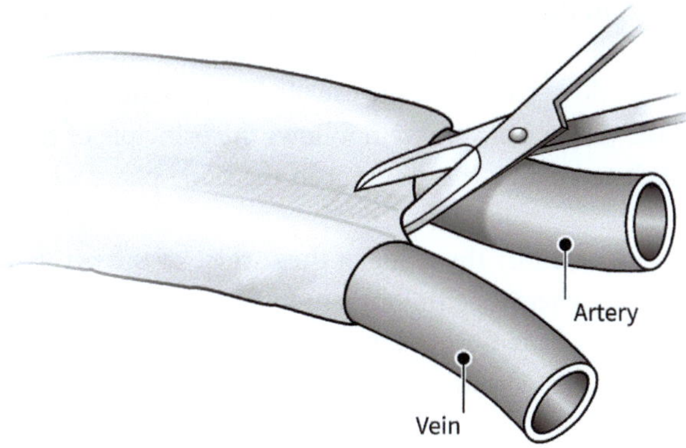

Figure 7.5.1 Schematic presentation of sub-dissection in the perivascular tissue (sheath) to separate the pedicle artery from the accompanying vein.

recipient artery is the facial artery and the recipient vein is the external jugular vein quite low in the neck, then the pedicle vessels have to be separated at a relatively extensive length in order to allow the artery to join the facial artery and the vein to anastomose with the external jugular vein low in the neck without tension on the pedicle.

Particular care must be given to flaps that have a VC (vena-comitans) system (radial, fibula, ALT) as these tend to have several interconnecting branches which need to be dissected and ligated with caution.

In most flaps the artery is accompanied by two main VCs that have numerous interconnecting venous tributaries and connecting vessels to the artery. More specifically, different flaps have different structures:

- Radial forearm free flap: the venae-comitantes of the radial artery form many interconnections and have many side branches connecting the venous system with the radial artery. Flap pedicle vessel preparation has to be meticulous and thorough.
- Latissimus dorsi: the thoracodorsal artery has usually only has a single accompanying vein with relatively few interconnecting vessels. The artery and the vein are connected with very loose connective tissue and the separation of the artery from the vein is quite quick and easy.
- Fibular free flap: the peroneal artery has two accompanying VCs that are quite voluminous with many interconnecting veins usually the separation of the artery of the vein can be quite laborious with the need for many divisions of side branches and interconnecting veins.

If the artery can be separated from the two joint VCs, that can reduce the effort of separation. In ideal circumstances, choose a recipient vein sited close to the recipient artery so the extent of separation of the artery from the vein should not be too long.

- DCIA—the deep circumplex artery has a few interconnecting branches with a single accompanying vein. The preparation has to be meticulous with extremely fine handling of the vein. The vein is extremely thin walled and easy to injure, and any mistake will not be forgiven in these extremely delicate vessels.

Separating the artery from the vein(s) follows the principles of meticulous dissection using the triangulation method, as described earlier. Any side branch identified MUST be controlled with liga clips; we do not advocate the use of bipolar diathermy.

The dissection of the artery from the vein follows the principle of triangulation. It is important that the pedicle is held by the assistant in the same plane within the same level of depth of focus.

The main operator will identify the plane of the surface of the perivascular sheath in the 'underbelly' of the pedicle, where the minimum number of interconnecting vessels cross over (Figure 7.5.2). This plane is quite fibrous but correct identification will allow a longitudinal cut through, like unzipping the sheath, that will offer an initial good inspection of the whole artery (Box 7.5.1).

The main surgeon holds the jeweller's forceps with the left hand to pick and pull the pedicle in order to stabilize it while with the right hand controls the micro-scissors to cut through the connective tissue that holds the vessels together.

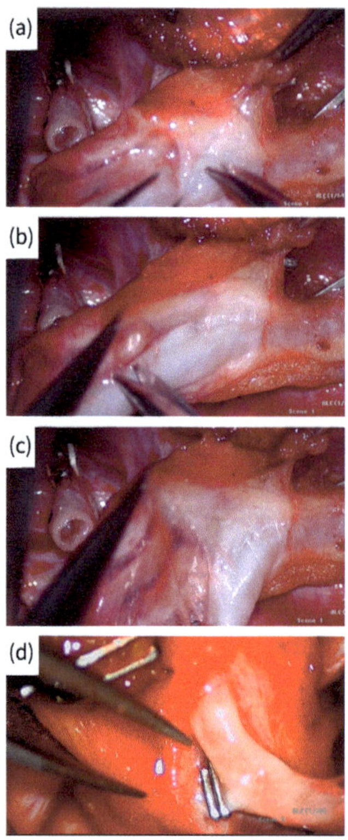

Figure 7.5.2 a. Separation of the radial artery from the accompanying venae-comitantes (VCs). The vascular plane ('underbelly') of the pedicle has been identified. This is the (narrow) corridor where the least risk of damaging the VCs and the least amount of interconnecting veins between the VCs exist. Following that plane in that narrow corridor avoids inadvertent injury to the vessels. b. Careful opening of the perivascular sheath continues alongside the radial artery. c. With the triangulation technique, the assistant tends the perivascular tissue open to allow easier further dissection and recognition, preparation, and separation of any arterial branches. d. Arterial side branch identified, dissection, and ligated with two Liga clips.

Box 7.5.1 Important tip in microvascular dissection of flap pedicle

Every pedicle and especially pedicles with two VCs has usually at its back (belly) an avascular plane where an incision can be easily and longitudinally propagated in order to separate the artery from the vein.

The assistant's role is crucial in this stage as it is important to 'foresee' where the next dissection move is going to be and pull the tissues with one forceps (jeweller's) to stretch the pedicle straight and stabilize it and with the other to provide countertraction in order to pull the tissue in such a way that will produce a 'see-through' view and clear identification of any side branches.

When a side branch is found, the team of two stop the LOGITUDINAL dissection and focuses on its obliteration. Again, the assistant with one hand offers traction and with the other either chooses to assist in the blunt dissection around the vascular branch or pulls the main artery to provide a gentle stretch and LENGTH for the main operator to place TWO micro-ligaclips prior to taking the micro-scissors and dividing the vessel. The 2× micro-ligaclips are placed on the arterial side—and we recommend TWO for safety (Figure 7.5.3), while the venous side will not require ligation. The venous side, due to its low-flow nature, will spontaneously close and not cause any bleeding.

Further dissection proceeds circumferentially with identification of any side branches or interconnecting venous tributaries.

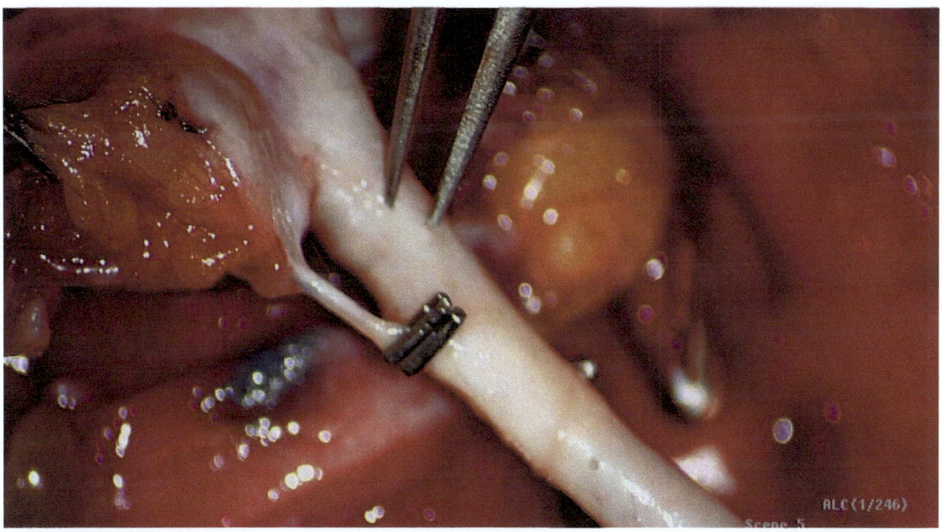

Figure 7.5.3 Another microscope photograph demonstrating ligation of an arterial side branch with two Liga clips prior to separation. It is not mandatory to place a clip on the venous side, as the contralateral side or the venous side is a low-pressure system and the likelihood of bleeding is minimal or practically zero.

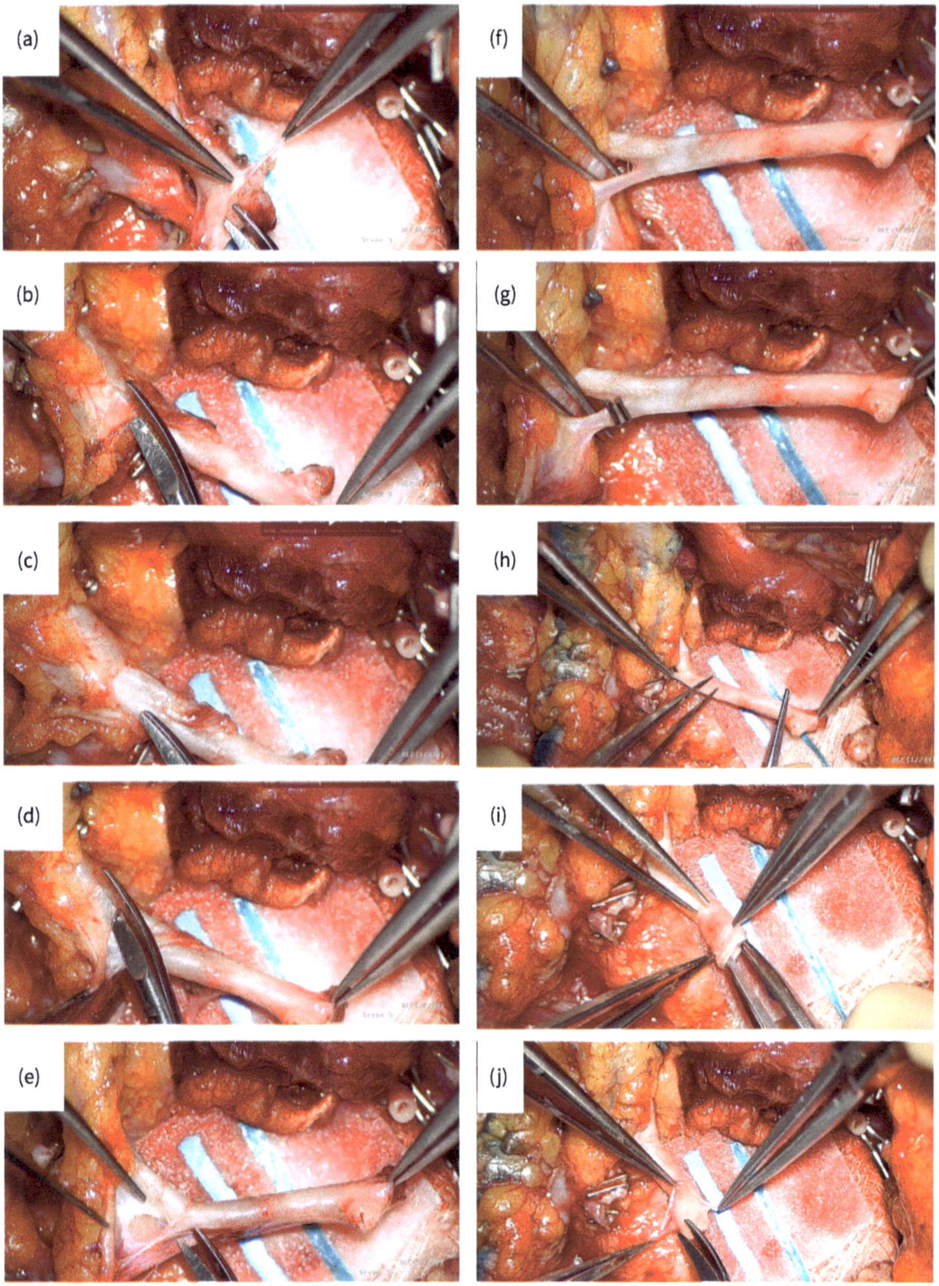

Figure 7.5.4 Summary of the sequence in preparation of the pedicle artery. a. Identification of the pedicle artery and triangulation for crude perivascular dissection. b. The perivascular sheath is gradually opened, and the artery progressively released. c. Identification of the narrow vascular corridor in the 'underbelly' of the flap pedicle on the opposite side of the VCs' course with the multiple interconnecting veins and side branches. d. Sharp dissection to open the perivascular sheath in the underbelly of the flap pedicle. e. Identification of side branches using the triangulation technique. The side branches are carefully dissected. f. The arterial side branch is cleaned and ready for ligation. g. Two liga clips are placed on the arterial side of the side branch. The other (venous) does not require ligation for the sake of time; this will not cause bleeding. h. When an adequate length of artery has been released, the vessel is immobilized as described in the previous chapter. The assistant holds firmly the end of the vessel, and the operator performs the arteriotomy perpendicular to the axis of the vessel. i. Careful dilation of the vessel. j. Fine adventitia dissection and trimming after dilation of the vessel is the last stage prior to commencement of microvascular suturing.

The dissection follows the pedicle length distally up to the defined point that has been predetermined. There is no requirement for fine adventitia dissection and only removal of the loose perivascular tissue is adequate.

Once the desired length of the artery is reached, care should be given to position the artery—the dilemma is always whether to go above or below the venous part of the vascular pedicle. The previously described dotting/marking of the pedicle on the donor side is valuable guidance on this matter.

Following separation of the artery from the veins, the vessel is prepared close to its edge as described in Chapter 7.2, and a clean arteriotomy is performed (Figure 7.5.4). The vessel lumen is inspected and dilated and a cannula is gently inserted for flushing of the pedicle.

Flushing of the pedicle constitutes a crucial step prior to the anastomosis as described in Chapter 7.4. Flushing is performed with papaverine and with heparinized saline. That aims to release any vessel spasm of small arterials and open up all the vascular channels to allow optimum profusion of the flap. Flushing removes any debris and microthrombi. It cleans the whole microcirculation system.

Flushing of the pedicle is important because it allows the operator to obtain tactile feedback of the microvascular system resistance and the required pressure to flush (perfusion pressure) through the pedicle.

While flushing the pedicle it is important to observe the outflow of heparinized saline through the veins. This initially is blood-stained but with further irrigation clears up.

The outflow should be passive and equal volume of fluid has to flow as injected. The whole pedicle is observed as the saline is following through. Any resistance or twisting motion of the pedicle should alarm the operator that the orientation may not be correct.

Flushing of the pedicle should allow the artery to obtain its relaxed, passive, and natural configuration and resolve any possible twists.

For soft tissue flaps, we recommend a minimum of two or three 20 cc syringes for flushing, whereas for composite bony flaps, additional flushing may be beneficial.

At the end of flushing the artery, the final confirmation of its orientation is made and the artery is dotted with methylene blue in order to maintain the optimum orientation and avoid twists prior to the alignment and anastomosis.

7.6 **Pedicle orientation and vessel alignment for anastomosis**

Introduction

This consists of the final stage of the artery preparation prior to the anastomosis. This is a crucial step for anastomosis.

If the vessel alignment is incorrect then no matter how technically perfect the microvascular suturing technique the pedicle will be subject to twisting, aberrant blood flow and likely thrombosis and failure.

This chapter explains in simple steps the technique to ensure that the pedicle and the recipient artery are properly aligned prior to the commencement of the anastomosis.

Technique

Assuming that all the previous steps have been conducted appropriately and uncomplicated, the operator should now have a fully prepared recipient artery with flow and pressure checked, and with marking dots to depict its orientation. Similarly, the pedicle artery would be completely prepared with clean edges, dilated lumen, and marking dots to signify its orientation.

The crucial steps in recipient artery and pedicle preparation are repeated here to remind the reader:

1. Recipient artery (flow/pressure check performed prior to committing to vessel preparation):
   a. Perivascular tissue excision and ligation of side branches
   b. Adventitia dissection
   c. Arteriotomy and dilation
   d. Lumen inspection (flow/pressure check can be confirmed at this point)
   e. Fine adventitia dissection
   f. Orientation marking
2. Donor artery:
   a. Vessel separation: artery from veins
   b. Adventitia dissection
   c. Arteriotomy and dilation
   d. Lumen inspection

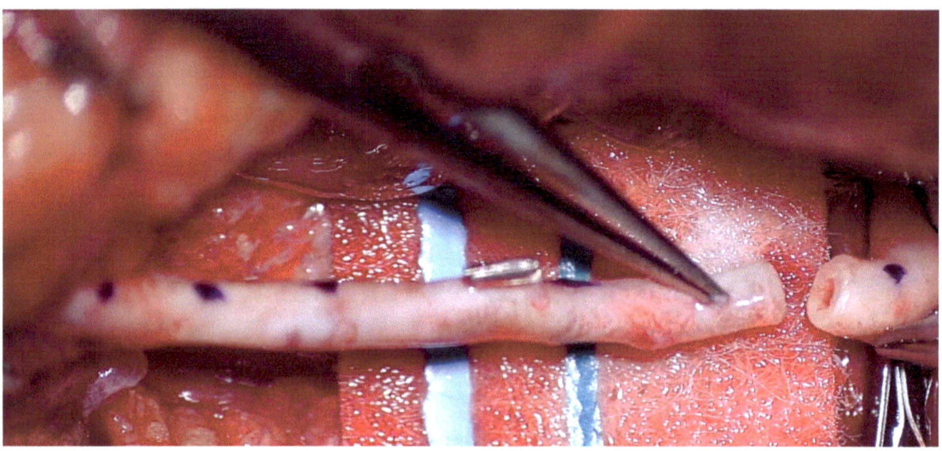

Figure 7.6.1 Pedicle and recipient arteries alignment prior to microvascular suturing. Note the dotted marks that signify the correct orientation of the vessel in its natural passive position. It is important that these dots are aligned, as if any possible twist (torsion) of either vessel during microvascular suturing will cause flap kinking, turbulent flow, and likely ischaemia and thrombosis.

e. Fine adventitia dissection
f. Orientation marking

The marking dots should correspond (Figure 7.6.1) and should point towards an identical predetermined plane. For example, if the agreed direction towards the marking dot pointing at is the superior surface, then it would be expected that upon the vessel's approximation these marking dots should match.

The arteries have been flushed and dilated using a background material of choice, the operator will approximate the vessels.

In our experience a neuro-patty (see Chapter 1.4) offers a satisfactory background but also a soft padded surface that absorbs fluids.

If possible, the ideal set-up is to bring both vessels at the same horizontal plane and perform anastomosis horizontally pushing the needle from right to left (for a right-handed operator) but any microvascular handling is as effortless as possible.

In less common circumstances (such as in a contralateral anastomosis or in cases of short arterial facial artery stump), the anastomosis can only be performed in a vertical fashion. This can be extremely challenging. It will rely on a skilled assistant to stabilize the vessels approximated for the operator to join them with micro sutures.

A vertical anastomosis on a short facial artery stump may also be further impaired by the lower border of the mandible, and a second assistant is required to retract the mandible superiorly (cephaloid) in order to open the surgical field and avoid obscuring it by the shadow of the mandible.

As the vessels sit relaxed and aligned prior to anastomosis a final check with the magnification zoomed out is performed in order to confirm that there are no vascular twists. At this stage it is important to check and provisionally predict the course of the veins.

In two system flaps such as in a radial forearm free flap with radial venae-comitantes and a cephalic vein it is important to determine that the artery is not passing through a venous loop.

Inadvertently failing to notice that may expose one vein above the level of the artery compromising the venous anastomosis at a later stage. It is preferable to confirm at this point that the artery is passing below the veins or at the correct course and is not entangled because if there is a problem after the anastomosis the only solution would be either to accept taking the risk or repeating the anastomosis.

In flaps with long pedicles such as a radial forearm free flap where the pedicle is forming a loop some temporary suspension of the vessel loop may be required in order to clear the field where the anastomosis is taking place and remove any hanging vessels that obstruct the view or frustrate the operator.

Once all the appropriate checks in low and high magnification have been conducted, then the anastomosis should begin as described, as in Chapter 8 with no further delay.

Once this is achieved, each component can be secured to the desired position/orientation. Several techniques have been proposed for this task; we prefer securing vessels either with the use of a micro-sutures or with 6-0 round-bodied prolene vascular sutures. Although Tieseal has been suggested as an easy, safe solution to stabilize the vascular pedicle, it will make a potential exploration attempt extremely difficult or even impossible and we don't advocate its use.

Important highlights in vessel orientation are summarized in Box 7.6.1.

Box 7.6.1 Vessel orientation: important reminders

- Prior to commencement of the anastomosis, spend some time deciding the optimum vessel position and the anastomosis layout (pedicle orientation, course of blood flow).
- It is preferable to aim for horizontal anastomosis by laying the vessels opposite to each other, resting on an appropriate padding (neuro patties or background).
- A horizontal anastomosis is always far more preferable than a vertical anastomosis.

Further reading

Ardehali B, Mehrara B, Cordeiro P, Mosahebi A. Painting the pedicle: a twist-proof marking method. *J Reconstr Microsurg* 2011;27(3):207–8.

Cai A, Horch RE, Arkudas A. The impossible anastomosis: intima-to-adventitia suture technique for microanastomosis of severely calcified arteries. *Plast Reconstr Surg Glob Open* 2021;9(10):e3866.

Cho AB, *et al.* A reinforcement of the sutured microvascular anastomosis with fibrin glue application: a retrospective comparative study with the standard conventional technique. *Microsurgery* 2017;37(3):218–21.

Couteau C, Rem K, Guillier D, Moris V, Revol M, Cristofari S. Improving free-flap survival using intra-operative heparin: ritualistic practice or evidence-base medicine? A systematic review. *Ann Chir Plast Esthet* 2018;63(3):e1–e5.

Kemler MA, Kolkman WF, Slootweg PJ, Kon M. Adventitial stripping does not strip the adventitia. *Plast Reconstr Surg* 1997;99(6):1626–31.

Kim JT, Kim YH, Kim SW. Effect of fibrin sealant in positioning and stabilizing microvascular pedicle: a comparative study. *Microsurgery* 2017;37(5):406–9.

Kim EK, Maldonado AA, Jeong WS, Hong JP, Song DH. Microvascular vessel preparation: What are we really removing during adventitial stripping? *J Plast Reconstr Aesthet Surg* 2015;68(11):1568–73.

Lohman R, Siemionow M, Lister G. Advantages of sharp adventitial dissection for microvascular anastomoses. *Ann Plast Surg* 1998;40(6):577–85.

Macias D, Kwon DI, Walker PC, Peterson NR. Local intraluminal irrigation with argatroban during free flap repair in a patient with heparin-induced thrombocytopenia. *Ann Otol Rhinol Laryngol* 2017;126(5):407–10.

Mücke T, Wolff C, von Düring M, Mitchell DA, Ritschl LM, Fichter AM. Form and size matter: increased risk of thrombosis in microvessels with surgically created endothelial lesions. *J Reconstr Microsurg* 2017;33(1):40–4.

Pafitanis G, Kyprianou K, Chen HC. Microvascular anastomosis in atherosclerotic vessels: Technical challenges and recommendations. *J Plast Reconstr Aesthet Surg* 2021;74(7):1633–701.

Rumbolo PM, Cooley BC, Hanel DP, Gould JS. Comparison of the influence of intralumenal irrigation solutions on free flap survival. *Microsurgery* 1992;13(1):45–7.

Sinclair S. The importance of topical heparin in microvascular anastomoses: a study in the rat. *Br J Plast Surg* 1980;33(4):422–6.

Stenmark KR, *et al.* The adventitia: essential regulator of vascular wall structure and function. *Annu Rev Physiol* 2013;75:23–47.

8

Techniques for anastomosis

Artery

Phil Pirgousis, Basim E.S. Dawoud, Leandros Vassilios F. Vassiliou, Panayiotis Kyzas, and Nicholas Kalavrezos

8.1 **Vessel alignment and orientation**

Introduction

The success of arterial anastomosis is dependent upon the preparation and set up of the microsurgeon, which has been discussed in detail in Chapters 1, 4, and 7.

Anatomically, the head and neck is a challenging area to perform anastomosis due to the complex anatomy in the region.

Chapter 8 discusses in detail the step-by-step process of performing the arterial anastomosis. In this sub-chapter, the importance and sequence of bringing the two arteries together prior to micro-suturing is explained.

Orientation

Once the vessels are prepared for anastomosis, the surgeon must turn their attention to the orientation of the donor vessels. This is a crucial concept to understand in order to maximize the success of microvascular surgery.

Orientation of the donor vessel is the three-dimensional spatial positioning and configuration at which the vessel is passively placed within the neck.

The operating microscope for microvascular reconstruction can be up to ×20 magnification. As the magnification power of the operating microscope increases, the operating field narrows, and the depth of focus (the area above and below (range of depth) the point of perfect focus where sharp focus is maintained) will decrease. That means that once the microsurgeon starts suturing, which will require higher or maximum magnification due to field narrowing and 'tunnel vision', they will lose a wider view (perspective) of the vessels' configuration, and any twist of the vessels will be missed. This is why the orientation of the vessel is crucial to be correct from the outset, otherwise the surgeon may carry on the completion of an anastomosis that may be destined to fail due to incorrect vessel alignment.

As discussed elsewhere in the text, the surgeon must be positioned in a passive, comfortable manner to minimize distracting movements during microsurgery. The entire circumferential ends of the vessels, both the recipient and donor arteries, must be within view to allow for successful microvascular surgery.

Consideration should be given to the orientation of the recipient artery (for example, the facial artery) prior to its ligation. The ideal set-up is adequate (a minimum of 1 cm) length of the recipient artery so that it can be gently bent downwards (caudally), allowing the anastomosis on a horizontal plane. If the artery is too short from its take-off from the external carotid artery, then the anastomosis may have to be performed in a vertical plane, which will be more challenging as described in subchapter 8.4. The danger is that when the recipient vessel is coursing the neck vertically, the surgeon will be unable to safely view the edges of the vessel and therefore the possibility of poor approximation is greater.

As mentioned, the vessels ideally must be passively seated in a horizontal plane, which will maximize the surface area the surgeon is able to view (Figure 8.1.1).

- Ensuring the correct horizontal orientation of the vessels also allows for efficiency of surgery by improving the economy of movements.
- Easier movements when holding instruments, as when working on the same plane, the hands are rested and supported and only the fingers move. This resembles the writing position with precise, minimal fingertip movements and better control.
- The level of focus required remains the same, as moving the working level up and down (vertical anastomosis) will displace the objects out of the field of depth of focus, requiring multiple interruptions for frequent focus adjustments.

By maintaining this horizontal arrangement, the surgeon is able to perform microsurgery seamlessly with minimal interruptions.

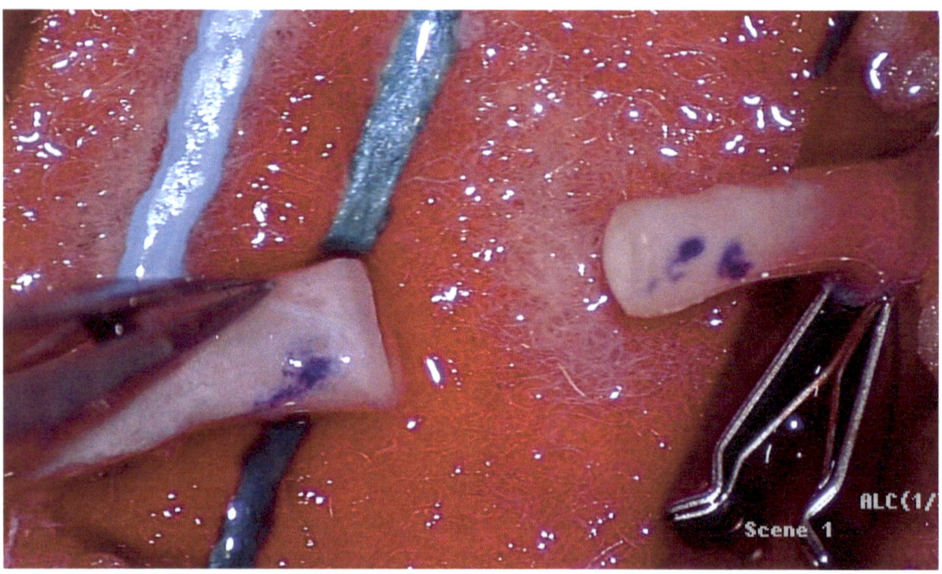

Figure 8.1.1 Approximation of the arteries about to anastomosed. After checking the correct orientation of the recipient vessel and the pedicle position, the corresponding marking dots are brought opposite each other when the vessels are approximated. It is important to maintain alignment of the dots to avoid twisting during anastomosis.

Should the orientation of the vessel be suboptimal, the surgeon will likely need to perform micro-adjustments in their positioning, which will translate to large movements under the microscope, ultimately reducing the efficiency of surgery. Furthermore, the risk of misalignment is greater and the inadvertent malposition of sutures.

Sequence of vessel approximation

At this stage, as discussed in Chapter 7 and above, the vessels are prepared according to the following sequence:

1. Recipient artery (flow/pressure check performed prior to committing to vessel preparation):
    a. Perivascular tissue excision and ligation of side branches
    b. Adventitia dissection
    c. Arteriotomy and dilation
    d. Lumen inspection (flow/pressure check can be confirmed at this point)
    e. Fine adventitia dissection
    f. Orientation marking
2. Donor artery:
    a. Vessel separation: artery from veins
    b. Adventitia dissection
    c. Arteriotomy and dilation
    d. Lumen inspection
    e. Fine adventitia dissection
    f. Orientation marking

The vessels are washed of any remaining blood and approximated in preparation for the anastomosis.

As emphasized earlier, every effort should be made to maintain both vessels in a horizontal alignment and at the same plane. The use of a background contrast material will improve the visibility, especially the fine configuration of the vessel ends, but it will also offer a level platform for the vessels to rest.

Various contrast materials (Figure 8.1.2) have been described in Chapter 1, but in our preference, we use a neuro-patty as it has a white surface that favourably reflects a light, fluid-absorbent consistency and soft, non-slippery surface.

Ensure that the dots placed at the stage of vessel and pedicle orientation are opposite to each other.

The next steps will depend on the experience, preference, and the coordination between the microvascular surgeon and the assistant.

A choice has to be made as to whether the assistant will be actively suspending the vessels during the micro-suturing process or a double clamp will be used.

Double clamps (Figure 8.1.3) are described next and have certain advantages and disadvantages. The main benefit is that due to the adjustable position of the clamps on the bar, the distance between the vessels can be adjusted. They can be used in the absence of an experienced assistant.

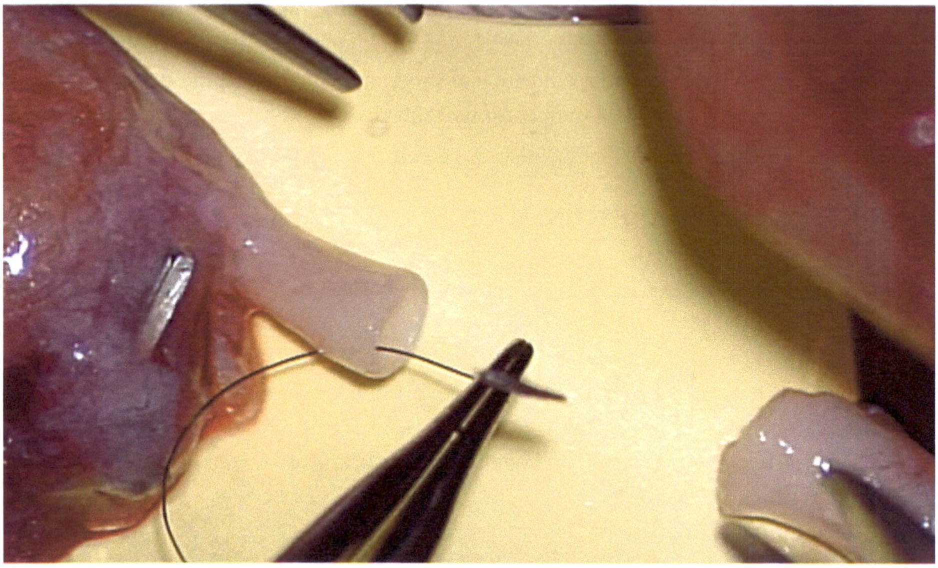

Figure 8.1.2 Contrast medium for optimum visibility. A bright coloured silicone sheet can offer a good contrast and also a working platform for the vessels to be anastomosed.

The order of micro-suture placement is another key factor which underpins the success of arterial anastomosis. There are a variety of techniques described (see subchapters 8.2 and 8.3) with surgeons adopting their own preference for the sequence of suturing, as discussed further in this chapter.

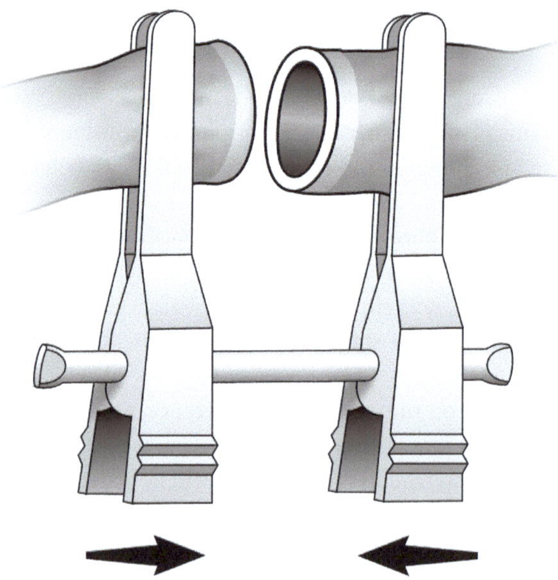

Figure 8.1.3 Double vascular clamp device schematic representation with the two arteries clamped. The clamps can slide alongside the bar in order to achieve optimum distance between the vessel edges and facilitate the anastomosis.

All approaches are designed to allow equal and passive vessel wall approximation:

- Even distribution of sutures.
- Elimination of vessel size (calibre and/or thickness) mismatch.
- Critically avoiding an inadvertent suture through the back wall of the vessel.

Therefore, from a technical perspective, any technique used should efficiently achieve vessel approximation while minimizing the risk of catching the backwall during microvascular anastomosis.

Double clamp as an adjunct to microvascular anastomosis

There are a number of adjuncts to microvascular anastomosis which have been designed to aid the operator. These particular instruments are of use when the assistant lacks the surgical experience to aid the surgeon. One of these tools is the double clamp approximator. This consists of two microvascular clamps which sit on a shared single rail, which allows both clamps to slide up and down accordingly. One of the clamps forms the proximal end and occludes the end of the vessel (recipient vessel) and the other the donor vessel.

Advantages

The clamp serves two purposes: the first is to occlude blood flow and therefore ensure a clear operating field. The second is to aid the approximation of both vessels by sliding the clamps up or down the frame. This allows passive seating of the vessel ends adjacent to one another. If the surgeon chooses to alter the vessel position within the clamp, then they must make sure they do not slide the clamp with the vessel *in situ* under tension.

Rather, the vessel can be fed into the clamp to allow the introduction of excess tissue distal to the clamp, allowing passive approximation. In addition to this, the clamp can be flipped 180 degrees, revealing the back wall of the lumen and therefore allowing complete circumferential approximation of the vessel walls.

The double clamp has the advantage of maintaining both vessels at the same level and preventing any movement up or down that will bring the vessel edge out of focus.

There are certain double clamps with a frame that has small metal projections that will allow the first stay (retention sutures) to be suspended on those hooks in order to maintain tension and keep the vessel mouth open as a better visual aid to the anastomosis.

Disadvantages

Double clamps also have disadvantages, mainly that they cannot fit in short-stumped vessels. That particularly refers to the recipient artery when sometimes the facial artery is cut down to the point of its take-off from the external carotid artery, hence not leaving enough stump length for the double clamp to adjust.

Double clamps also cannot fit on a vertical anastomosis. Again, in scenarios of short recipient arteries or contralateral anastomosis, as they create shadows, they obscure the field, and they may hang and tangle, causing disruption and frustration.

The concept of a double clamp is also that rotation of the whole frame will expose the back wall of the vessels, which assists better in the triangulation technique. That double clamp frame rotation can be quite traumatic in delicate, small, or atherosclerotic vessels, and again the rotation would be technically impossible for short recipient arteries.

Technique of approximation

When using a double clamp, initially bring the frame into the operating field with the clamps moved as far to the end of the bar away from each other as possible. Using the clamp applicators, open the clamps, and with jeweller's forceps, gently bring the vessel into the clamp prior to gently closing it. Allow a good length of the vessel to be exposed.

The same for the other clamp. Assess the length of the vessel which is available for manipulation and, if required, open the jaws of the clamp and pull a little bit more of the artery inside.

With mosquito forceps, gently squeeze the two clamps to move alongside the bar in order to approximate the vessels in the optimal distance (approximately one vessel width apart from each other).

As a rule of thumb, the starting position will be the distance approximately equal to the width of the vessels. In cases of calibre mismatch, that will be the diameter of the smallest vessel.

8.2 **Principles of microvascular suturing and triangulation techniques**

Introduction

This and the next subchapter focus on the most common techniques of microvascular suturing in arterial anastomosis. The techniques described refer to end-to-end anastomosis. The authors avoid end-to-side anastomoses for arteries as this is more suitable for larger vessels than the ones encountered in the neck region. End-to-side arterial anastomosis may propagate turbulent blood flow and predispose to thrombosis.

It is of crucial importance to emphasize that the microvascular anastomosis is not only about fine microsurgical skills and dexterity, but also and most importantly of judicial assessment of the situation, concentration, and strategical planning of how each suture is placed.

The best chance for a successful anastomosis is the first chance and the most the microsurgeon has strategically planned every move and every pass of the needle the least the chances of errors and failure.

Vessel edge orientation for explanatory purposes

As this chapter focuses on suturing the vessel ends, it is best to set an orientation 'map' to facilitate better understanding. For this purpose, the vessel's end cross-section will be seen as a clock with the most superficial and closest to the operator spot marked as 12 o'clock and the deepest, innermost point of the back wall seen as 6 o'clock (Figure 8.2.1).

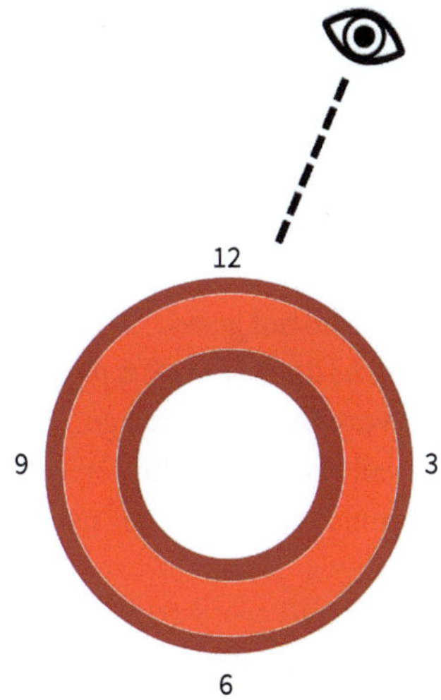

Figure 8.2.1 Basic vessel orientation 'map'. Note that the most superior point closest to the microvascular surgeon represents the 12 o'clock point. The rest of the vessel is mapped arithmetically in a clockwise manner.

Principles of microsuturing

Basic techniques for microvascular suturing have been discussed in Chapter 1.5. The main principles of vessel microsuturing are the following:

- *Vessel handling for optimum eversion.*
  During vessel suturing, it is important to evert the vessel edges. This facilitates perpendicular trajectory of the needle through the wall.
  For this purpose, the vessel edge can be either lifted upwards or supported from inside the lumen and gently pushed outwards.
- Lifting upwards: Choose a spot of the vessel where there is some thin adventitia layer in a distance ideally from the vessel edge ideally to evert the edge successfully but also not to obscure the fill from the passing the needle. Pinch this gently with jeweller's forceps and gently lift the vessel edge.
- Supporting from inside the lumen: Dilators can be gently inserted into the lumen and gently lift the vessel edge upwards. That also provides counter pressure when the needle is passed through the vessel wall, also protecting the vessel from collapsing and hence endangering the needle to impinge the back wall. It is important to avoid injuring the endothelium of the vessel with the tip of the forceps. The dilators with blunt tips are better used for this task as the jeweller's have sharp edges and may inadvertently damage the intima.
- *Plan carefully the entry point.*
  Carefully assess and judge the vessel's size, calibre, and also the vessel wall thickness. Usually, the optimum entry point should be approximately the same size as the vessel wall thickness.

- *Always pass the needle in a perpendicular direction to the vessel wall.*
  This will avoid enlarging the suturing hole that may precipitate bleeding and also avoid tearing the vessel which could be detrimental to the anastomosis.
- *Develop sensitive tactile feedback sense.*
  Feel the give when the needle is passed through the vessel wall.
- *Don't lose the needle tip off your sight.*
  Always be able to see the needle—do not guess.
- *Pull the needle completely out of the lumen once it is passed through the first vessel.*
  Avoid passing through both vessel walls in one go. The vessel lumen may be narrow and that may prohibit the needle acquiring the correct angle to pass through the exit point in a perpendicular fashion. Also passing the needle in one go risks impinging the back wall.
- *Plan carefully the exit point.*
  This requires calculation, judgement, and strategic assessment. It has to factor in any mismatch in calibre or vessel thickness.
- *Square knots.*
  Always place the knots flat and square to regulate the optimum tension and stability of the knots. Control the tightness of the knots. It is important to develop a tactile sensation in the working fingers. Once a knot is tightened enough to approximate, gently the vessel edges but without squashing or strangulating them develop a tactile memory to remember the 'sense' of this degree of tension. This has to be recapitulated in the further sutures to come.
- *Plan the spacing of the sutures.*
  Aim for equal distance between the sutures within each respective vessel.
  Aim for equal distance from the edge (size of bite) for each respective vessel.

The principles of micro-suturing are summarized in Box 8.2.1.

Box 8.2.1 Principles for microvascular suturing

Vessel walls must be everted when suturing. To achieve this:

- Gently grasp the adventitia close to the vessel end and pull so that the vessel edge is everted
  or
- Insert dilator forceps in the lumen and push outwards. This offers counter-resistance when the needle passes from out in.

Carefully plan and target the needle entry point.

Always pass the needle perpendicular through the vessel wall.

With practice, develop a sensitive fingertip tactile feedback sense. This helps to feel the 'give' when the needle penetrates through the vessel wall.

Never lose sight of the needle tip. Eversion of the vessel walls is important for this.

When the needle is through the first vessel, pull it out completely. Avoid passing the needle through the second vessel at once.

Carefully plan and target the needle exit point.

Always tie square knots.

Plan and space the sutures evenly.

Combination of the aforementioned principles in a sequence of moves

Bringing these rules into motion, the general course of the needle should have the following sequence: to facilitate perpendicular entry and exit of the needle it is important to utilize tactile feedback. Once it is felt that the needle is through the vessel wall, the needle is gently curved parallel to the axis of the vessel, and once the exit point is targeted again the needle is rotated so that it exits in a perpendicular course through the lumen wall.

In order to achieve this '90-degree trajectory' through the vessel wall, a gentle 'bent' of the vessel edge may be required. This will avoid inadvertent injury of the back wall of the endothelium.

Entry point

This at entry point is achieved by inserting a pair of forceps inside the lumen and gently lifting the vessel edge up while pushing with the needle through till the tip is visible through the wall.

Exit point

For the needle exit as the needle tip is pushed from the lumen and through the wall outwards a pair of forceps can be placed outside the vessel wall at a point slightly distal (away from the edge) to the targeted exit point. The tips of the forceps are kept slightly open and gently pushing downwards as the needle is pushing out to come through and by this counteracting action the edge of the vessel is everted and the course of the needle at a right angle to the wall.

It is important to avoid oblique passage of the needle through the vessel wall as this may lead to tears that may be detrimental to the whole anastomosis.

Flushing the anastomosis prior to tying the last stitch

Regardless of the suturing technique used (triangulation or back-wall-first as described in subchapter 8.3), it is important to mention that when placing the one before the last suture on the anterior wall, without tying the knot, cut the thread leaving adequate length to return later with the needle holder and form a loop (approximately 2 cm). Place then carefully the last suture and tie a square knot. Now the only suture left untied in the previous one (one before the last). Through the remaining opening advance the irrigation tip within the lumen of the anastomosis and irrigate with papaverine and heparinized saline.

Flushing the anastomosis prior to tying the knot on the last suture serves important purposes:

- Flushing 'inflates' the anastomosis ('hydrodistension'), offering a view of how balanced the distribution of the sutures is and how symmetrically the anastomosis expands.
- As papaverine irrigates the flap microcirculation it pre-empts the possibility of any media tunica vessel spasm. The papaverine and heparinized saline will help relax the vessel's smooth muscle and prevent spasm. The heparinized saline will flush all the vascular micro channels.
- As the residual fluid post irrigation is leaking through the suture gap prior to the tying the knot, it will flush away any possible trapped debris and any possible trapped adventitia.

- With the flow of the fluid outwards, the lips of the vascular edges will be everted so that during the time of the last stitch (as there is no further ability to visualize the lumen past this), they will have the maximum chance of eversion.

Common pitfalls

Distribution (spacing) of sutures

It is important to achieve equidistant distribution of sutures. The other concern with unequal suture placement is unequal tension across the vessel walls and anastomotic junction. By having a poor distribution of the forces across the anastomosis, the vessel can be prone to asymmetrical expansion or leaks.

The first may lead to turbulent blood flow which creates the possibility of endothelial damage within the tunica intima and subsequent clot formation.

Gaps between sutures may cause leaks and bleeding after the clamps are released.

The greatest concern with unequal bites is the increased risk of a 'through stitch' where the opposing wall of the vessel is caught, occluding the anastomosis.

As the vessel is approximated, and more sutures are placed, the view within the lumen diminishes. Furthermore, unequal bites of the vessel walls compound this problem and lead to even less intraluminal visibility. This therefore increases the risk of inadvertently catching the opposing wall with a suture, which would lead to occlusion of the vessel and subsequently microvascular anastomosis failure.

As stated earlier in the text, it is the pass on exiting the lumen which dictates whether the suture is equidistant from one another, so the surgeon should take extra care during this part.

Tightness of knots

An important component which contributes towards tension across the edges of the microvascular anastomosis is how tight the thread material is tied across the junction.

It is crucial that the tension across the junction is enough to approximate the vessel edges, but not to strangulate the tissue. Excessive force of approximation across the anastomotic junction may lead to additional damage to the delicate layers of the vessel walls. In addition to this, in particular with older patients with atherosclerotic vessels, there is a greater chance of dissection within the layers of the vessel.

Care should always been taken to approximate vessels gently and with enough tension across the thread to avoid strangulation of the vessel edges.

Triangulation suturing 120 degrees

The method of triangulation suturing was one of the first techniques published in Lyons Medical by Alexis Carrel in 1902 for microvascular repair of small vessels. He described a technique for end-to-end anastomosis for blood vessels, which forms the foundation of triangulation stitching.

Fundamentally, this classical method of suturing involves the placement of three 'stay' sutures 120 degrees apart from each other. This is usually at the position of 10 and 2 o'clock as the first 'stay' sutures followed by 6 o'clock (midpoint of back wall) (Figure 8.2.2).

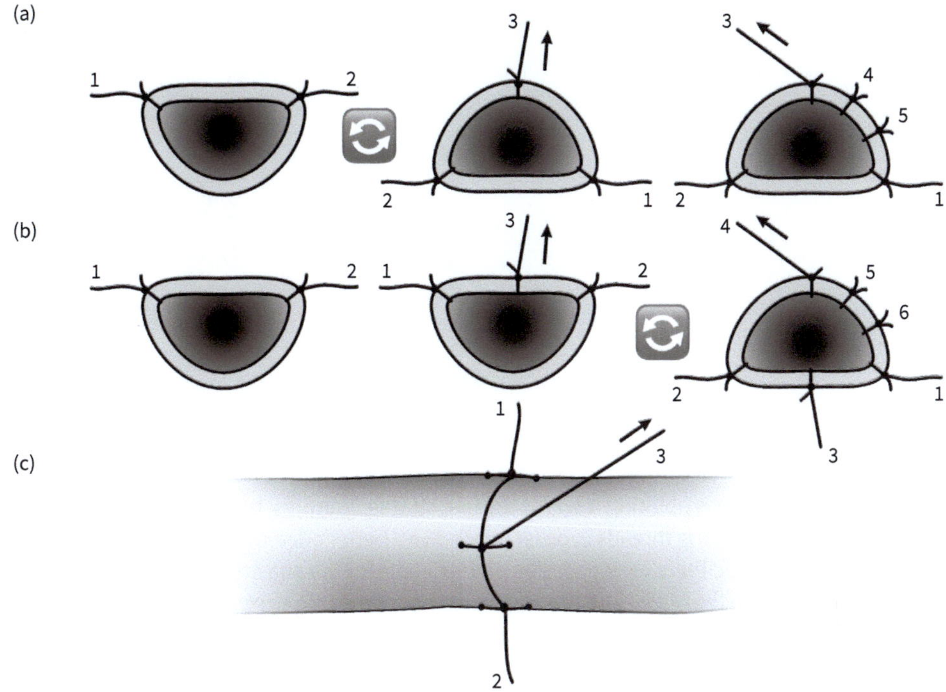

Figure 8.2.2 Sequence of suture placement based on triangulation techniques. a. The first two sutures are placed in positions 1 and 2, 120 degrees apart. Note that the back wall is left free hanging. At this point, the vessel is reversed, and a midpoint suture in position 3 of the back wall is placed. Suture number 3 is then used for retraction and gentle vessel wall tenting in order to allow subsequent sutures numbers 4 and 5 to be placed. The procedure is continued until completion with all the sutures circumferentially and equidistantly placed. b. This is a modification of the previously described technique. After sutures 1 and 2 are placed 180 degrees apart, a third stitch is placed at the midpoint of the anterior wall. Following that, the vessel is now reversed and the back wall is sutured as described previously, with a midpoint stitch at position 4 to allow retraction and gentle tenting, followed by sutures 5 and 6, onwards. c. This is an overview of the two vessels being sutured with the stitches in positions 1 and 2 (120 degrees apart). The stitch in position 3 is used for gentle (pulling) for retraction and vessel wall tenting.

Using this nomenclature, the 6 o'clock corresponds to the back wall of the vessel (furthest away from the microvascular surgeon). The near sidewall corresponds to 10 o'clock and 2 o'clock being between the anterior wall (opposite the back wall) and the sidewall superiorly.

By using this technique, the assistant is able to use two adjacent stay sutures to lift the segment of the wall being sutured.

These stay sutures are strategically placed to allow the surgeon to rotate the vessel symmetrically, therefore allowing placement of additional sutures safely while mitigating the risk of inadvertently catching the intima of the back wall. Nevertheless, caution should be paid when lifting the vessel wall and approximating the other end, as it is possible to rotate or create a vessel mismatch (Figure 8.2.3).

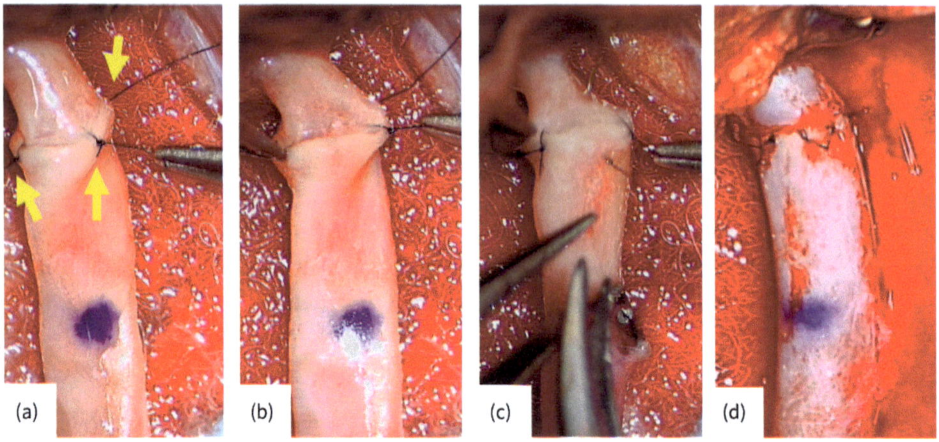

Figure 8.2.3 a. Initial three sutures placed according to the triangulation 120-degrees technique. Note the arrows pointing towards the first strategic sutures. b. The assistant is pulling differentially the long threads in order to achieve a better edge-to-edge apposition of the vessel ends and facilitate easier passing of the needle for the anastomosis. c. Note the needle passing through the vessel and the equal distance of the bite sizes. d. Completion of the anastomosis and release of the vascular clamp. The artery, especially at the site of the anastomosis, has symmetrically expanded. Note the equal position of the sutures. This is the sight of a healthy arterial anastomosis.

Triangulation suturing 180 degrees

The evolution of this method led to the development of the 180-degree suturing technique where stay sutures are placed at 9 o'clock and 3 o'clock (Figure 8.2.4).

This is the most basic form of microvascular anastomosis. Once these two sutures are placed, the microvascular surgeon places additional stitches, completing the anterior (wall closest to the surgeon) first.

Upon completion, the vessel is flipped 180 degrees to expose the back wall. The suturing then continues in a methodical manner from the back wall.

Usually, the next sutures are placed, halving the distance between the existing ones; for example, at a 6 o'clock position, leaving one thread long to pull, then another one or two in the distance left between, and so on.

Great care and attention must be taken when suturing this side as the view of the lumen gradually diminishes with progressive vessel approximation, thereby carrying the greatest risk of catching the opposing wall intima. The jeweller's forceps in the non-dominant hand become pivotal in the protection of the opposing wall intima. The reader can refer to these techniques as they are described elsewhere in the text.

The need to flip the vessel and suture the back wall is the major disadvantage due to the risk of opposing intimal vessel wall suturing and vessel damage. Of further consideration for this technique, additional length of the vessel is required to allow safe 180-degree rotation of the vessel without excessive tension across the sutures *in situ*. As discussed elsewhere in the text, atherosclerotic vessels are particularly at risk of dissection and tearing when using this approach to microvascular anastomosis.

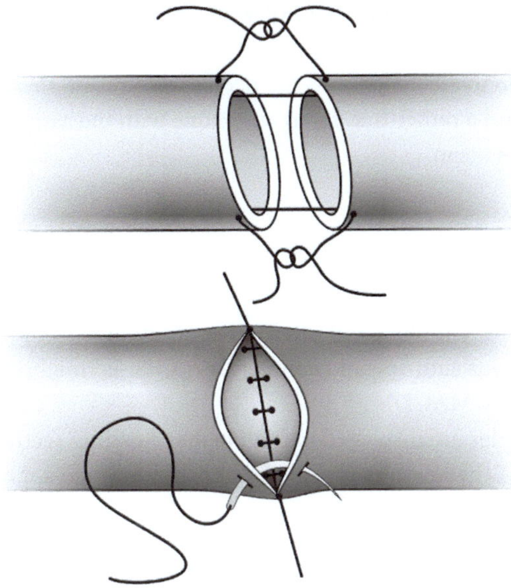

Figure 8.2.4 Triangulation 180-degree technique. Note the two stay sutures at the corners that suspend the vessels close together. It is good practice to first close the back wall and leave the anterior wall until last.

Microvascular double clamp

A slight modification of this tool is the same instrument but with a frame attached around the double clamp. These frames have small hook-like extensions which allow the securing of the suture material, thereby providing a means of retraction to the vessel walls. There is a particular way these hooks should be used in relation to the thread material to optimize their use. Once a suture has been placed, the tail end of the suture must be kept long enough to allow it to be secured to the hooks. The thread is brought over the frame and between the two hooks. It is then passed down over the frame and around the posterior or anterior edge of one of the hooks. It is then passed in a horizontal fashion towards the opposing hook, passing the suture on the same side as the frame. Then the suture material is passed around the hook in the opposite direction to the opposing hook. The thread is then tightened slightly, ultimately leaving a figure of eight throw around the hooks.

The method of approximation usually follows the 180- or 120-degree triangulation technique that is discussed earlier in this chapter. This is because the hooks on the double clamp with frame approximator suit starting microvascular surgery at the 9 o'clock and 3 o'clock (180-degree technique), or 10 o'clock and 2 (120-degree technique) o'clock position. The threads, once secured to the hooks on the frame at the top and bottom of the vessel, effectively hold the vessel edges in a linear fashion while circumferential suturing takes place.

These adjuncts to microvascular surgery can be useful and certainly have a place in anastomosis. Nevertheless, the neck is a unique anatomical environment with a complex interplay between hard and soft tissue structures. As discussed elsewhere in the text, typically the facial artery is used as the recipient vessel for which the path of the artery is somewhat tortuous. In addition to this, the space to perform microvascular surgery can be limited and near and under the mandible, with other structures such as the hyoid bone, supra-, and/or infra-hyoid musculature hindering a horizontal field of work. Therefore, the use of these sometimes-bulky adjuncts often occupies additional space, which minimizes the available room for the microvascular surgeon to efficiently pass the needle. As a result, these adjuncts are not often used by the authors and a rather free-hand technique with the assistance of a second microvascular surgeon is the norm.

Other suturing techniques

The literature offers an abundance of alternative anastomosis approaches from 'mattress' techniques to continuous suturing and coupler device-based methods (microvascular anastomosis coupler devices, MACD).

Representative articles are displayed in the Further Reading section. The authors analyse in this subchapter and the next the most validated and fail-safe approaches that have stood the test of time.

8.3 **Back-wall-first or 'one-way-up' anastomosis**

Introduction

This subchapter describes another anastomosis approach where the first suture is placed at the 6 o'clock position, essentially the innermost point of the posterior (back wall). Again, and as disclosed in Chapter 8.2 this technique describes an end-to-end arterial anastomosis as the authors do not favour end-to-side anastomosis for arteries in the typical head and neck setting. With this technique the posterior wall approximation is completed first (Figure 8.3.1).

It is of crucial importance to emphasize again that the success of the microvascular anastomosis is depended on careful meticulous strategic judgement of where its single suture is placed and the precise execution of this using fine dexterity and fingertip skills.

The best chance for a successful anastomosis is the first chance and the most the microsurgeon has strategically planned every move and every pass of the needle the least the chances of errors and failure.

Technique

First and 'strategic' stitch

It is the authors' preference to place the back wall (suture furthest away from the surgeon) stitch first. This first stitch should be considered the 'cornerstone' stitch during microvascular suturing (Figure 8.3.2).

By the precise placement of this first suture, the surgeon mitigates the risk of inadvertently catching the backwall of the vessel during the further process of the anastomosis (Figure 8.3.3).

The first step is to ensure correct vessel orientation, which has been discussed in detail elsewhere in the text.

(a)

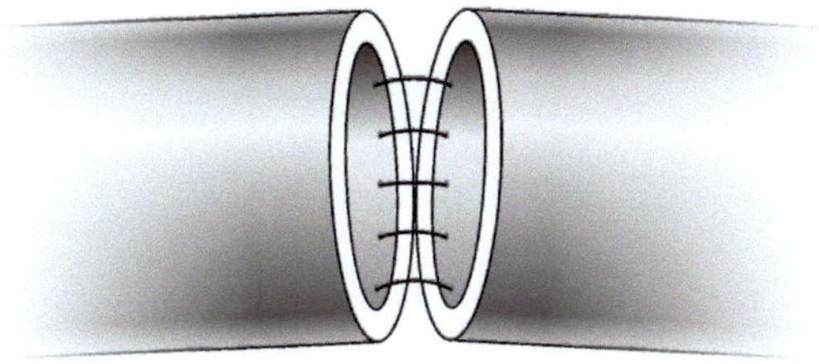

(b)

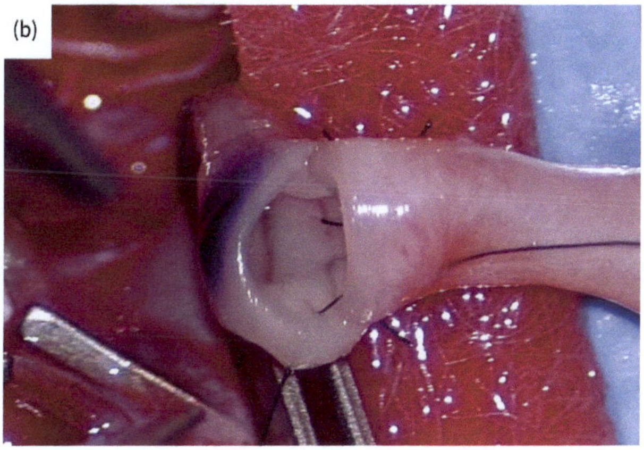

Figure 8.3.1 Back-wall-first or one-way-up anastomosis. a. Schematic representation of microsuture placement at the back wall first. b. Real anastomosis pictures showing closure of the back wall first. It is much easier to close the hemi half (hemi circumference) of the vessel when the posterior wall is already completed. That offers excellent control of the back wall and visualization of the whole lumen in both arteries.

The needle tip must be placed parallel to the side of the vessel while it is handled by the adventitia only. It is crucial to avoid holding the vessel wall directly, as all techniques are designed to minimize microtrauma to the intima of the vessel and thus decrease the risk of thrombosis.

The vessel must then be lifted by the adventitia so that the lumen can clearly be seen. The needle is then passed from the outside of the vessel entering the lumen under direct vision. The needle is then carefully brought to the part of the opposite vessel for which exit is planned.

The exit 'bite' is crucial as this determines how the vessels will subsequently approximate and the tension across the anastomotic junction (Figure 8.3.3a).

Using the jeweller's forceps in the non-dominant hand, the vessel wall is supported externally to encourage the needle to pass smoothly in a curved pattern exiting the vessel. It is vital that the bite on the side where the needle is exiting is equidistant from the edge of the vessel as the side of entry into the lumen. It is crucial that the greatest care is taken to ensure this otherwise there will be unequal approximation of the vessel. It is therefore true that it is the second bite (exiting pass of the needle through the lumen) that dictates the uniformity of the vessel approximation. In addition to this, should it be felt the bites are unequal or inadequate, the

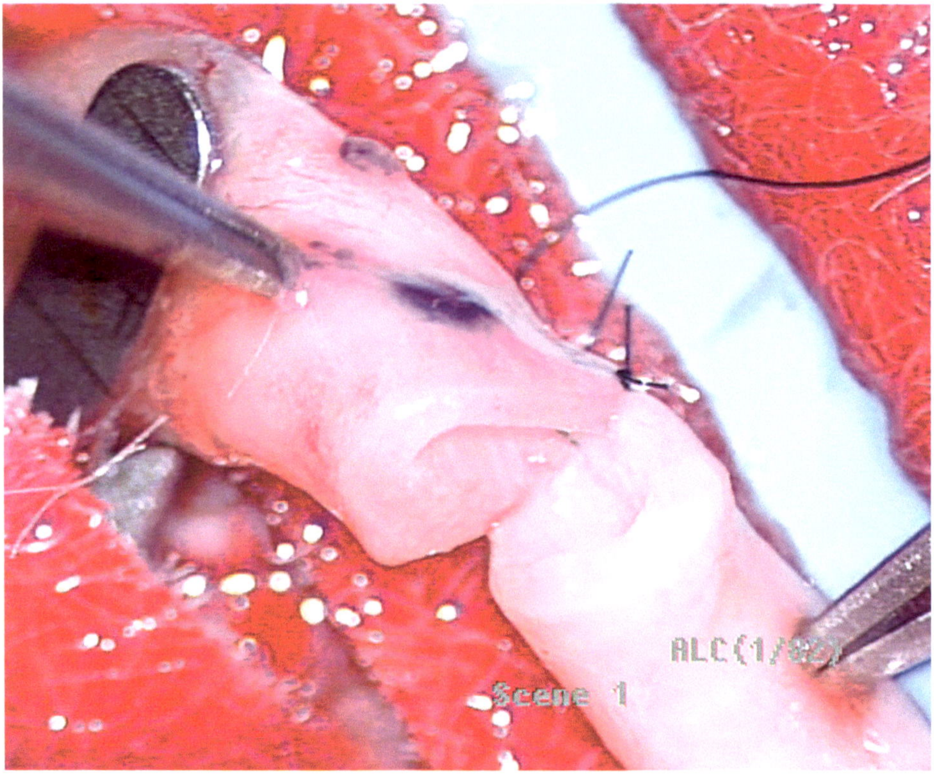

Figure 8.3.2 Demonstration of the first two strategic sutures in the back-wall-first anastomosis. Note the precise approximation of the vessel walls and the smooth transition from one lumen's intima to another. These two strategic sutures are decisive for the course of the whole anastomosis and set the foundation for any elimination of size (calibre) or thickness mismatch. It is important that the sutures are placed accurately in the position of vessel dots as mentioned in Chapter 8.1 to avoid contortion (twisting).

subsequent removal of the suture will leave damaged intima behind. This endothelial damaged surface then carries potential for a prothrombotic formation of a platelet plug which could lead to catastrophic failure.

For the backwall stitch to be placed first this must be done in a reverse fashion with the lumen visualized throughout (Figure 8.3.3b). Once the thread is passed through a double throw is made to secure the thread down flat.

It is recommended that the first backwall stitch is placed as a 'double throw' (Figure 8.3.3c) of the thread to control tension of approximation, as with a single throw the vessels may slip apart. By placing a double throw for the first suture, the surgeon is able to align the vessels with better stability and tension in the thread and minimize the risk of the walls collapsing or migrating away from one another. This is because this first suture has the greatest tendency to 'slip' as it typically carries the most tension across the thread and vessel walls.

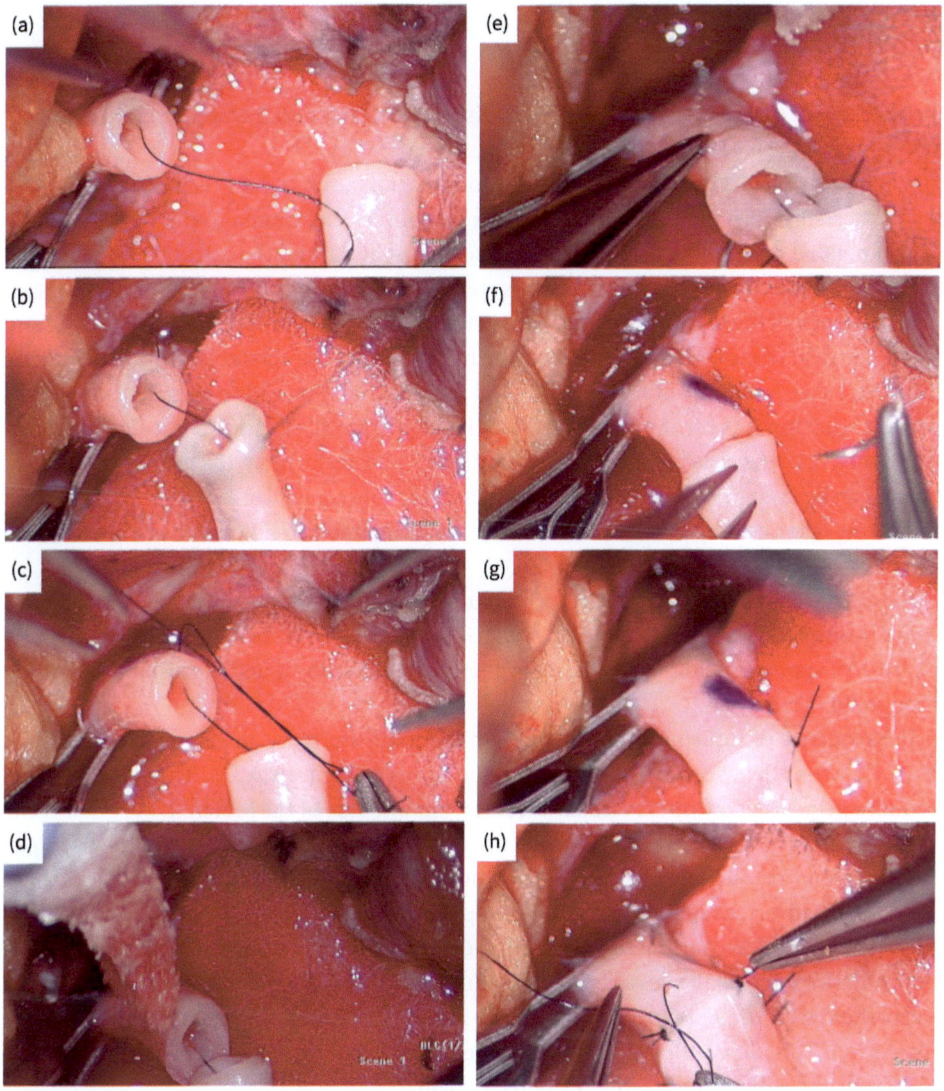

Figure 8.3.3 Sequence of back-wall-first anastomosis. a. Passage of the suture first through the posterior wall of the recipient artery. B. Careful approximation of the arteries in a 'mouth-to-mouth' or 'kissing' fashion. The input of the assistant in aligning the vessels is crucial. c. Double thread prior to tying the knot. d. Careful tying of the knot with optimum tension (not too loose, but not too tight) to crush or strangulate the vessel edges. The input of the assistant is crucial at this point in order to bring and hold the vessels together ('kissing' position). e. Placement of the second posterior wall suture. The vessels have now achieved a good primary position that will make the rest of the anastomosis much easier. f. Continuation of sutures with good position of the two vessels. g. Transition towards the back wall. Placement of the suture in the 9 o'clock position. h. Completion of the anterior wall with a good position of the sutures. The anastomosis is perfectly conducted.

Propagation of anastomosis

The subsequent sutures are passed in an equidistant fashion for each vessel, circumferentially continuing on the back wall.

When suturing it is essential that the surgeon pays attention to how the knot is being laid down externally onto the vessel wall. The aim is to minimize trauma to the vessel wall and have a knot that does not 'slip'. Therefore the knots must be flat and the surgeon must carefully assess the knot as it is being thrown to ensure this objective is achieved. In order to maximize efficiency of the throws, it is best to keep the tail end of the suture reasonably short and within the field of view throughout. By ensuring the tail of the thread is short, the surgeon maximizes their economy of movement, as all the material required to complete the microvascular stitching is present in front of them. Furthermore, it means that the needle holder does not have to travel as far to pick up the tail end while performing the throws. The placed sutures can be used to aid positioning of the vessel for subsequent sutures, so the tail end can be left long when cutting the stitch, so that the assistant is able to hold it for manipulation of the vessel.

These sutures can be placed in the normal single alternating throw until the 9 o'clock and 3 o'clock positions. With each subsequent stitch, it is essential the surgeon carefully assesses the progressive approximation of the vessel wall ensuring a uniform and consistent apposition throughout.

The sequence of suturing continues circumferentially until the anterior wall (side of the vessel closest to the operating surgeon) is to be sutured (Figure 8.3.3h). The authors would recommend passing the microvascular needle from one side of the lumen to the other using two separate passes rather than one single pass. If the surgeon chooses to pass the needle in one pass from one side of the vessel to the other, the chances of unequal, asymmetric bites along with inadvertent approximation of the opposing wall of the vessel are greater.

The microsurgeon continues to approximate the vessel wall circumferentially towards the most superior edges of the vessels. Corner sutures can be kept long to aid closure of the front wall of the vessel. The assistant can use these to manipulate the vessel to maintain a transverse orientation. This allows the microsurgeon to enter and exit the vessel perpendicular to the vessel wall and enhances the economy of movement.

As approximation progresses, the ability to see within the lumen gradually diminishes. Therefore, it is at this stage that the surgeon has the greatest chance of inappropriately catching parts of the vessel wall and compromising the anastomosis. Therefore, the non-dominant handle, which typically holds the jeweller's forceps, becomes a key instrument. The forceps (or preferably dilators with blunt tips) are passed within the lumen, gently tenting up the inside of the vessel through which the needle is to be passed. By doing this, the surgeon protects the side of the vessel which would be at risk of being caught during the passage of the suture. The needle is then passed in the usual fashion from the external side of the lumen to the internal side between the beaks of the dilator or jeweller's forceps.

The risk of catching the side or backwall of the vessel is greatest upon the needle entering the lumen and as such the greatest care must be taken for this particular part of the stitch.

Jeweller's instrument does have a sharp end and can traumatize the intima so great care must be taken with its use or preferably use a dilator for this task.

Furthermore, as discussed, this risk increases the more sutures are placed as the view within the lumen reduces. The core principle for the use of any surgical instrument is that if you can't see the end of your instrument, you cannot be sure where it is and thus iatrogenic trauma is possible. The same is true for microvascular anastomosis. Do not guess or assume you know where the needle tip lies, as this carries the greatest risk of 'through-stitching' of the back wall and subsequent anastomotic failure.

When placing the one before the last suture on the anterior wall, without tying the knot, cut the thread, leaving adequate length to return later with the needle holder and form a loop (approximately 2 cm). Place the last suture carefully and tie a square knot. Now the only suture left untied in the previous one (one before the last). Through the remaining opening, advance the irrigation tip within the lumen of the anastomosis and irrigate with papaverine and heparinized saline. This will inflate the anastomosis, offering a view of how balanced the distribution of the sutures is and how symmetrically the anastomosis expands. The papaverine and heparinized saline will help relax the vessel's smooth muscle and prevent spasm.

Once this step is complete, the knot is tied, and the clamp can be released to allow the anastomosis to run and be assessed.

A 'back-wall-first' anastomosis is demonstrated in Video 8.3.1.

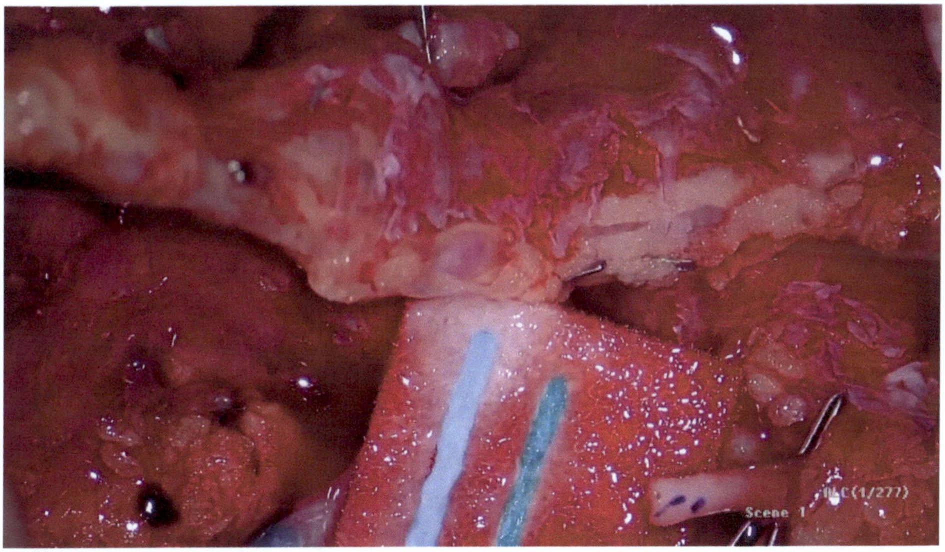

Video 8.3.1 Back-wall-first anastomosis. Demonstration of arterial anastomosis via the back-wall-first fashion.

See this video online by searching for this book's title or ISBN at https://academic.oup.com/

Reproduced courtesy of Leandros Vassiliou, Manchester University NHS Foundation Trust, Manchester, UK.

8.4 **Difficult anastomoses**

Introduction

Microvascular surgery is a highly technical skill and as such the success of the surgery is highly operator dependent. As discussed elsewhere in the text, the chances of increasing success of this surgery are correlated to the preparation given towards the procedure in terms of set up, lighting, and vessel orientation. All these components, which form the foundation of microvascular surgery, have been discussed. Nevertheless, despite optimal set-up and preparation there can still be operator-dependent techniques which can affect the outcome.

- Vertical anastomosis
- Vessel calibre mismatch
- Vessel wall thickness mismatch
- Vessel global size mismatch
- Atherosclerotic vessels

Vertical anastomosis

Vertical anastomosis is challenging as often demands hands on the air that tests steadiness and stability (Figure 8.4.1).

The occurrence of vertical anastomosis is most often met in the following scenarios:

- Short recipient artery stump.
- Contralateral anastomosis.
- Pedicle coming lateral to the mandible, such as lateral defects (face, parotid, scalp, or some maxillectomy defects).

Vertical anastomosis is challenging due to the following main reasons:

1. Poor visibility of the vessels' lumen.
2. Inconvenient seating of the vessels for the operator to pass the needle through the vessels' walls.
3. Difficulty working in high magnification as the target object easily moves out of focus.

In order to overcome the aforementioned challenges, the operator must follow steps to convert the vertical anastomosis to horizontal, both transiently and as soon as possible.

The key is to follow the back-wall-first anastomosis technique and place the first strategic suture in the most 'obscure' point (Figure 8.4.2):

- If the recipient artery is the facial artery and the pedicle comes from below, then the inferior-most stitch (3 o'clock, based on the orientation set in Chapter 8.2, Figure 8.2.1) needs to be placed first.

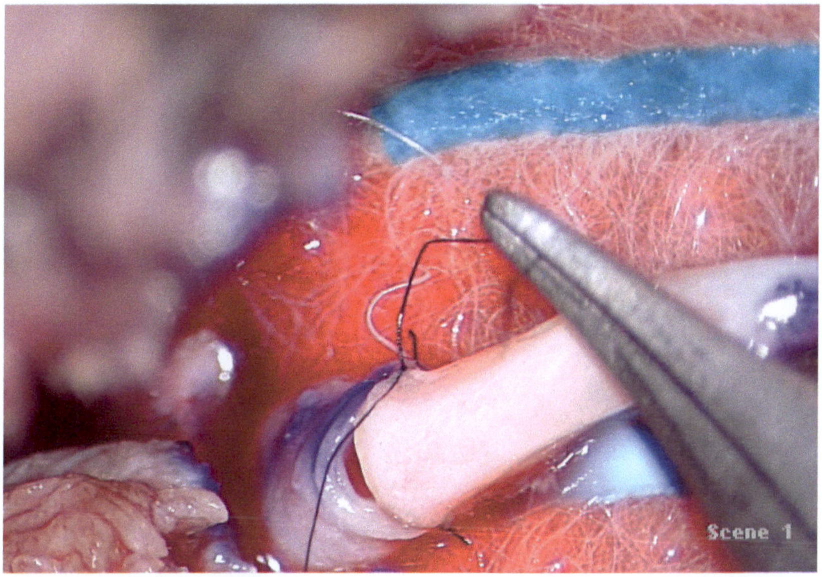

Figure 8.4.1 Vertical anastomosis. Note the vertical position of the short stump of the recipient artery. The donor artery is opposed in a 'kissing' position. The ventral wall is performed first which equals the back wall, when the vessels are in the horizontal position which allows gentle bending of the vessels when performing the rest of the anterior hemi circumference suturing. That gradually transforms the vertical into horizontal anastomosis. Note the position of the mandible in the top left corner. Suturing the anterior hemi circumference first would have to overcome significant space constrictions due to the position and the obscuration caused by the mandible.

- If the recipient artery is the facial artery and the pedicle comes from above (lateral to the mandible), then superior-most stitch (9 o'clock, based on the orientation set in Chapter 8.1) needs to be placed first.

This will allow the anastomosing vessels to 'bend' downwards and horizontally for the next sutures, slowly converting the vertical anastomosis to a horizontal working plane one (Figure 8.4.2).

The sequence of the following sutures is continued as described in Chapter 8.3, and the last two sutures are placed in an almost horizontal anastomosis.

An example of vertical anastomosis is demonstrated in Video 8.4.1.

Calibre mismatch

Calibre (diameter) mismatch is the discrepancy of the diametrical size between the two arteries that have to be anastomosed.

Imprecise suture placement is one of the most common pitfalls encountered by an inexperienced microvascular surgeon. Equal suture placement from the proximal to the distal vessel with equidistance entry and exit points of the needle is vital for success.

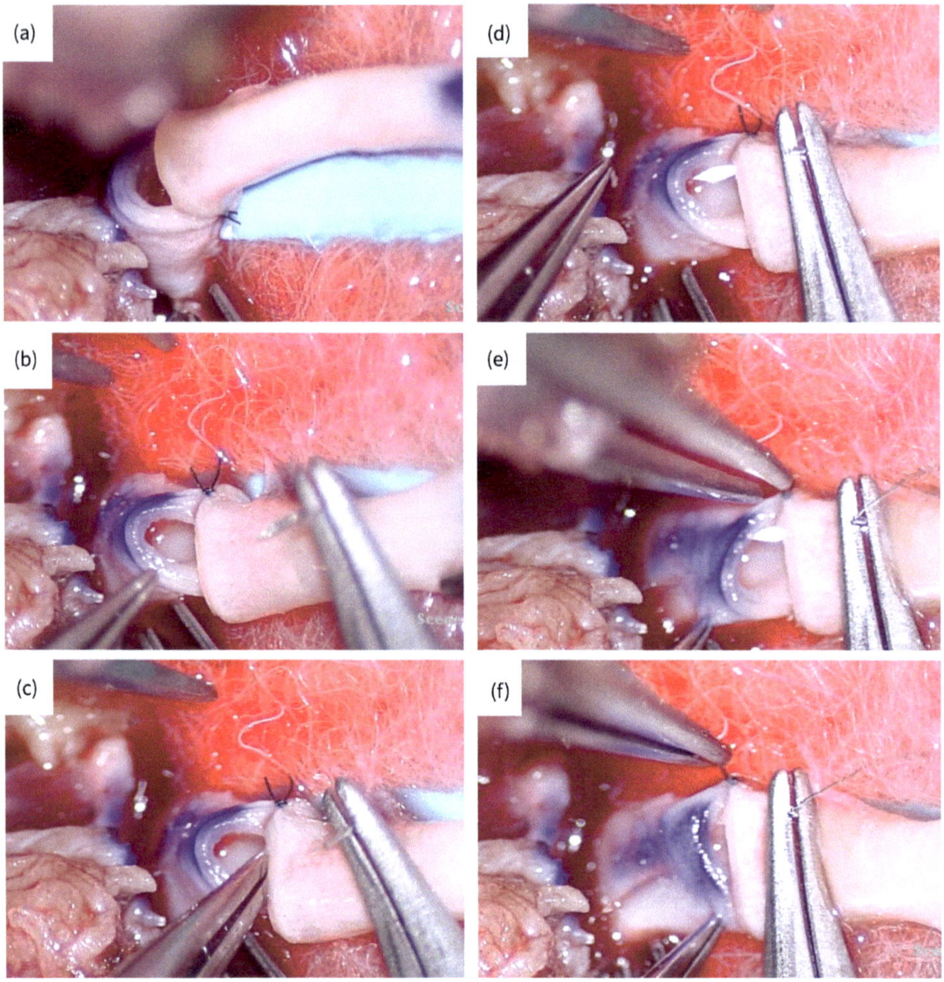

Figure 8.4.2 Sequence of vertical anastomosis. a. The initial first sutures were placed in the ventral wall (equivalent to the posterior wall). b. Careful passing of the needle, one vessel at a time, in order to better control the trajectory of the needle. c. Receiving the needle tip from the inside lumen of the donor artery. d. Change of angulation of the needle in order to pass perpendicular through the wall of the recipient artery. e. Careful calculation of the exit point. f. Note the needle point protruding through the exit point. It is important to calculate the correct bite size to eliminate any mismatch. g. Gentle push perpendicular through the vessel wall. h. Suturing completion of the knot. i. Completion of the lower (ventral or posterior hemi circumference) vascular anastomosis. j. Gradual transition into the anterior wall. k. Placement of the last suture. Note that the penultimate suture isn't a completed knot. l. The former allows for an irrigation cannula tip to pass through the suture gap and irrigate the vessel lumen with papaverine and heparinized saline. m. Note that after irrigation that the residual fluid is coming out, pushing the lips of the vessel edges outwards and cleansing the lumen of any debris. n. Completion of the anastomosis by tying the knot of the last suture.

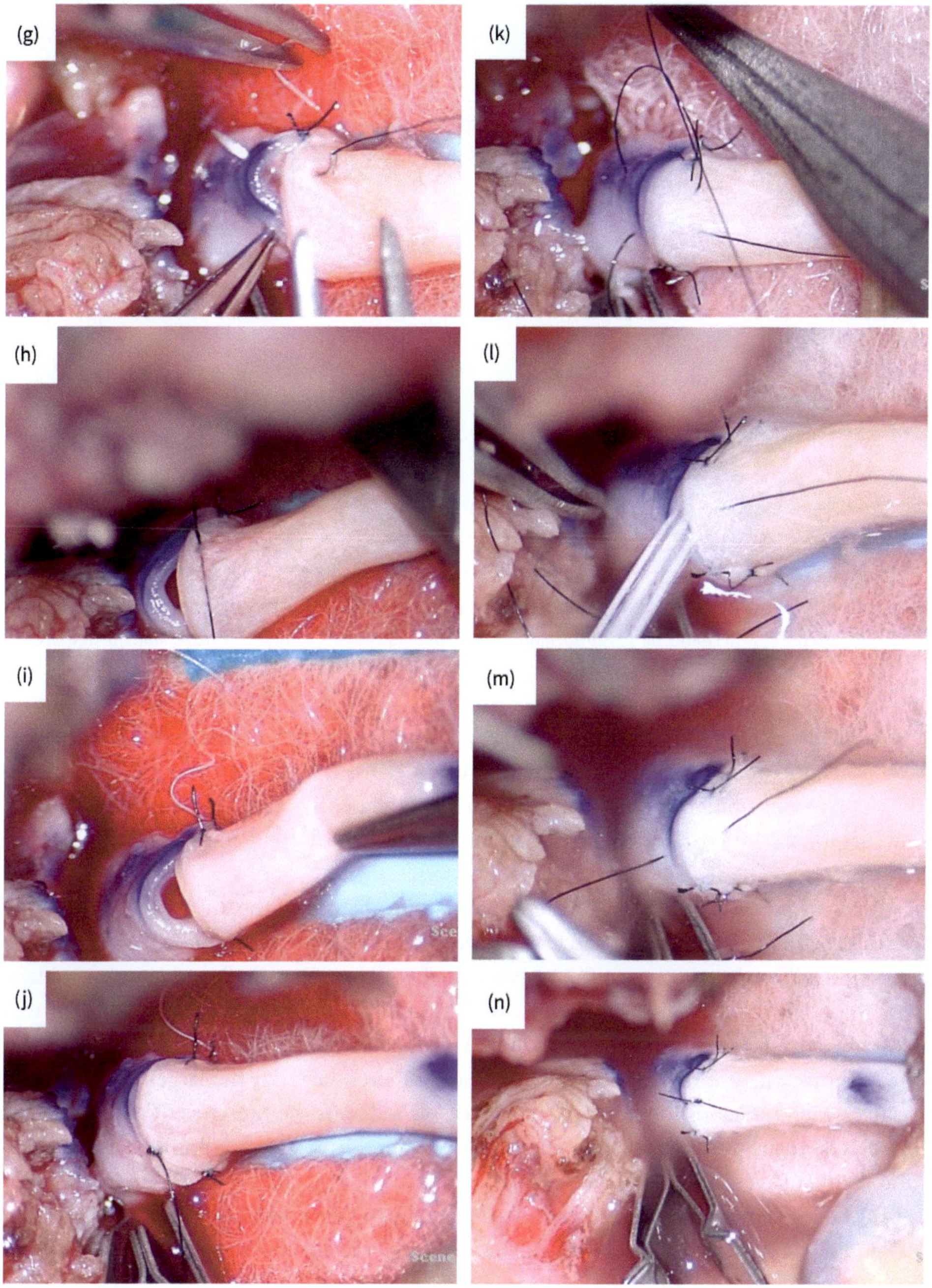

Figure 8.4.2 Continued

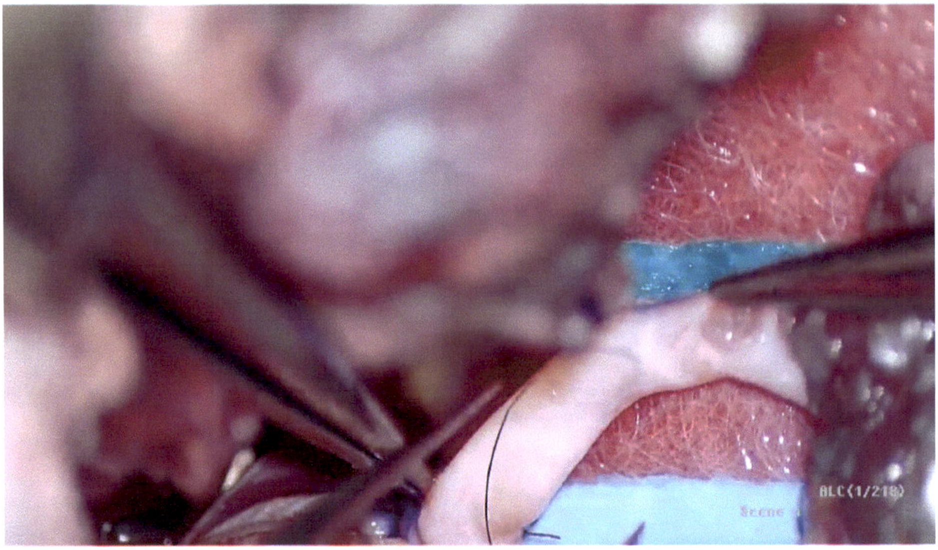

Video 8.4.1 Vertical anastomosis.
See this video online by searching for this book's title or ISBN at https://academic.oup.com/
Reproduced courtesy of Leandros Vassiliou, Manchester University NHS Foundation Trust, Manchester, UK.

Vessel mismatch can be mitigated by carefully selecting recipient and donor vessels, however is not uncommonly encountered. This is where either the recipient or donor artery is not of the correct or similar calibre (diameter) each another. This creates a technical challenge to the surgeon as this creates difficulty in alignment and increased likelihood of gaps, leaks or telescoping.

As discussed earlier in the text, when the anatomical layers of the vessels are not matched correctly with one another, this can lead to microtrauma of the intima and ultimately thrombosis and failure. In addition to this, mismatched vessels can create flow dynamic problems with turbulent blood flow, which can cause intima layer damage. Another concern with vessel mismatch is the haemodynamic imbalances across the anastomotic junction. Due to the difference in size there is usually a pressure differential from the larger to the smaller vessel, which increases the pressure on the vessel walls. In the presence of atherosclerotic disease, this can have a catastrophic consequence, with the pressure leading to tears or dissection within the vessel walls.

The first step to avoid vessel mismatch is in fact during the neck access (or neck dissection, depending on the surgical case). During the neck surgery, attempts should be to identify suitable vessels of equivalent calibre to the donor vessel on the flap. Normally, the facial artery is used; however, if a larger calibre vessel is required then it is possible to use distal end of the external carotid artery. The other potential vessel of choice is the lingual or superior thyroid artery branches.

Despite best efforts, it may not be possible to select vessels with the correct orientation, axis, and position which is a suitable calibre match therefore techniques should be utilized to mitigate this.

Different flaps have different sizes of donor arteries. In principle, if we take as the recipient standard the facial artery (most commonly used neck artery for flap anastomosis) then the radial forearm free flap, lateral thigh, and latissimus flaps display relatively small calibre mismatch. The fibula free flap usually has a large-bore artery and the DCIA flap has a small artery.

Calibre mismatch <1:2

In principle, with up to a 1:2 ratio calibre mismatch, the discrepancy can be evened out by differential distribution of the sutures. That means that if one artery is larger in calibre by factor 'l', then the space between the sutures on the bigger artery has to be wider by the same factor 'l' compared to the small artery (Figure 8.4.3).

That requires experience and visual judgement. For the less experienced surgeon then triangulation techniques will help with anchoring the edges of the vessels and then the following sutures will have to be placed in a fashion, slowly addressing any discrepancies.

An example of calibre mismatch anastomosis is demonstrated in Video 8.4.2.

Calibre mismatch 1:2 up to 1:3 ratio

'Slit' arteriotomy or 'fish-mouth' technique

When larger calibre discrepancies then an arteriotomy in the shape of a slit is often required in the smaller vessel. That will increase the opening of the lumen in a 'fish-mouth'-like configuration and help adapt the vascular edges of the smaller vessel onto the larger one (Figure 8.4.4).

It is important to emphasize that the arteriotomy (slit) has to be one single, clean cut, preferably with straight adventitia scissors or with sharp eye (Iris) scissors. This cut can be modified in length to achieve the desired size for anastomosis.

The end point of the arteriotomy must be very carefully sutured to the opposed edge of the larger vessel (Figure 8.4.5). In other words, the 'slit' cut results in an apex of the cut forming the most proximal part of the longitudinal arteriotomy. This is effectively the make-or-break

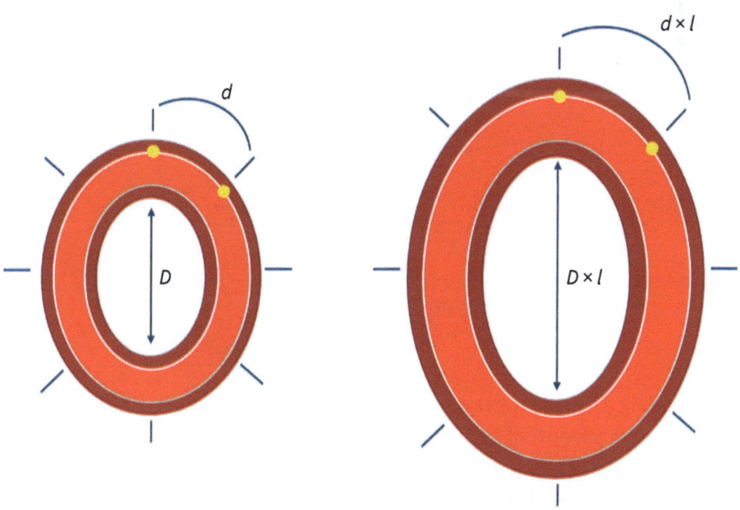

Figure 8.4.3 Schematic representation of the formula used to adjust the distance (gaps) between the sutures. If the calibre of the vessel (diameter) 'D' have a size difference (discrepancy) by factor 'l' then the distance 'd' between the sutures in the larger vessel has to be 'l' × wider than the distance between the sutures in the smaller vessel.

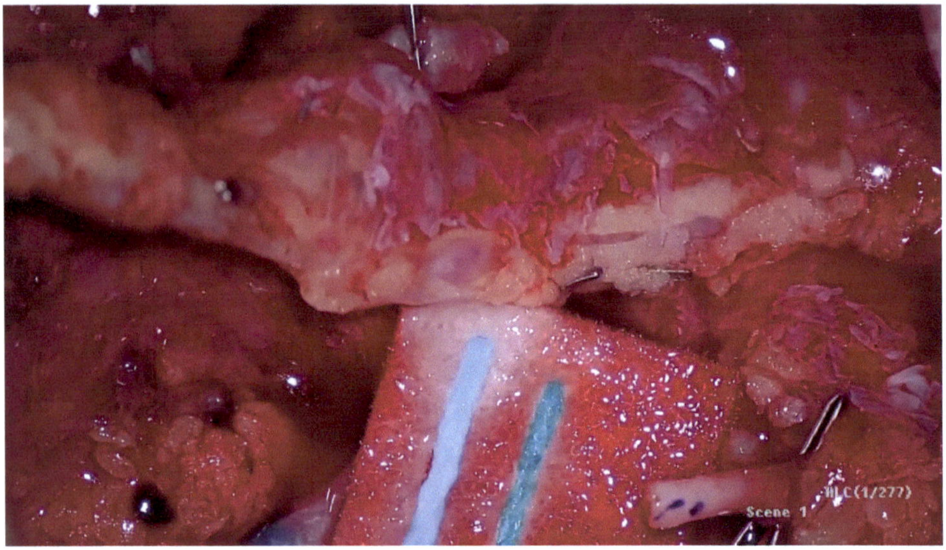

Video 8.4.2 Management of calibre mismatch.
See this video online by searching for this book's title or ISBN at https://academic.oup.com/
Reproduced courtesy of Leandros Vassiliou, Manchester University NHS Foundation Trust, Manchester, UK.

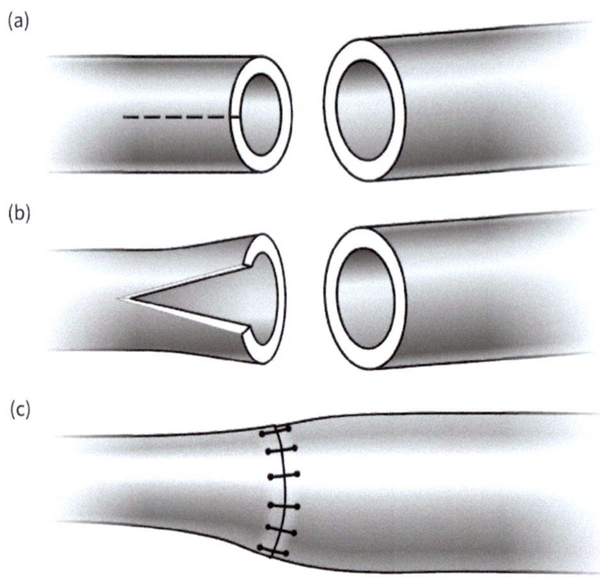

Figure 8.4.4 Managing a calibre mismatch over 1:2 ratio. a. Arteriotomy, a slit vertical cut performed with straight adventitia scissors. b. The artery is cut through full thickness, allowing this additional V-shaped cut to align with the opposing vessel wall. c. Completion of the anastomosis. In this technique, the end anastomosis will be funnel-shaped.

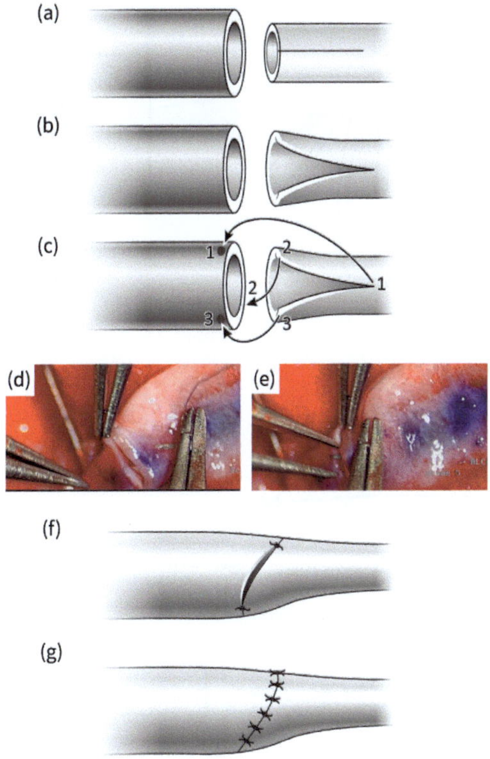

Figure 8.4.5 Further illustration of the technique of arteriotomy slit or 'fish-mouth' anastomosis. Note the position of sutures. a. Slit arteriotomy design. b. Full-thickness arteriotomy. c. Note the position of the crucial sutures. The corner sutures on each side of the slit arteriotomy (2 and 3) are crucial to eliminate the calibre mismatch. d. Suture number 1 is crucial to correctly oppose the vessels. e. The suture has to be passed separately from each vessel each time in order to better control the perpendicular trajectory and avoid suturing the back wall. f. Position of the vessels prior to completion of the anastomosis. g. Funnel-shaped product anastomosis.

of the anastomosis, as failure to oppose that edge of the vessel into the opposing artery may compromise the fate of the anastomosis.

When the vessel is advanced to meet the larger recipient, two flaps will envelope the larger vessel and such trimming may be required to allow approximation. The procedure then proceeds in the usual fashion as described earlier, achieving vessel anastomosis. Ongoing trimming of the vessel with the arteriotomy may be required throughout the anastomosis to ensure a balanced circumferential union, avoiding all the potential pitfalls described earlier in the text.

Bevelled-end arteriotomy

Another technique to overcome small to moderate-sized calibre discrepancies is to cut the smaller vessel in a bevelled fashion (Figure 8.4.6). The diameter of the vessel edge increases

(a)

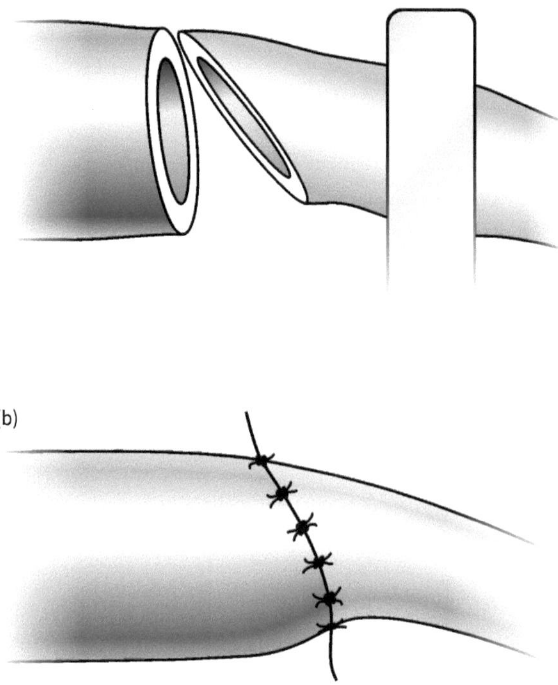

(b)

Figure 8.4.6 Managing a mismatch anastomosis with a mismatch ratio of 1:2 bevelled anastomosis. a. Note the bevel cut on the smaller vessel. The wider the angle of the bevel, the bigger the diversion in the axis of the anastomosis. b. Funnel-shaped anastomosis end product.

proportionately to the angle of the arteriotomy and may decrease or eliminate the calibre mismatch.

It is important to mention though that the bevelled arteriotomy will create an 'angle' in the final anastomosis, possibly diverting the blood flow and even risking formation of turbulent flow.

The bigger the angle of the arteriotomy (the more bevelled the edge) the more angulated the anastomosis will be. For this reason, the authors are not in favour of this approach for large vessel size discrepancies.

Calibre mismatch of a ratio more than 1:3

Such significant differences of over 1:3 ratio between the donor and recipient arteries are unusually met in the head and neck setting.

In this case, an arteriotomy will not work as it is in danger of rupturing the vessel completely or even causing an anastomosis blow out if the arteriotomy is carried out on the flap pedicle artery due to the significant amount of incoming pressure. It is best to partially suture the redundant opening of the larger vessel, forming a gracious 'funnel-shaped' anastomosis (Figure 8.4.7).

(a)

(b)

(c)

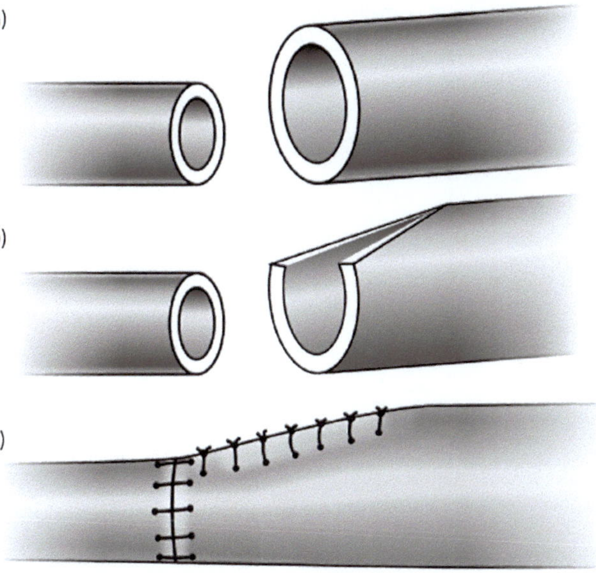

Figure 8.4.7 a. Management of calibre mismatch anastomosis over 1.3 ratio. b. Note the vessel wall arteriotomy on the larger vessel that will allow vertical suturing in order to eliminate the excess of tissue. c. The technique is similar to removing 'dog ears'.

Thickness mismatch

Vessel edge thickness mismatch is another common challenge encountered in arterial anastomosis. As different arteries from different flaps have variable tunica media, the vessel edge thickness may vary significantly.

If the bites of the vessel wall are uneven, the approximation will also be uneven. This can lead to telescoping of the vessels, where the side with the larger bite telescopes over the side of the smaller bite. This therefore leads to the vessel effectively narrowing its patency, as the entire vessel wall of the side with the smaller bite now sits within the lumen of the side with the larger bite. This typically creates turbulent and reduced flow within the vessel and ultimately flap perfusion. Furthermore, the intima of the side which has received the telescoped vessel is in direct contact with the tunica externa of the telescoped vessel. This may lead to microtrauma of the tunica intima and subsequent clot formation and catastrophic failure of the artery with thrombus formation.

The thickness mismatch is important to be addressed appropriately, as failure to do so may cause telescoping of the vessels or lumen obstruction with a potential detrimental impact on the success of the anastomosis.

It is important when addressing thickness mismatch to try and visualize the effect of every suture in the configuration of the lumen. In other words, the way that the thickness mismatch is dealt with or addressed will directly affect the shape or configuration of the endothelial wall's position.

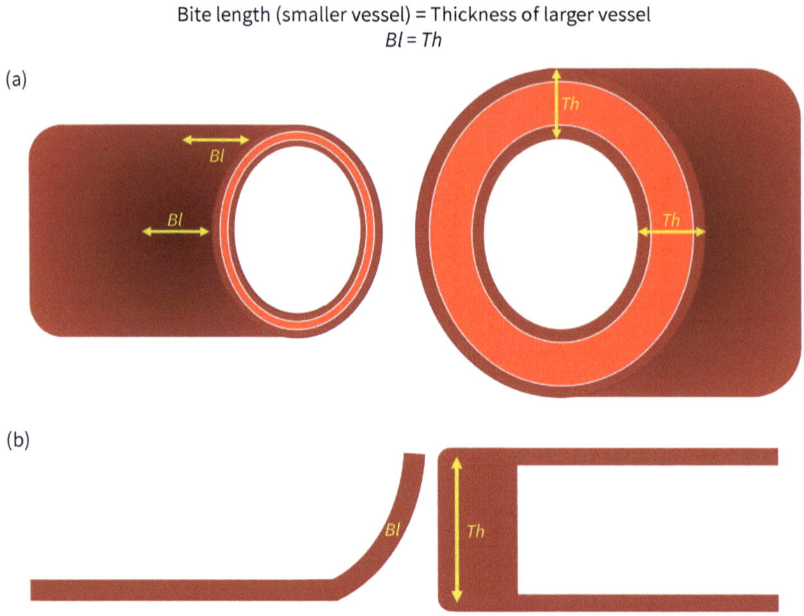

Figure 8.4.8 Managing thickness mismatch. a. Carefully calculate the vessel thickness mismatch. If the thickness of the wider vessel is 'Th', then the size (length) of the bite 'bl' on the smaller vessel has to equal the thickness of the larger vessel. b. Sagittal view of end vessel position demonstrating the small, thinner vessel edge wall laid out against the thick wall of the larger vessel. This is why 'bl' has to equal 'Th'.

It is important that the vessel with the thinner wall is sutured in such a fashion that its walls are laid against the thick edges of the larger vessel.

It is also important to first pass the needle on the thinner vessel so that when tying the knot, the thinner vessel is pulled against the thick wall of the larger vessel and gently aligned across its thick wall edge.

This is better displayed in Figure 8.4.8.

In order to achieve this, if the factor *Th* is the size of the larger vessel edge thick wall, then the suture bite length *Bl* on the thinner vessel (distance between vessel edge and needle entry or exit point) has to equal the same factor *Th* (Figure 8.4.8).

This being repeated in every suture around the 360-degree perimeter of the vessel will create a perfect position and a symmetrical funnel-shaped anastomosis. By doing so, the endothelium is protected, promoting a linear blood flow and preventing turbulence or areas of asymmetrical pressure (Figure 8.4.9).

An example of thickness mismatch anastomosis is demonstrated in Video 8.4.3.

Global mismatch

It is a common scenario that when the vessel sizes vary, then the mismatch involves both the calibre as well as the thickness. With experience and practice, a combination of the elements discussed in the predominantly 'calibre mismatch' and predominantly 'thickness mismatch', in the preceding paragraphs, will mitigate the issue (Video 8.4.4).

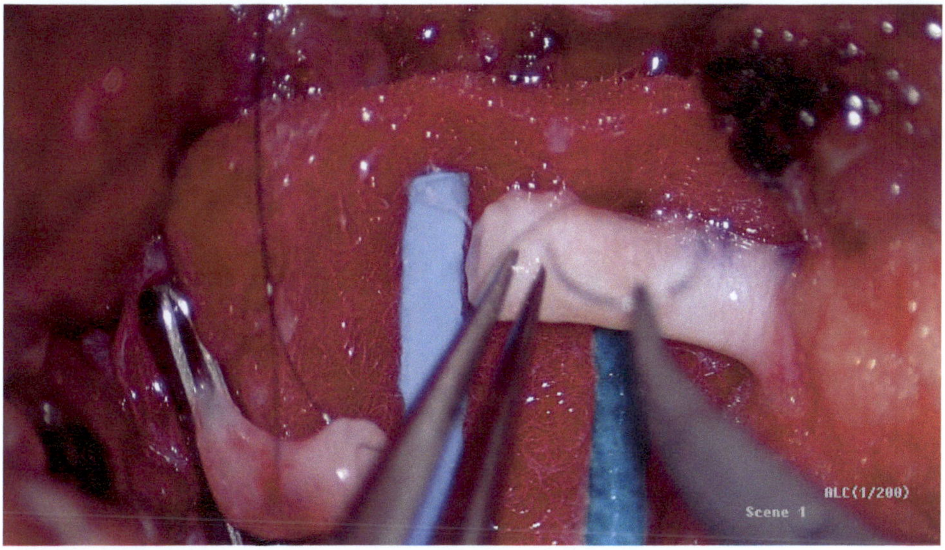

Video 8.4.3 Management of thickness mismatch.
See this video online by searching for this book's title or ISBN at https://academic.oup.com/
Reproduced courtesy of Leandros Vassiliou, Manchester University NHS Foundation Trust, Manchester, UK.

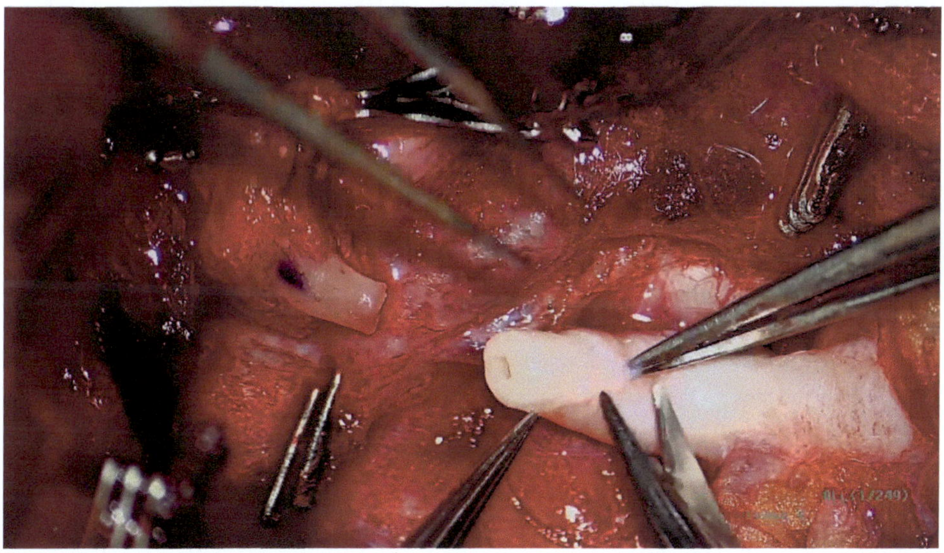

Video 8.4.4 Management of global size mismatch (calibre and thickness).
See this video online by searching for this book's title or ISBN at https://academic.oup.com/
Reproduced courtesy of Leandros Vassiliou, Manchester University NHS Foundation Trust, Manchester, UK.

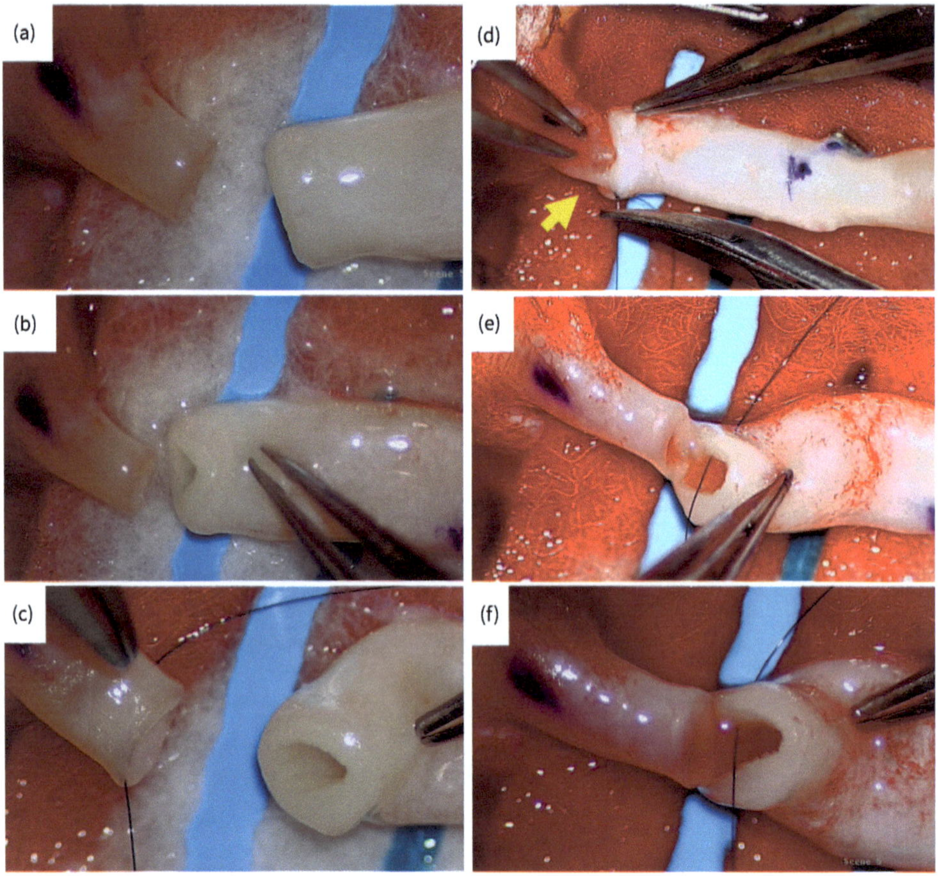

Figure 8.4.9 Sequence of managing vessel mismatch. a. Arteries are positioned prior to anastomosis. b. Note the significant calibre and mismatch. c. Suture passing first through the recipient vessel. The bite length equals the thickness of the larger vessel. d. Careful positioning of the vessels in order to tie the first sutures. e. Back-wall-first anastomosis demonstrating the placement of the first two strategic sutures. f. Note how the jeweller's forceps of the operator slightly pulls the adventitia of the larger vessel in order to visualize the lumen of the vessels. g. Carefully note the exit point of the needle in the thinner, smaller vessel (yellow arrow). That equals the principles that have been discussed in the previous chapter. h. Careful tying of the knot with the optimum tension without crushing the vessels. i. Gradual transition into the anterior wall. j. Tying square knots is crucial. k. Note the bite length between the two vessels, aiming to eliminate the size mismatch. l. Note the careful positioning of the jeweller's forceps by the assistant (yellow) in order to achieve vessel edge eversion and suturing of the thinner wall against the wall of the thicker, larger vessel. m. Last suture placement. Note that the penultimate stitch does not have a complete knot. That allows careful pulling of the knot of the adventitia in order to evert the vessel edge and control the lumen when placing the last stitch. n. Cannula and irrigation of the anastomosis through the untied penultimate stitch. o. The redundant fluid is coming out, achieving aversion of the vessel edge prior to tying the last knot (yellow arrow). p. The anastomosis is now running. Carefully note the symmetrical expansion and the healthy shape of this successful anastomosis.

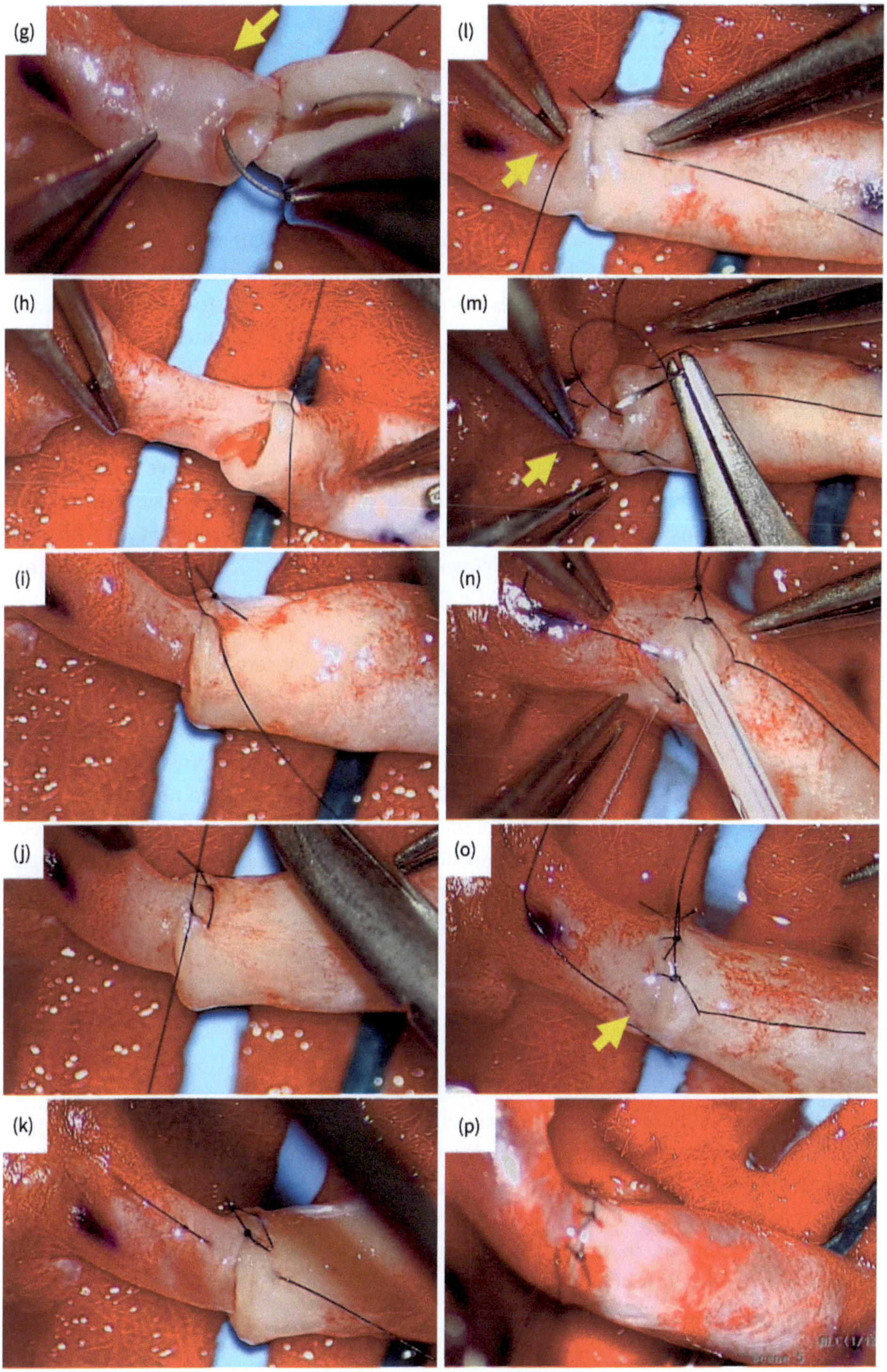

Figure 8.4.9 Continued

Atherosclerotic vessels

Atherosclerotic vessels represent a different challenge to the microvascular surgeon. Patients who are now fit to undergo microvascular surgery are often elderly with comorbidities. The ageing population brings with it new operative challenges for the microvascular surgeon, in particular with atherosclerotic vessels.

Atherosclerosis leads to increased calcification, a thickening of the vessel walls, which ultimately reduces compliance of the vessels. In addition to this, the thickened wall typically leads to a narrower lumen, which reduces blood flow distal to the anastomosis and increases the risk of thrombosis. The microvascular surgeon must pay careful attention to these factors, as suboptimal suturing techniques can lead to catastrophic failure of microvascular anastomosis.

Atherosclerotic vessels have fibrotic tunica media and are far less compliant and far more rigid when being handled by microvascular instruments. As a result, excessive force upon approximation of these vessels leads to intima dissection, tears, or complete avulsion of tissue. The surgeon must consider the patients' tissues and handle atherosclerotic vessels with extra care and attention as they are far less forgiving and have a higher risk of anastomotic failure.

Minimal vessel handling

Firstly, the surgeon must handle these vessels gently with great care as they are more fragile and prone to tearing.

Next, the surgeon must visually inspect the intima of the vessel to assess for atherosclerotic plaques. These plaques involve the tunica intima and media and appear as a raised area within the lumen of the vessel, typically with a fibrous cap. They should not be removed as any handling of the plaque leads to intimal damage and subsequent clot formation. Instead, the surgeon should remove the affected portion of the vessel, until there is a section visually inspected to be satisfactory with less atherosclerotic plaque. It is unlikely to find a part of the vessel unaffected by atherosclerotic disease, as this represents a systemic condition which will affect the vasculature throughout. Every stage of the microvascular suturing carries risk. From the outset as mentioned earlier, the vessel handling must be gentle with minimal manipulation.

Gentle dilation

Next, attention must be given to how much dilatation is performed within the vessel lumen. As discussed elsewhere in the text, vessel dilation is an important part of preparation; however, in the presence of atherosclerotic disease, this should be kept to a minimum due to the inelastic vessel walls increasing the likelihood of tears. The atherosclerotic plaque leads to abnormal tunica intima and media morphology and thus the risk of arterial intima dissection is highest when the needle is being passed through the layers of the artery.

Suturing technique

The author's preference to mitigate against the risk of intima dissection is to pass the suture in reverse from 'in' to 'out'. By adopting this approach, the suture effectively splints the intima and compresses the layers of the vessel. This tamponades any potential space for dissection and ensures a safer approximation of the vessel ends. By considering all this, the surgeon can mitigate against the risk of anastomotic failure in atherosclerotic disease. The aggregation of these factors is what leads to failure rather than any individual stage. By having an awareness of patients who are likely to suffer with atherosclerotic disease (peripheral vascular, ischaemic heart disease or previous transient ischaemic attacks or strokes) the surgeon is able to approach the surgery with caution and maximize their chances of success.

Further reading

Acland RD. *Practice Manual for Microvascular Surgery*. St Louis, MO: C.V. Mosby Company, 1989: p. 134.

Adam D, Broderick D, Kyzas P, Vassiliou L. Microvascular anastomotic coupler devices versus hand-sewn technique for arterial anastomosis: a systematic review. *Br J Oral Maxillofac Surg* 2021;59(5):524–33.

Ahn CY, Borud LJ, Shaw WW. Analysis of suturing techniques in the microvascular anastomosis of vessels of unequal diameter. *Ann Plast Surg* 1994;32(5):469–73.

Alghoul MS, *et al*. From simple interrupted to complex spiral: a systematic review of various suture techniques for microvascular anastomoses. *Microsurgery* 2011;31(1):72–80.

Aviles AJ, Theodorou S, Sekosen M, Schraufnagel D, Ramasastry S. Challenging Alexis Carrel: a study in alternate microvascular techniques. *Neurol Res* 2004;26(8):809–15.

Aygün H, Yildirim OS. Vertical mattress suture technique: an alternative vascular anastomosis. *J Reconstr Microsurg* 2008;24(6):397–404.

Blackburn CW, *et al*. A comparison of the minimal-touch technique and the eversion technique for microvascular anastomosis in a rat model. *J Reconstr Microsurg* 2017;33(2):97–102.

Chen YX, Chen LE, Seaber AV, Urbaniak JR. Comparison of continuous and interrupted suture techniques in microvascular anastomosis. *J Hand Surg Am* 2001;26(3):530–9.

Isogai N, Fukunishi K, Kamiishi H. Use of fibrin glue to minimize bleeding of microvascular repairs in hypertensive rats. *Microsurgery* 1992;13(6):321–4.

Krag C, Holck S. Microvascular anastomoses: a comparison of the end-to-end and the telescoped techniques in rats. *J Microsurg* 1980;2(1):3–10.

Lykoudis EG, Spyropoulou GA, Liadakis GN, Papaliodi ET. A new combined 'interrupted-continuous' microvascular anastomotic technique. Experimental study and clinical application. *J Reconstr Microsurg* 2008;24(2):79–84.

Rickard RF, McPhaden AR, Hudson DA. Healing of two microarterial anastomoses with diameter mismatch. *J Surg Res* 2014;191(1):239–49.e3.

Simşek T, Eroglu L, Engin MS, Kaplan S, Yildiz L. End-to-end microvascular anastomosis in the rat carotid artery using continuous horizontal mattress sutures. *J Reconstr Microsurg* 2006;22(8):631–40.

Sullivan B, Zoppo M, Yao A, Henderson PW. Simple interrupted microvascular anastomosis: review of four sutures placement sequences. *J Reconstr Microsurg Open* 2020;5:e101–6.

Tetik C, Unal MB, Kocaoglu B, Erol B. Use of continuous horizontal mattress suture techniques in microsurgery: an experimental study in rats. *J Hand Surg Am* 2005;30(3):587–95.

Topalan M, Bilgin SS, Ip WY, Chow SP. Effect of torsion on microarterial anastomosis patency. *Microsurgery* 2003;23(1):56–9.

Watanabe H, Ueda K, Ohkouchi M, Kajikawa A, Suzuki Y. Posterior-wall-first continuous suturing combined with conventional interrupted suturing for microvascular anastomosis. *J Reconstr Microsurg* 2006;22(8):617–23.

9
Techniques for anastomosis

Vein

Basim E.S. Dawoud, Phil Pirgousis, Leandros Vassilios F. Vassiliou, Panayiotis Kyzas, and Nicholas Kalavrezos

9.1 **Considerations in venous anastomosis: Vessel selection and orientation**

Introduction

The stages of venous anastomosis should not be considered a repeat of the arterial one (Chapter 8). There are fundamental differences in the anatomy and function of veins, and these require a completely different mindset and skillset than the arterial anastomosis.

The main differences between veins and arteries derive from their distinct functional purpose which translates to structural differences in the vessel wall. Veins are in principle low-pressure blood vessels, the blood flow in neck veins is directed caudally, and there are a number of valves especially in the junctions of tributaries.

The vein is almost always anastomosed after the arterial anastomosis is completed, which means that blood is flowing through the vessel and this either inevitably will obscure the field of the anastomosis, or the vessel has to be transiently clamped, which means the venous anastomosis has to be performed quickly.

All those differences dictate modifications not only in vessel handling, but the whole preparation and execution of anastomosis.

Structural differences from an artery

In general, the wall of the vein is far thinner (as they function under lower pressure) than the artery. However, in contrast to the artery, the venous tunica externa is thicker with a larger amount of connective tissue.

The tunica media is considerably thinner or almost non-existent than the artery. There are fewer smooth muscle and elastin fibres within the wall. Due to how little smooth muscle tissue the vein wall has, they are collapsible but also dilate easily.

Due to the wall's poor ability to maintain its shape and structure, identifying the lumen can be challenging.

The intima also is very thin and due to the nature of the vein to shrink or dilate is often rich in folds. This can risk inadvertently catching the back wall with the micro-suture.

There is also rich perivascular loose tissue but quite adherent venous adventitia. This is entirely different to arterial adventitia and for the beginner microsurgeon, challenging to identify the correct plane for dissection during dissection and preparation. Without due care and caution, it is easy to wrap the vessel within the perivascular tissues, thereby obliterating the lumen.

This structure of the vessel renders the walls prone to damage, in particular to the delicate intima and media layers.

It is therefore essential that vessel handling is kept only to the adventitia, and instrumentation of the intima is kept to an absolute minimum. Extra care should be taken to carefully identify the vessel walls and edges, otherwise anastomosis could fail due to incorrect vessel approximation.

Timing—clamping

The venous anastomosis differs from the arterial, in the sense that it is often performed under time pressure and duress.

This is because it is the general practice of the microsurgeons to first perform the arterial anastomosis.

This is completely justified as one of the markers or indicators for the success of a patent arterial anastomosis is the volume and rate of blood outflow through the non-anastomosed veins.

It is also sensible to perform the arterial anastomosis first to minimize ischaemia time and get the flap perfused as soon as possible.

This, and in flaps with one vein only (radial forearm free flap with a conjoined single vein, latissimus dorsi/scapula, ALT, DCIA) means that during the vein anastomosis the venous outflow the vein has to be clamped and hence the flap outflow is transiently blocked. For many, this carries the risk of flap congestion and damage to microcirculation. For this reason, some surgeons prefer to perform the venous anastomosis first. There is no literature evidence that one technique is superior to the other; what matters most is the technical perfection of both anastomoses.

The duration of venous clamping has to be kept to a minimum. The venous anastomosis must be performed as soon as possible, speed is of the essence, but this should not compromise the precision and quality of the anastomosis.

This is one of the reasons why the venous anastomosis must follow a step-by-step systematic approach in order to be standardized, reducible, and hence after a learning curve and some practice formed efficiently and with time economy.

When the anastomosis takes longer or when the vein seems visibly engorged medial to the clamp, then transient release of the clamp to allow the blood to drain for a few minutes and then re-clamping of the vein with irrigation to resume the anastomosis is a possibility.

For flaps with more than one vein (radial forearm free flap or fibula free flap) then clamping one of the veins does not carry this concern.

Valves

Valves can be recognized as vessel wall baloon-like dilations at the junctions of confluent veins. This is important during the vessel selection and preparation for the anastomosis.

It is not uncommon to think that an adequate length of IJV tributary has been left for an end-to-end anastomosis, only to find out when cutting the edge of the vein that this stump contains a valve and hence the anastomosis cannot be performed on the site of the valve.

Another important fact regarding venous valves is that when the valves are present due to their structural and functional purpose, they prevent blood returning backwards. This refers to microvascular surgeons that during the vessel preparation and vessel check in order to ascertain patency expect to see blood flowing through the vein. In the presence of a venous valve more distally in the junction of a tributary to the IJV or further caudally in the external jugular vein, the surgeon may perform the venotomy and with a vein unclamped, expecting to see the blood returning with no result. This shouldn't discourage the surgeon from forming the impression that there is a vessel obstruction.

The lack of black blood return is most likely due to the presence of a valve. In order to test the patency, a heparinized syringe with a cannula is inserted into the vascular lumen and heparinized saline is pushed through the vein. if there is no resistance, then that confirms the patency of the vessel.

Passive flow—low pressure

Of crucial importance is the vessel's propensity for large thrombus formation even with small insults to the intima. The flow through the vein is slower and thus platelets readily stick to any site of endothelial injury and will subsequently rapidly propagate a thrombus. Any inaccuracy in suture placement can lead to trauma and ultimately endothelial damage with thrombus formation and ultimately venous failure. It is important to note that the placement of the sutures can be circumferentially further away from one another than in the artery. As the venous system is under lower pressure, the vessel doesn't require a tighter intersuture approximation.

It is important to understand that the veins are low-pressure systems. They do not actively pump blood, such as the arteries, but instead passively receive and divert it as passive drainpipes towards the heart. The veins are passive drains, and they lack structural stability (lack of vessel wall stability) and are easy to collapse and kink. The microsurgeon has to consider every possible parameter on interrupted blood flow when choosing the correct site and vessel for the anastomosis.

The recipient vein must always sit more caudally than the position of the pedicle (donor) vein, and the anastomosis must encourage a direction of blood flow from cephalad to caudal. This is to avoid any anti-gravity direction of blood flow that may result in stasis, thrombosis, and failure.

The above does not refer to flaps with long pedicles, where the pedicle can gently curve low in the neck prior to forming a lazy 'S' configuration upwards, reaching the site of the venous anastomosis slightly higher up. It refers to the actual anastomosis, not sitting higher than the pedicle (donor) vein, and the direction of the blood flow should point downwards (see Figure 9.1.1).

Transferring those to the surgical reality, good recipient veins could be the following:

- For relatively short pedicles or contralateral anastomosis is the facial vein (unless care has been taken as described in Chapters 6 and 7 to form a gracious curvature of the pedicle).

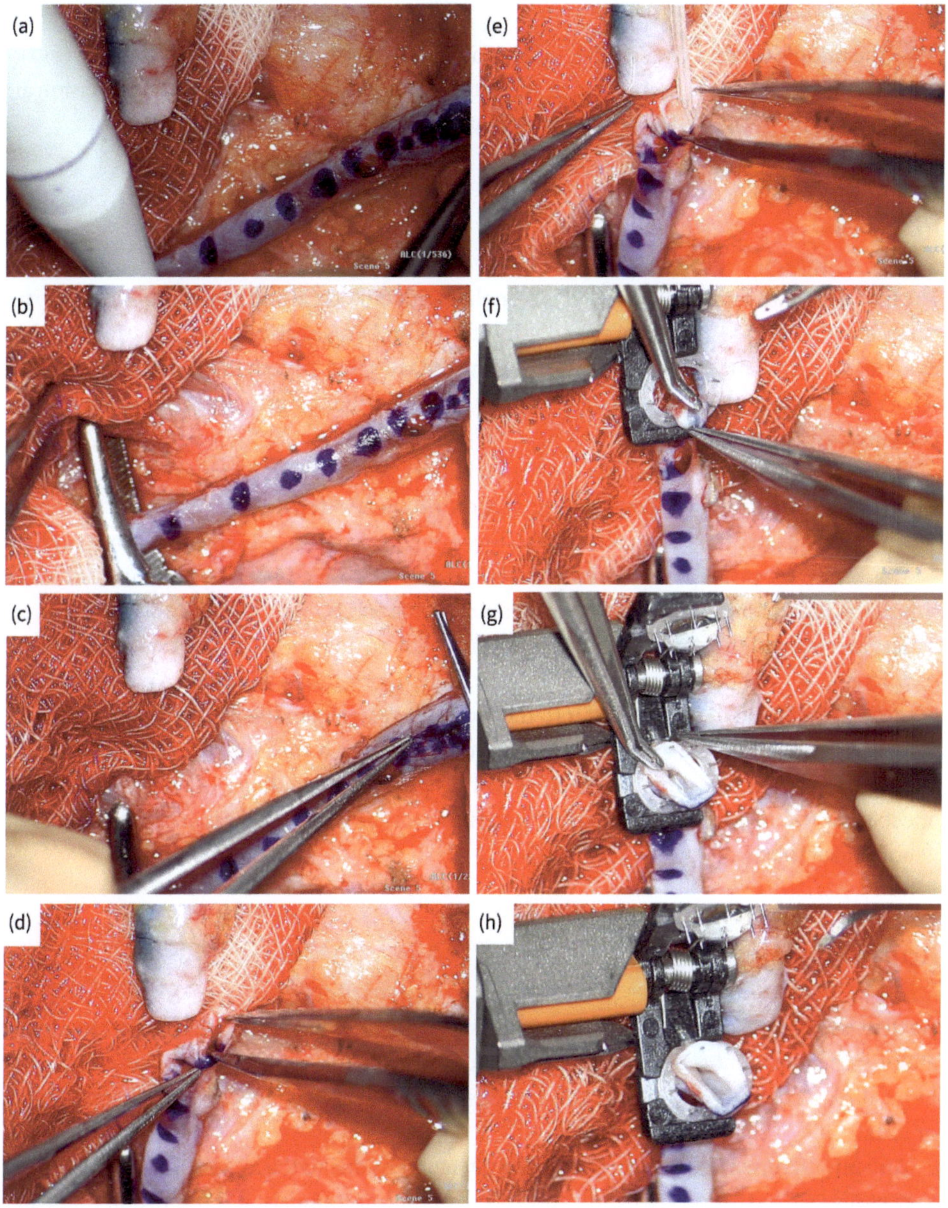

Figure 9.1.1 a. The external jugular vein is selected as the recipient vein. The length of the vein prior to division is dotted to mark the correct orientation and position at passive rest of the vessel. b. A small bulldog clamp is applied prior to division. c. The vessel is prepared for division. d. The vessel has been divided and is slowly rotated to approximate the donor vein (above). In this figure, a gentle dilation of the vessel end is demonstrated. e. Irrigation with heparinized saline to clean the lumen of the recipient vessel. f. Maintenance of the correct orientation is crucial. Note the dotted surface of the vein as the vessel end is carefully passed through the coupler ring. It is important that the pin that the superior vessel edge is fixed will not cause any twist of the vessel. g. Progress of pinning the vessel edge on the coupler. h. Pinning of the vessel is almost complete. Note the correct orientation of the vessel and the maintenance of the position as shown on the dots. If the dots were not present, it would be easy for the operator to inadvertently twist the vein, that would cause compromise of the anastomosis.

- The middle thyroid or an end-to-side anastomosis at that level (of the middle thyroid).
- If the anastomosis is performed in the external jugular vein (EJV), then EJV division at a low point in the neck may fulfil the above criteria.

Physics

The blood flow within the blood vessels complies with biological and molecular biology principles but also obeys the laws of physics. In physics and engineering fluid dynamics, hydrodynamics, or fluid mechanics describe the physical laws that govern the flow of fluids. These refer to a complex system of laws and actions that describe the principles of flow velocities, pressures, and tubing configuration.

One of the main law of physics is the Venturi Effect, which is the reduction in fluid pressure when fluid flows through a constriction section which also termed as a 'choke'. The Venturi Effect is named after the Italian physicist, Giovanni Battista Venturi in the eighteenth century.

The Bernoulli principle essentially describes that the speed/velocity for fluid increases simultaneously with the decrease of its pressure (static) or its energy.

The meaning of the above is that in the context of an anastomosis, the leaner flow of the recipient vessel and the partial restriction due to the anastomosis will cause a partial vacuum that will allow blood to be pumped into the recipient vessel from the flap outflow.

This in principle protects the venous anastomosis from a thrombosis, as apart from the positive outflow of pressure that emerges from the flap outflow, there is a negative pressure effect from the recipient vessel that acts against venous stasis, risking and predisposing a venous thrombosis.

Approximation

As discussed in the previous chapters, approximation and correct orientation of the vessels about to be anastomosed is of crucial importance. For the venous anastomosis it is even more important, as the veins, for the reasons described above, are easy to collapse, rotate, or kink.

Any misalignment of the veins, which easily happens due to the lack of structural stability, may easily lead to torsion (twisting) and failure of the anastomosis. It is important that when the recipient base vein is chosen prior to division, it is marked and dotted in its original position (Figure 9.1.1). After a vein is ligated and divided, it is very easy for the vessel to twist, and it's very difficult to identify its original configuration and orientation.

If the EJV is the candidate recipient vein, then we strongly advise to avoid dividing it until the time of the anastomosis. This will maintain the integrity of the orientation of the vessel and will avoid any twisting. If the vein is divided and left long during neck dissection, as the field often gets dry it is very likely that it will sustain an element of twisting and hence it will be very difficult to find the exact orientation prior to performing the anastomosis.

Any candidate recipient veins are advised to be dotted and maintain markings of the correct orientation during the neck dissection.

For end-to-side anastomosis onto the internal jugular vein (IJV) the venotomy is ideally placed along the line of the IJV tributaries. As for an end-to-side anastomosis, the IJV has to be completely mobilized and with the clamps will sustain some degree of twisting.

It is important that the venotomy site from a sagittal plane perspective is demarcated by a line that passes through all the tributaries.

Double clamps

Double clamps are useful for performing venous anastomosis, especially for the less experienced microvascular surgeon.

The vascular clamps for end-to-side anastomosis can easily suspend the two vessels. Care should be taken to leave enough length for the vessels to be handled.

If the triangulation technique is used, then the vascular clamp maintains the optimum distance between the vessels. Due to the nature of the vein's structure for an end-to-end anastomosis, it is easy to flip the clamp as the veins are more flexible and accept a transient twist more easily than the arteries.

9.2 **Hand-sewn techniques: End-to-end anastomosis**

Introduction

The microvascular surgeon should be aware of the challenges associated with venous anastomosis which are unique to this vessel over the artery.

From the outset, extra care and attention should be paid during vessel preparation to ensure the correct layer is being dissected out.

Overhandling the vein leads to tears, intima injury, and thrombus formation far easier than in the artery. In addition to this, the vessel is prone to in-rolling due to the thinner walls and lack of smooth muscle meanings the walls do not hold their structure well.

With careful attention to these common areas of challenges and a methodological step-by-step system in performing the anastomosis, the microvascular surgeon is able to maximize the chances of success.

Preparation for the anastomosis—the concept of 'hydrodistension'

As discussed in the text earlier, preparation of the vessels should be done carefully with correct orientation, alignment, and matching of vessel calibre. Using contrast material as a background can often help with the identification of the lumen.

During placement of clamps on the vein, ensure enough vein tissue is introduced distal to the clamp in order to allow passive approximation of the tissues.

The first step is to gently rinse the vein lumen with heparinized saline. As the vein walls are collapsible, without good irrigation, the walls will no longer be clearly apparent. Maintaining a generous amount of irrigant in the surgical field will keep the walls slightly distended and thus easier to identify and begin suturing.

Once the set-up is complete, introduce a vessel dilator within the lumen and carefully dilate the wall. It may take time to identify the vessel wall and this stage should not be rushed, as this can cause micro trauma to the intima. If the dissection around the vein has been done correctly, there should be almost no adventitia remaining. Take care to trim off any loose pieces of adventitia, rather than allowing them to fall within the lumen.

Due to the structure of the vein wall and the partial moist of the surgical field, the vascular edges of the veins tend to collapse. The most frequent technical errors in venous anastomosis are the following:

- Inadvertent capture of the back wall;
- Inversion of the vessel wall edges into the lumen; or
- Inclusion of adventitia.

All these are as a result of the poor visibility and ability of separation of the vessel walls because of the collapsibility of this type of vessel.

In contrast to suturing arteries—and this is the principle different between arterial and venous anastomosis—the venous anastomosis needs to be conducted in a wet environment. This can be achieved either with frequent irrigation with heparinized saline or creation of a small 'pool' around the anastomosis site, where this can be flooded with heparinized saline and leave the two veins to be anastomosed, floating within transparent liquid.

The liquid environment helps the vessel walls to separate and unstick. They remain open and hence more visible and accessible for the process of microsuturing.

Hydrodistension: Irrigation within the lumen of the anastomosis of heparinized saline under mild pressure distends the vessel and expands the vessel walls, making the target vessel edge much clearer to see (Figure 9.2.1).

The liquid medium also makes any loose adventitia tissue float rather than stick onto the vessel wall, and hence it becomes identifiable to the microsurgeon for this to be trimmed and not allowed to be caught by accident within the anastomosis.

Using a syringe of heparinized saline, the lumen of the veins is frequently irrigated with a little bit of pressure so that the vessel walls expand, which allows for a far more precise calculation of the distances between the sutures and also a safe assessment of the back wall and the process of the anastomosis as sutures are placed circumferentially.

Hydrodistension, especially towards the last sutures, will help evert the lips of the vessel edge and flush out of the lumen any redundant hanging adventitia tissues.

Triangulation techniques

It is important to emphasize that the size of the bite when performing a venous anastomosis has to be a very small, almost one or two times the thickness of the thin wall. The veins are low pressure systems therefore big bites are not required as only approximation of the vessel edges is needed. Big bites carry the risk of inadvertent inversion or crushing of the vein edges. The thin bites facilitate better expansion of the vessel wall for precise approximation of the vessel walls.

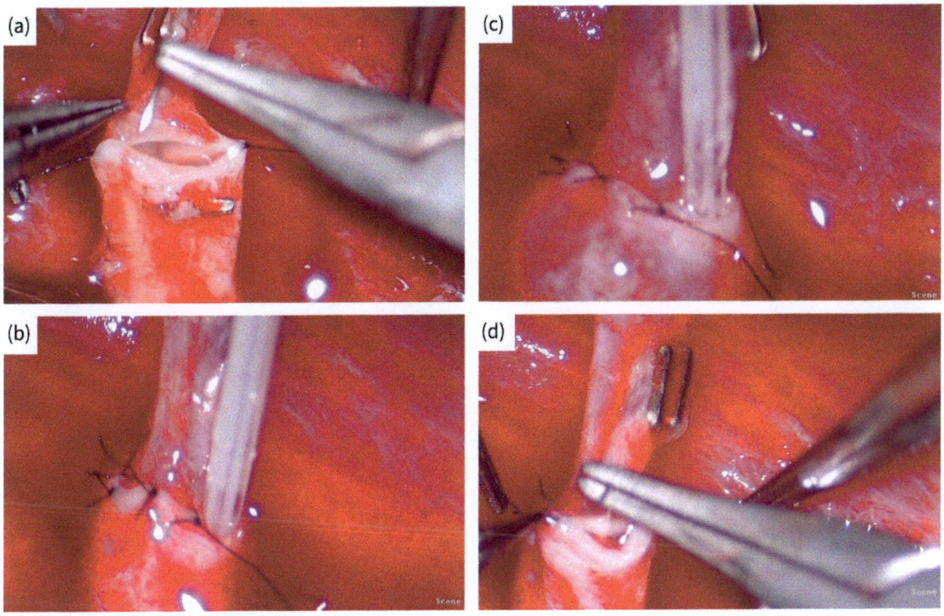

Figure 9.2.1 Technique of 'hydrodistension'. a. This venous end-to-end anastomosis is being performed using the technique of hydrodistension. Note the 'wet' environment with ample fluid to prevent collapse of vessel walls and to allow visibility of the vessel edges. The technique of 180 degrees is used. b. Further suturing has commenced. Note the tip of the heparinized saline cannula, which is introduced into the lumen of the vessels in the remaining gap between the sutures. c. As heparinized saline irrigates the lumen of the vessels with gentle pressure, the veins distend. That allows the operator to assess the anastomosis for any gaps and of course any impinged intima. d. As the fluid slowly flows out of the vessel after the hydrodistension, the vessel edges spontaneously evert outwards to allow the last sutures to be placed. The transparency of the clear fluid also allows good visibility for the operator to pass the needle through both vessel edges.

Triangulation techniques are very useful when performing venous anastomosis (Figure 9.2.2). The first two sutures suspend the opposite sites and help establish the base for the anastomosis. The suture edges remain long for the assistant and the operator to be able to rotate the vessel and access the back wall. Rotation of the vein, especially in an end-to-end anastomosis, is much easier as the veins are principally much more stretchable and flexible.

As the first suture is about to be placed, double-check that you can clearly see the vein wall, and there is a clear path of entry and exit of the needle. Do not rush the first suture, as incorrect placement here can compromise the remaining sutures. Most of the time, any faults with vein anastomosis come from not clearly seeing the vessel edge. This therefore leads to inaccurate placement of the suture. In order to maximize the chances of passing the needle through the vessel wall ensure you have good lighting and sufficient magnification, along with a well irrigated surgical field.

Although liberal use of irrigant in the surgical field is encouraged, sometimes it can be counterproductive with the light from the microscope being reflected back up the lenses causing discomfort. If this is the case, then change the angulation of the microscope to reflect the light elsewhere.

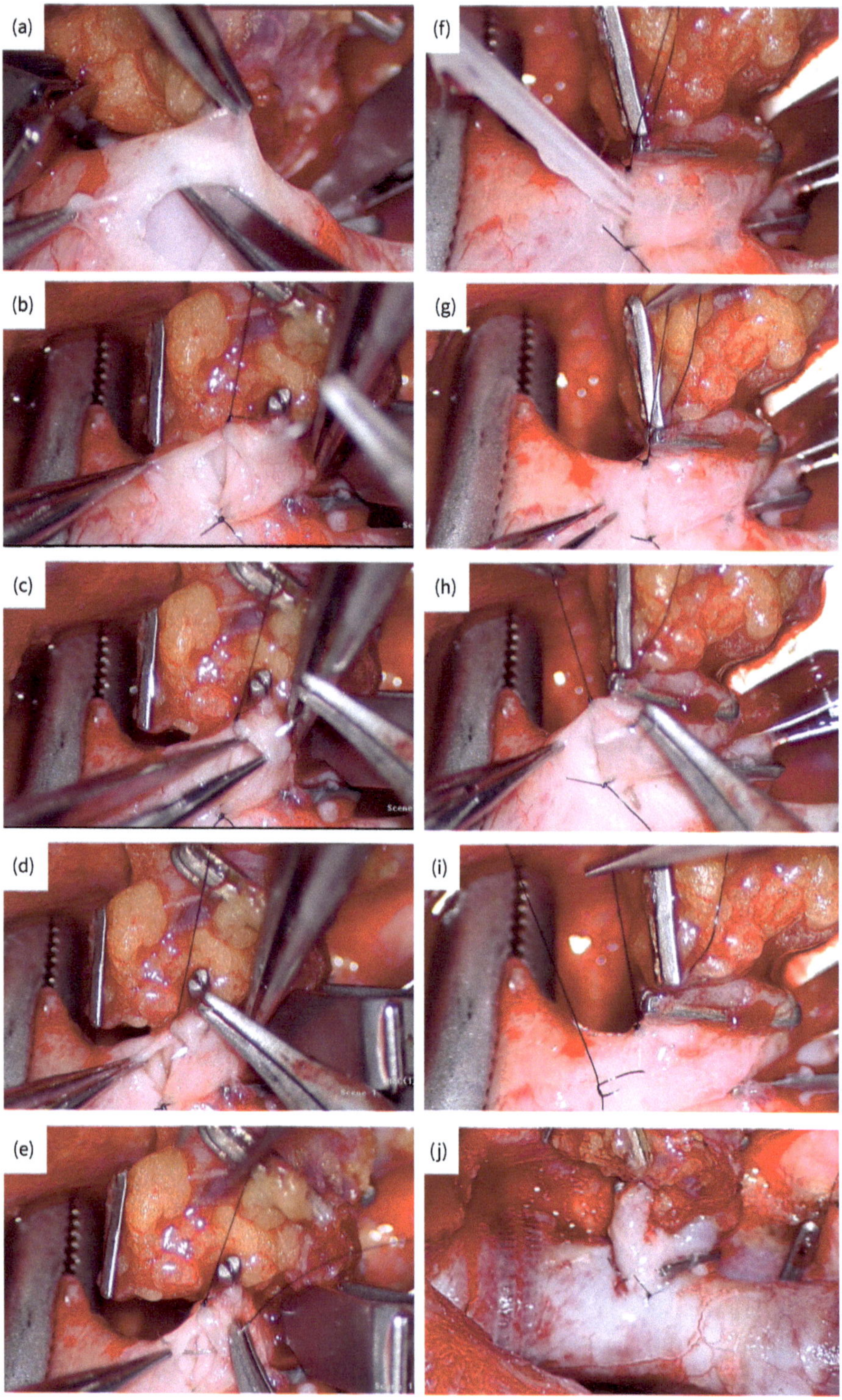

(a)
(b)
(c)
(d)
(e)
(f)
(g)
(h)
(i)
(j)

Figure 9.2.2 Sequence of end-to-end anastomosis utilizing the 120-degree triangulation technique. a. Note the adventitia preparation and the clean vessel edges on the recipient vein. The tip of the instrument is running on the inside of the vessel edge to allow assessment of the vessel wall thickness. b. The first two strategic sutures have been placed. c. With gentle retraction of the two sutures, further suturing of the anterior wall is commenced. Note that the dilator is gently introduced and tenting up the vessel edge in order to allow smooth passing and better control of the needle. d. The needle to has to pass separately (in two goes) through the respective vessel edges. The operator is pulling away the vessel edge from the recipient vein to allow the needle to rotate outwards. e. The needle is now passed through the second vessel edge from inside out, with the adventitia suspended with jeweller's forceps. f. The technique of hydrodistension is utilized the vessels are 'ballooned' up with heparinized saline to allow targeting the next entry and exit points. g. The vessels are full of heparinized saline, and the vessel edges are spontaneously approximating, guiding the operator as to the passage of the next stitch. h. The needle is passed through one side. Note the silhouette of the needle inside the lumen through the thin wall of the donor vein. i. A square knot is tied. j. That is the end of the venous anastomosis, showing even placement of sutures.

The sequence of suture placement is the same as for artery suturing (described elsewhere in the text).

A variation of the triangulation technique is to suspend one corner (e.g. the cephalad one) to continue with suturing the posterior wall and when placing the suture in the inferior-most corner (3 o'clock), leave it long. With traction of the two corner sutures (the first one, 9 o'clock, and the inferior-most one, 3 o'clock) suturing of the anterior wall becomes much easier, especially with constant flushing of the lumen with irrigant and utilizing the principle of hydrodistension.

Back-wall-first anastomosis

Back-wall-first anastomosis can be used to suture the back wall first, as it is this side of the vessel that carries the greatest risk of 'through' suturing.

It is important that when performing the back wall, the principle of hydrodistension is applied, so that the back wall separates visibly from the anterior wall, the flaps are rolled out, and the vessel edges are much easier to control (Figure 9.2.2f).

Place the needle through the vein wall, entering the lumen, crucially under direct vision. The surgeon must ensure the angulation of sutures mirrors that of a 'forehand' stitch. This will allow the most ergonomic and efficient movements during suturing. The next bite is the exit of the needle from within the lumen on the opposing side, which must be equidistant to the entry bite. This ensures the correct approximation of the vessel edges without any bunching or telescoping of vessels. Care must be taken to ensure that the needle has entered the lumen and not just taken a bite of adventitia.

Due to the thicker layer of externa (compared with arteries) with a corresponding thin layer of intima and media, it is possible to partially pass the needle through adventitia, without actually entering the lumen. This therefore causes the vein wall to roll in on itself without correct approximation of the walls.

As you make the entry bite into the lumen, pass the tip of the instrument in the non-dominant hand within the lumen of the vessel to open it up and guard against taking a bite of the opposing wall. This also serves as a support to the vessel intima wall, aiming to slightly roll the edge of the vessel outwards (everting the edges), thus mitigating against 'in-rolling' of the vein wall.

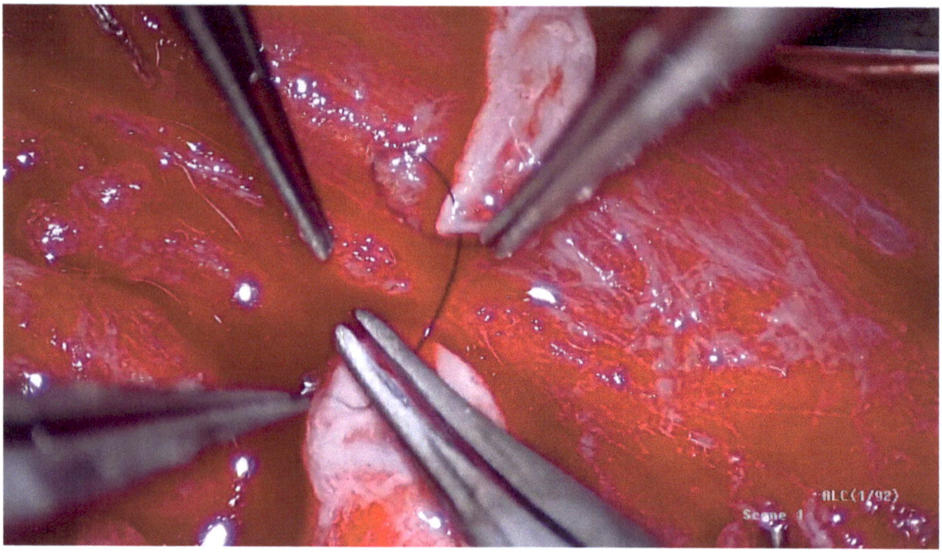

Video 9.2.1 Venous anastomosis. End-to-end with size mismatch and using hydrodistention technique.
See this video online by searching for this book's title or ISBN at https://academic.oup.com/
Reproduced courtesy of Leandros Vassiliou, Manchester University NHS Foundation Trust, Manchester, UK.

When exiting the vein wall, pass the needle slightly beyond the vessel edge. This will allow the vein wall to be everted slightly and once again will guard against in-rolling. Ensure the area is generously covered in heparinized saline and continue to inflate the vessel with the solution, to ensure the walls can be clearly seen.

As the suturing progresses and the view within the lumen diminishes, there should be liberal use of heparinized saline. This will allow dilation of the vein walls, which have a high propensity to adhere to one another without sufficient irrigant. It will also allow distention of the vein walls, allowing for an easier passage of the needle.

Prior to placement of the final sutures, it is possible to gently insert the blunt-ended tip of the irrigant solution container (usually the plastic sheath of a fine-bore cannula) and irrigate the junction. Check for equal distension across the anastomosis with filling both distally and proximally. When placing the final few sutures, ensure the vein is generously filled with the solution to try and minimize the chances of through suturing the back wall.

The sequence of an end-to-end venous anastomosis with global size mismatch is demonstrated in Video 9.2.1.

Completion of the anastomosis and release of the clamps

Upon completion of anastomosis the distal clamp is removed first, followed by the proximal. The vein walls should dilate instantly at the site of the anastomosis, if this is slow (assuming there is no arterial outflow obstruction) then there should be a low threshold for internally inspecting the vein due to the high chance of through stitching.

The usual check of vessel patency can ensue, with vessel uplifting where an instrument is gently placed under the vessel and moved proximally and distally. With the movement of the instrument, the vein wall is just lightly occluded and then released, allowing brisk filling of the vein behind the instrument.

This check should be performed both distal and proximal to the site of anastomosis. If there is a blockage of the vein, the filling test will be negative and the vein distal to the anastomosis will be more dilated than proximally. In addition to this, the blood will visibly become darker with time, reflecting blood associated with venous stasis.

9.3 **Hand-sewn techniques: End-to-side anastomosis**

Introduction

End-to-side anastomosis is not usually the primary method of choice when planning venous anastomosis. However, despite attempts to identify a suitable recipient vein of similar calibre it may not be possible to isolate a suitable match. As discussed in the text above, the identification of suitable recipient veins should be conducted throughout the neck dissection (or neck access) surgery. Any potential suitable veins should be kept as long as feasibly possible, including the external jugular vein that should remain undivided.

End-to-side is a technically demanding procedure, which typically involves utilizing the side of the internal jugular vein (IJV) (Figure 9.3.1). This is the most common vein used and the ensuing discussion will be regarding the IJV as the recipient vein.

Selection of site

The stages of this procedure start with the mobilization of the IJV. This is first done without the use of the microscope and can be done during the neck dissection (or neck access

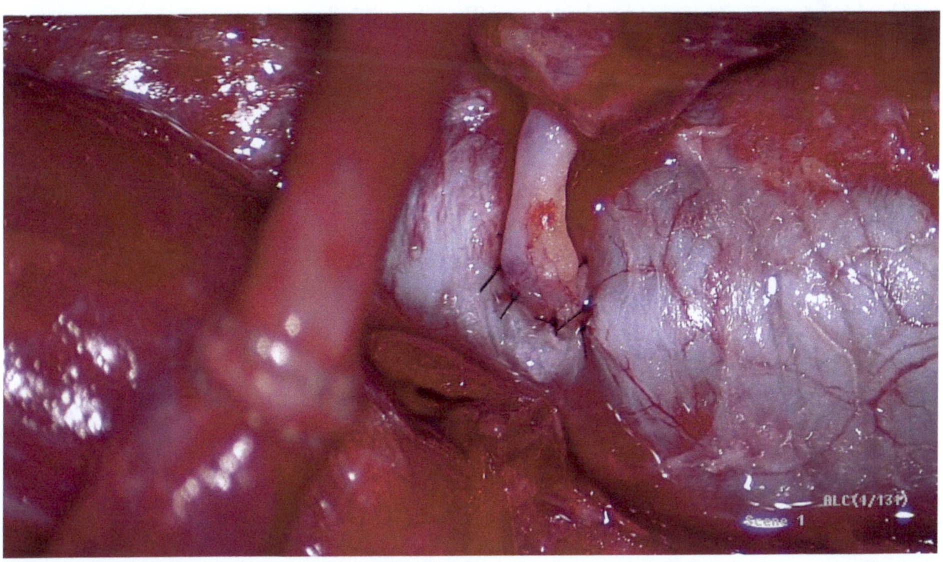

Figure 9.3.1 End-to-side anastomosis of a relatively small VC to the internal jugular vein at the centre of the picture. Note that above a second end-to-end venous anastomosis to the external jugular vein with couplers has been performed.

procedure). It is the authors' preference to circumferentially dissect around the IJV so that all sides of the vein can be controlled. It is worth ensuring this is done prior to the introduction of the microscope as this can be done using the usual surgeon's loupe magnification. This has the advantage that the surgeon is able to see the entire length of the IJV.

In addition to this, the IJV must be mobilized by ligation of all corresponding tributaries, in order to allow passive approximation of the donor vein to the side. Once the vein has been circumferentially isolated, with all tributaries that could impede venous anastomosis ligated, attention can then turn to preparing the donor vein under microscope magnification. The preparation for which proceeds in the usual fashion as described earlier.

The most frequent mistake of an end-to-side anastomosis is the performance of the venotomy when the IJV is twisted with the clamps, only to find out after completion of the anastomosis that the junction of the pedicle vein is kinked when the IJV returns back to its original formation.

The imaginary line that connects all the tributaries is the line where the veins transverse almost at a 45-degree angle anterolaterally in the neck, being protected from kinking or compression from the overlying sternocleidomastoid muscle structure.

Again, if performing end-to-side anastomosis it is advisable that the line that connects the tributaries is carefully dotted to guide after clamping of the IJV, the correct equator site for the venotomy.

Once the IJV has been mobilized and the donor vein prepared the surgeon must turn their attention to the planned site of venotomy. The advantage of the end-to-side anastomosis is that the microsurgeon can determine the optimum site for anastomosis. There are a number of factors which must be considered prior to making the venotomy on the IJV wall.

The first is by observing the optimal (and most passive) path of the donor vein to the IJV side wall. The donor vein must be laid out passively without any kinking or twists in the pedicle to see where it seats in relation to the IJV. It is preferable to not leave the course of the pedicle too short as turning of the head away from the site of anastomosis, can lead to excessive tension across the anastomotic junction. In contrast, a lengthy pedicle will lead to increased likelihood of twisting and kinking due to excessive redundant tissue. Therefore, it is dependent upon the microsurgeon to observe how the pedicle seats and reduce the length accordingly. In our experience, the usual length of pedicle seats approximately at the middle to distal third of the IJV to allow sufficient length for anastomosis without encouraging kinking or twists. Clearly the choice of flap will likely determine the site of venotomy as certain flaps such as radial forearm free flap have longer pedicle lengths compared to the shorter deep circumferential iliac artery free flap.

Vascular control and isolation of venotomy site

Once the optimal site for venotomy is identified, the IJV is carefully clamped along its longitudinal axis. There are a number of clamps that can be used for this purpose but all are designed to give the same aim of allowing enough space for anastomosis while atraumatically occluding the IJV.

Satinsky

The other commonly used clamp is the Satinsky Debakey clamp which also achieves the required aims, but has a longer ratchet handle applied for control of the vessel further away from the site of surgery. Other surgeons may prefer this clamp as it allows continued flow through the vein during anastomosis. This would be of benefit where the contralateral IJV has been resected to allow venous outflow mitigating against the risk for the development of cerebral oedema (unlike Bulldog clamps which cause complete occlusion). The problem with these clamps in head and neck reconstruction is that they are typically too large as they occupy too much space in an already confined area.

Bulldog clamps

It is the authors' preference to use the spring-loaded Bulldog clamps. These are small enough to allow both surgeon and assistant to work around while reliably occluding the vessel. In addition to this, they are lightweight and easy to handle while the surgeon is looking down the microscope. Due to their smaller and more compact size they allow for highly precise clamping of the IJV.

This is particularly important in the head and neck where end-to-side anastomosis is performed in close proximity to other critical structures. The IJV runs within the carotid sheath which also encapsulates the internal carotid artery and vagus nerve. Careless application of a vascular clamp would lead to iatrogenic damage to either of these structures.

Now that the IJV has been mobilized, site of venotomy planned and successfully clamped, the next step is to perform the venotomy. This calls for absolute precision. Any error here can create a challenging anastomosis even more difficult creating additional layers of complexity. Firstly, for the planned site of venotomy, the adventitia must be carefully cleaned off. As discussed earlier, the plane of dissection for the adventitia is challenging to correctly identify so the surgeon should take time to perform this task carefully and diligently (steps on how to perform this have been covered elsewhere in the text). The area to be cleared of adventitia is usually at least twice the size of actual venotomy. If liberal removal of adventitia is not performed, there will be a tendency for the tissue to creep within the venotomy thus compromising the anastomosis.

The final consideration for site of venotomy should be the side of the vessel wall planned for venotomy. Veins are prone to external forces of compression, causing subsequent occlusion with thrombus formation and this should be considered when laying the donor and recipient vessels side by side. It is therefore crucial for the donor vein to have a 'straight' course to the recipient vein without the need to overlay or cross over the recipient vein. Equally the site of the venotomy should not be on the 'side' otherwise this will lead to anastomosis to be performed at an angle. The optimal site for venotomy is usually the side of the vein closest to defect (as thus closest to the course of the pedicle) however it should be made slightly further around the vein circumferentially between the side and anterior wall (the side closest to the surgeon facing superficially). This will ensure the course of the pedicle is straight to the recipient vein while minimizing the chance of pressure, kinking or twisting, while also allowing a more suitable placement for ease of anastomosis.

Venotomy

The venotomy is made with two scissor cuts from opposite directions as close to 45 degrees of angulation as possible to the vessel wall. Prior to making this cut it is wise to practice this technique a few times ensuring the angulation and set up is correct with the microscissors.

Plan the venotomy hole to be 1.5× times the size of the donor vein as it sits passive after dilation. This will allow a gentle 'funnelling' outwards of the anastomosis and will prevent constriction.

Gently pick up the side wall of the vein by the adventitia only (Figure 9.3.2). Once held securely, perform the angulated cuts from both sides at 45 degrees in relation to the vein as

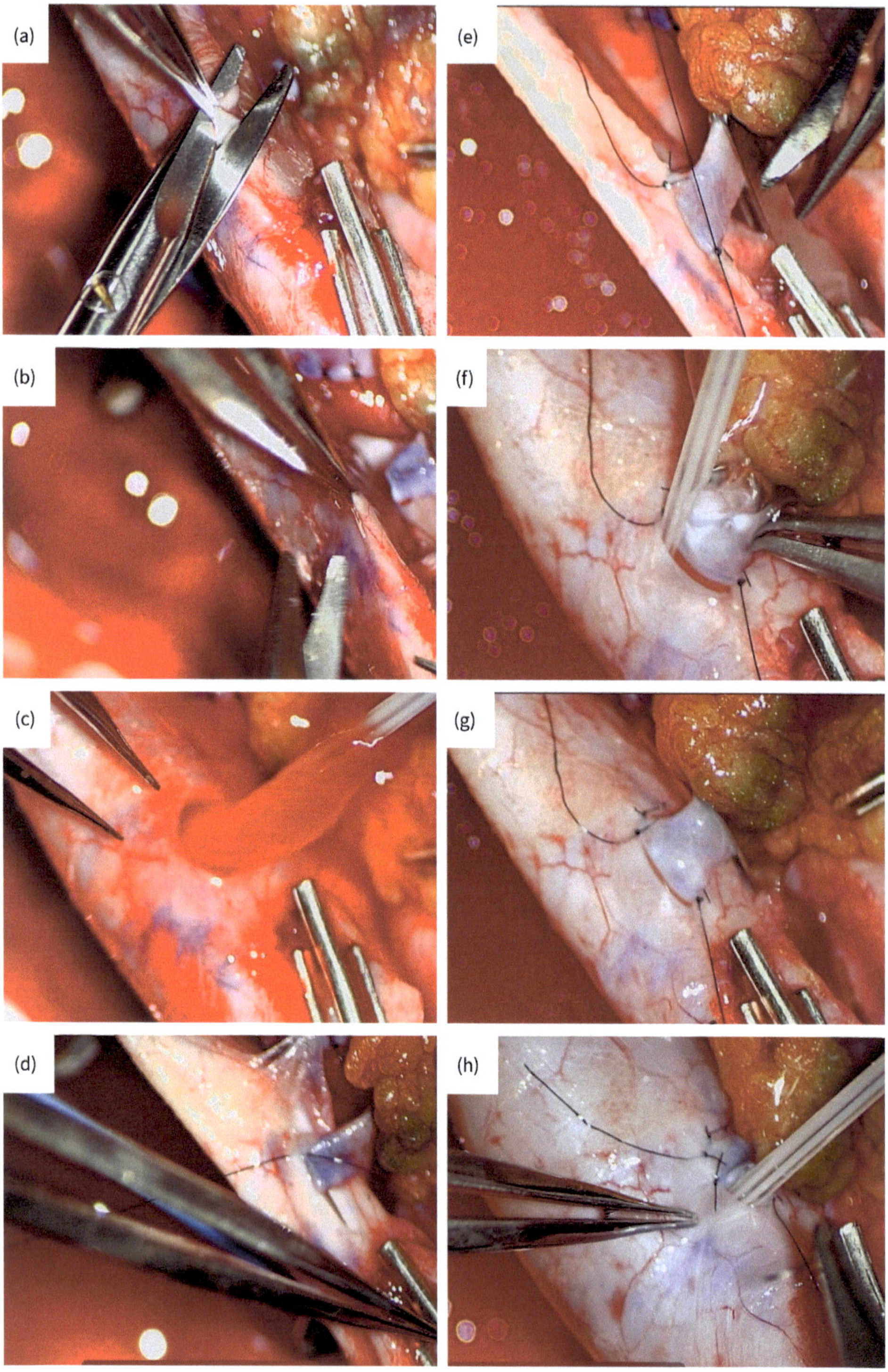
(a)
(e)
(b)
(f)
(c)
(g)
(d)
(h)

Figure 9.3.2 End-to-side anastomosis. a. Conduction of venotomy. Note that after preparation and dissection of the adventitia, the side of the venotomy has been selected and the IJV wall is pinched and pulled outwards with the jeweller's forceps. Adventitia scissors are prepared to perform the first part of the venotomy. b. The second part of the venotomy is being performed. c. Notice the 'gush' of blood after the hole is created, while the isolated segment of the IJV is emptying the blood. If the Satinsky clamp has not been placed properly, blood will continue to flow through the hole. The operator should not panic but carefully reapply the Satinsky to effectively block the vessel. d. The end-to-side anastomosis is via the 180-degree triangulation technique. The top suture has been placed. Note that the venotomy hole is 1.5× times the diameter of the donor vein. e. The bottom suture is placed, allowing gentle stretch of the donor vein in order to achieve a 'funnel-shaped' anastomosis. f. The technique of hydrodistension is applied. The vessels are ballooned with heparinized saline that gently stretches the vessels and allows better visibility of the vessel edges and calculation of the site of the next suture placement. g. After hydrodistension as the heparinized saline is flowing out through the suture gaps, the vessel edges are everted, allowing seamless anastomosis. h. The anastomosis has now progressed, and prior to placement of the last sutures, hydrodistension is applied.

stated. It is important that the size of the cut closely correlates with the calibre of the planned donor vein. The first cut passes halfway along the planned size of venotomy.

Once this first cut is made, flush the incised site with heparinized saline. The angulation of the second cut should proceed directly opposite to the first, thereby completing the venotomy. Prior to making the second cut, the surgeon should consider the angulation and shape of their first cut and make any adjustments accordingly. The most common correction is in relation to the length of the vessel cut. Usually the first cut in the vein can be larger than planned, thus the second cut would need to be shorter in length. Ideally the venotomy from each side of vein should be half the length of the planned venotomy size. The pattern of the microscissors angulation cut usually resembles that of a 'V' directed towards the vein wall. Once the cut is made, wash the venous blood within the clamped portion of the vessel out with heparinized saline immediately. This will ensure that there is no residual clot within the lumen which could potentially occlude the anastomosis upon resumption of venous flow across the join. An alternative technique to perform the venotomy is by placement of a microsuture at the central site of the planned cut. This suture is then used to tent up the wall of the vein and allow for the venotomy cut in a slightly more controlled fashion as this will allow control of the vein wall without overzealous use of jeweller's forceps on the delicate vein wall.

Anastomosis

Once the venotomy is made following clamping and the incised portion of vein has been liberally flushed with heparinized saline, attention can move to the commencement of venous anastomosis.

The approach to suturing is usually done with the wall furthest away (the back wall) completed first (Figure 9.3.3). The donor vein is positioned adjacent to the venotomy site. The donor vein venotomy (and the required angulation for entry into the IJV have been discussed in Chapter 6.5, Figures 6.5.2 and 6.5.3) The needle is passed firstly into the recipient (IJV) lumen, roughly at the central-most position on the back wall edge of the venotomy site. In

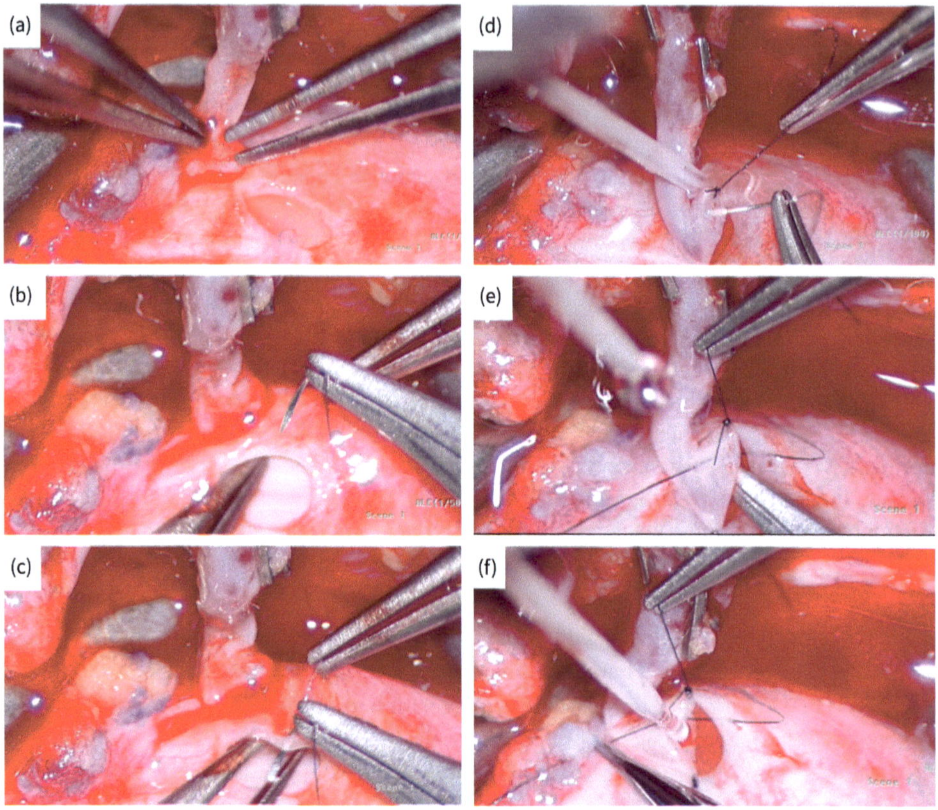

Figure 9.3.3 Another example of end-to-side venous anastomosis. a. Note that the venotomy hole has been created. The size (diameter) of the hole is 1.5× times the passive diameter of the donor vein. b. The back-wall-first technique is applied. Forceps are entering the inside of the IJV lumen to tent the vessel wall up and to receive the tip of the needle. c. Note the relatively small bite as the needle passes. The veins are low-pressure systems and thin-walled and in contrast to arterial anastomosis the bites have to be quite small and close to the vessel edge. d. The posterior stitch has been secured. One thread has been left longer to allow easier manipulation and rotation of the vessel. Note that the inner space of the vessel has been irrigated to allow eversion of the vessel edges (hydrodistension). e. The needle is passed through. Note the insertion of forceps inside the lumen to ensure avoidance of the back wall. f. Further hydrodistension is applied allowing better visibility of the inner lumen and eversion of the vessel edges.

a similar fashion to end-to-end anastomosis, it is important that the following bite on the donor vein be equidistant to the entry bite. The aim is to try and maintain a 'forehand' action of suturing and avoid the somewhat inaccurate and more uncomfortable 'backhand' motion of suturing. The ensuing suture is tied carefully ensuring the knot is flat. Using the same principles described elsewhere in the text, it is advisable to make the first through for this particular 'corner stone' suture a double throw. Once this is completed the recipient and donor veins will be connected allowing an assessment of the position and orientation.

The next suture is placed in the same way with entry into the IJV first followed by exit bite through the donor vein. The authors' preference is to continue to develop the suturing on the back wall, ensuring equally spaced sutures towards the medial and lateral edges (marking the halfway point of the anastomosis).

At this point, what remains is the front wall of the vein with the back wall entirely secured to the venotomy site. It is important to continue liberal use of the heparinized saline to ensure distension of the vein and also inspection of the anastomosis to ensure there has been no through stitch placed. What remains is the nearside (front wall) to be anastomosed. The placement of these sutures can be from the donor to recipient vein (until the back wall) as this will maintain a normal hand and wrist action of suturing during placement.

The role of the assistant is crucial here as they can gently tent the donor vein up while the surgeon passes the needle under direct vision through. It is advisable in a similar fashion to end-to-end suturing that an instrument in the non-dominant hand supports the intima and protects the back wall upon passage of the suture.

As the view within the lumen diminishes it is important for the surgeon to continuously flush the vein to ensure patency and distend the vein to allow easier passage of the suture. Remove the proximal clamp first and check for any obvious leaking of the anastomosis which can be corrected with additional sutures if required. This would require the proximal clamp to be re-applied and additional sutures placed as necessary. Following this, release the distal clamp and check the veins distend equally across the anastomosis. As discussed earlier, checking for patency can be done by up-lift and refill techniques.

The whole sequence of a venous end-to-side anastomosis is demonstrated in Figure 9.3.4.

Important highlights in end-to-side anastomosis are summarized in Box 9.3.1.

Additional considerations in end-to-side anastomosis

It is important to mention to areas which create additional difficulty for this procedure. By far the most common is too large a venotomy in the recipient vein. This will lead to added tension across the anastomotic junction and risk of profuse leakage.

Planning the venotomy carefully without rushing is vital to ensure an appropriate sized incision which matches the calibre of donor vein. Techniques described earlier will help facilitate this procedure without compromising the anastomosis. Insufficient clearing of adventitia can also shroud the view and lead to encroachment of this tissue upon the venotomy site. As stated earlier, it is important for at least twice the amount of adventitia be removed for the planned size of venotomy. This gives enough clearance for the surgeon to perform the anastomosis without any interference from the tissue.

The vein can tolerate sutures spacing slightly further apart from one another than the area. This is due to the lower flow within the vein walls and thus less likelihood of leakage. However, liberal spacing can lead to the incomplete anastomosis. Although this problem is simple to correct by the placement of additional sutures, the repeated clamping and unclamping of the delicate vein walls risk microtrauma and clot propagation. Therefore the instrumentation of the vein walls both externally and internally should be kept to a minimum and for what is absolutely necessary.

Lastly, with end-to-side suturing the suture must consider their orientation of the vessels. The most intuitive method of suturing a vein is end-to-end as the vein walls are sat opposing one another in a single axis. End-to-side changes the axis of suturing from a vertical donor vein to a horizontal orientated recipient. This challenging orientation creates the potential for unequal bites, through stitching and passage of the needle in an angle other than perpendicular to the vein edge. Therefore, the surgeon should ensure all the other variables

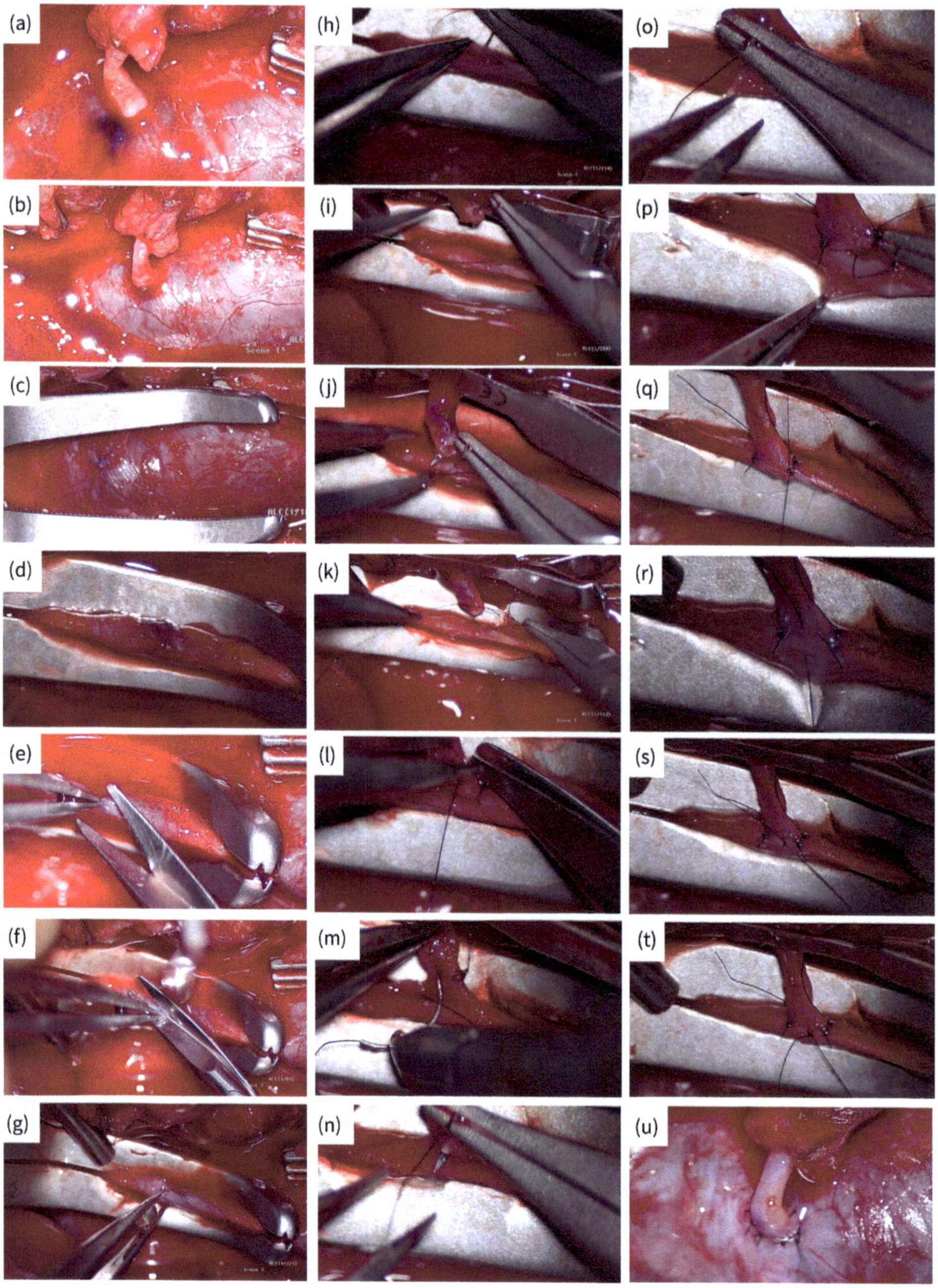

Figure 9.3.4 Sequence of end-to-side anastomosis. a. Selection of the venotomy site and marking of this with an ink dot. b. Confirmation of the position of the donor vein is order to confirm that there will be no twist, and a passive blood flow will be facilitated. c. Placement of the Satinsky forceps. d. Satinsky forceps have isolated the venotomy site. e. Performance of the venotomy first cut. f. The venotomy is performed under irrigation for better visibility. g. A small venotomy has been created. h. The back-wall-first technique is applied. i. The donor vein is approximated to the recipient vein. j. Suturing of the donor vein. k. The first thread is applied. l. The thread is left long to allow rotation of the vessel and easier manipulation. m. Further suturing ensues. n. Anterior wall suturing. o. Note the silhouette of the needle under the thin wall of the vein. p. Inferior suture of the anterior wall after completion of the back wall is placed. q. The penultimate suture is tied. r. The last stitch is placed after hydrodistension. s. Suturing of the last stitch is performed. t. Inspection of the anastomosis to confirm no further gaps. u. The anastomosis after removal of the clamp shows a passive flow and equal expansion of the vessels.

Box 9.3.1 Recommended tips for end-to-side anastomosis (IVJ)

- Always fully mobilize the internal jugular vein when performing an end-to-side anastomosis.
- Always mark the line of the IJV tributaries. The venotomy site should be located alongside this line.
- When performing a venotomy, always aim for a hole 1.5 times the calibre of the donor vein at rest. This will facilitate an opening funnel venous outflow as opposed to constriction and obstruction.

contributing to the microvascular anastomosis are controlled (surgeon and patient positioning, lighting, arm rests to eliminate tremor, etc.) in order to maximize the chances for success.

9.4 Microscopic anastomotic coupler device (MACD)

Introduction

The microscopic anastomotic devices (MACD), simply termed venous couplers (as they are mostly used for veins), are remarkable devices that have revolutionized venous anastomosis.

The venous coupler system with its holder and the detachable single-use frame that bears the ring-pin system has been described in detail in Chapter 1.6.

The advantages of venous couplers are reduced anastomotic time, requirement for less detailed and extensive vessel preparation in terms of adventitia trimming and stenting of the anastomosis preventing vessel collapse in the early days post-surgery.

Preparation for vessel couplers

It is important that couplers are used after careful and appropriate vessel selection. Short recipient venous stumps close to the take-off of the internal jugular vein may be challenging and may require clamping of the internal jugular vein with a Satinsky forceps.

Couplers are contraindicated in an end-to-side anastomosis and in a significant, more than 1:3 ratio, vessel calibre mismatch.

The prospective venous stumps are prepared. The optimum vessel orientation is marked with methylene blue dots to avoid twisting. The veins are clamped with 3V clamps or small bulldog clamps. In case of a short internal jugular vein (IJV) recipient vein, a Satinsky clamp or bulldog clamping of the internal jugular vein will facilitate fitting of the coupler device.

When 3V clamps are used, it is important that adequate vein length is left free to be handled through the coupler. The coupler device can be quite bulky so adequate vessel length for mobility and manipulation is of essence.

The prospective veins should not bear any Liga clips close to the edge as this may get trapped or jammed in the frame. Avoid having a venous valve close to the venous edge.

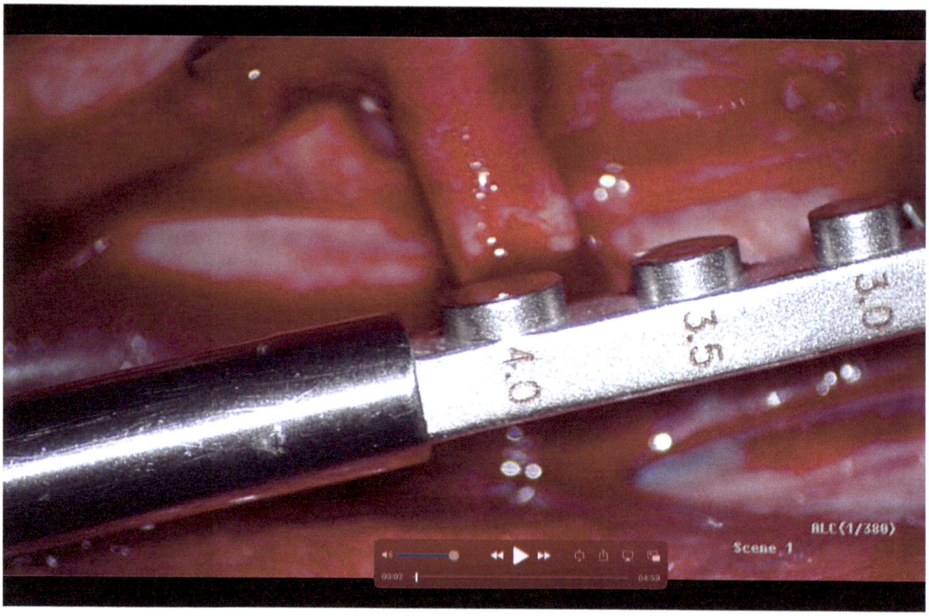

Figure 9.4.1 Approximation of the coupler sizer to a vessel edge to choose the correct size of MACD.

Choice of coupler size

After the vessels are prepared, irrigated, inspected and dilated then the coupler 'sizer' is approximated to the vessel's 'mouth' (Figure 9.4.1). The optimum size is the size of the knob that has the same (more or less) diameter of the vessel in a relaxed position.

It is not uncommon to have a calibre mismatch. The coupler of choice is the one that fits the smallest vein. If mismatch is approximately a 1:2 ratio, then half a size bigger than the smallest vein can be trialled as the veins are stretchable and elastic and with some effort a bigger coupler may fit a smaller vessel. The size of the coupler should be nearer to the size of the smallest vessel.

Mounting the frame

The frame can only be mounted in one direction. If forcibly pushed, it can be mounted in a reverse fashion; however, this will prevent the frame from closing. It is best mounted by the operator as erroneous mounting can be detrimental for the anastomosis.

The MACD handle is held by the operator's non-dominant hand. This will allow movement and rotation in the three spatial dimensions. As the coupler handle is quite long it is best held on the caudal aspect of the neck as holding it close to the head direction may cause obstruction due to the mandible and suboptimal angulation and entry into the operating field.

However, the operator will only have the dominant hand to use the microvascular instruments hence a trained assistant is important when this technique is used.

The assistant with one hand will irrigate the vessels and with the other will hold the hockey stick instrument to assist mounting and pinning the vessels on the rings.

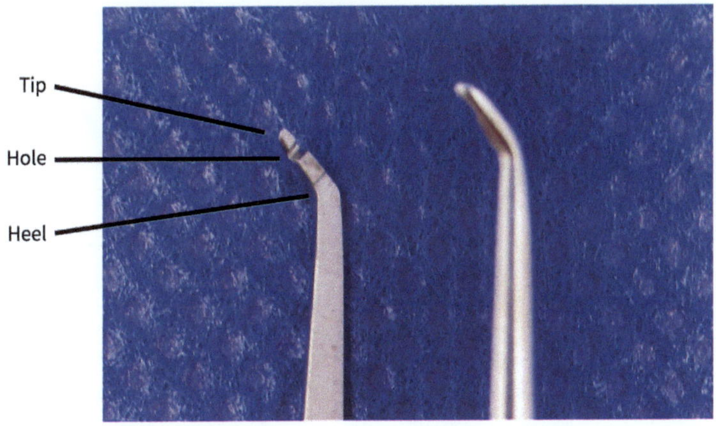

Figure 9.4.2 'Hockey-stick' forceps. The tip resembles a foot. Note the small hole that allows the foot-shaped end to press the pin through the vessel wall. The end of the instrument has a tip for finer handling of vessels and pushing the vessel wall through the tip of the pin only. The other end has a rounded, broader 'heel' that is also used to pass the vessel wall of thicker vessels through. Effectively, when pressing the whole vessel wall down to the base of the pin, use the full length of the instrument's 'foot'.

Pinning of the vessels

When commencing pinning the vessels into the coupler gently pull the edge of the vein through the coupler ring, ensure that the blue methylene marking dot faces the right direction and gently pin it on the first pin.

What is crucial is to familiarize with the shape of the 'hockey stick' coupler forceps (Figure 9.4.2) and the length of the pins.

Only suspend the vessel edge in the optimum length/depth of the pin (Figure 9.4.3). Initial suspension of the vessel will only require the pin tip to penetrate through the vessel wall until visualized. The vessel wall should not be pushed all the way to the base of the pin. This is because the distance component between the point of fixation and the diametrically opposite point will increase any vessels of the exact size or slightly smaller than the diameter of the ring will cause excessive stretch and likely tears (Figure 9.4.3).

Passing the vessel wall through the tip only of the pin can be facilitated either by pushing with the tips of the hockey stick foot only or with jeweller's or dilator forceps held tangent to the pin so that the tips do not damage the vessel endothelium.

From this point onwards, there are two different courses:

- One is to pin the vessel wall on the diametrically opposite pin. That will provide an estimate of how stretchable the vessel is and whether the vessel can adapt to the diameter of the ring. This process is almost like suspending a trampoline on the springs by pinning the vessel on a pair of oppositely seated pins. Again, it is important for borderline-sized vessels is to only pass the tip of the pin through the vessel edge to avoid excessive stretching and tears.
- Another legitimate course of action is to proceed with pinning the vessel wall and the successive neighbouring pins. When doing so, the operator will hold with the edge of

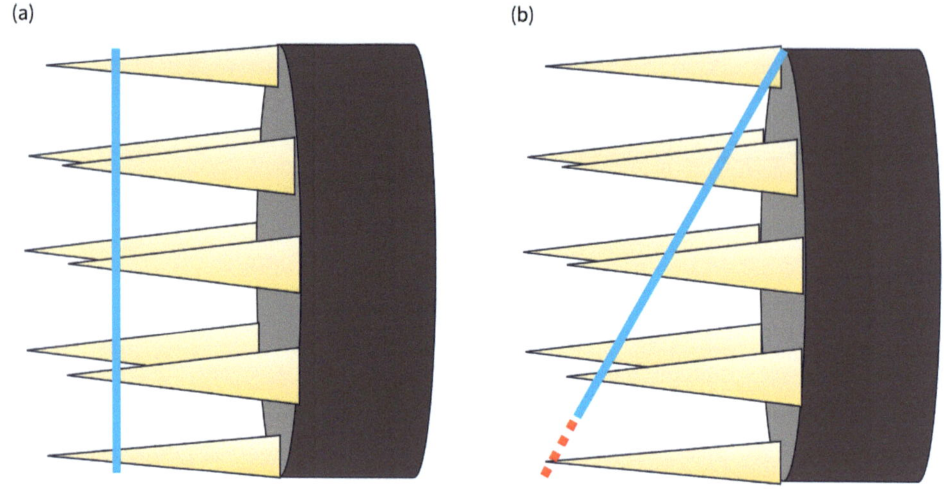

Figure 9.4.3 Schematic explanation of why, in a borderline size match between the vessel calibre and the coupler ring size, it is important to fix the vessel edges only through the tip of the pins. a. If the vessel under stretch is just about the size of the pin ring diameter, then it has to pass through the tips only, as shown in the figure. b. If in one or two points the vessel edge is pushed down to the pin, that will increase the needed diameter and will not allow passage of the vessel edge on the contralateral pins (opposite pins), potentially causing a detrimental tear. This is because the required length equals the hypotenuse of a right triangle, as per basic geometric principles and the Pythagorean theorem.

the vessel with the jeweller's forceps and will try to maximize the stretch before pinning it to the next pin. That way, the maximum stretchability of the vessel is utilized.

Once all the pins are through the vessel edge then the operator and assistant can use the hockey stick foot hole, or its heel, to push the vessel down onto the base of the pin in contact with the ring. By doing so by a gentle outwards stroking motion is exercised in order to gently evert the lip of the vessel edge and avoid areas of inversion or adventitia entrapment (Figure 9.4.4). Eversion of the vessel edges is important to avoid inclusion of adventitia that can precipitate thrombosis. If the vessel wall is to 'tight' and resists eversion then a small cut

Figure 9.4.4 Eversion of the vessel edges after the vein is suspended to the coupler pins. It is crucial to evert the edges to avoid inclusion of adventitia that may cause thrombosis. a. Note that the vessel edge is slightly stretched as the coupler ring is exactly or slightly wider than the vessel calibre. That causes some difficulty in everting the vessel edge towards passing the last two pins. b. The last two pins have just been passed but note that the resistance of the vessels is there, and there is a constriction ring that prevents eversion. c. Most prominent site of constriction of the vessel edge (arrow). d. A small cut will overcome the constriction where the arrow shows. e. After the cut is performed, using the hockey-stick tips, gently stroke the vessel edges across the periphery of the vessel to achieve eversion. f. The area where the vessel edge still resists is grasped with jeweller's forceps and actively everted. g. See the successful eversion of the vein after grasping the vessel edge with forceps to rotate it. h. Rounded 360-degree eversion of the vessel edge. The hockey-stick 'heel' can be used now to press the whole vessel edge down to the base of the pins.

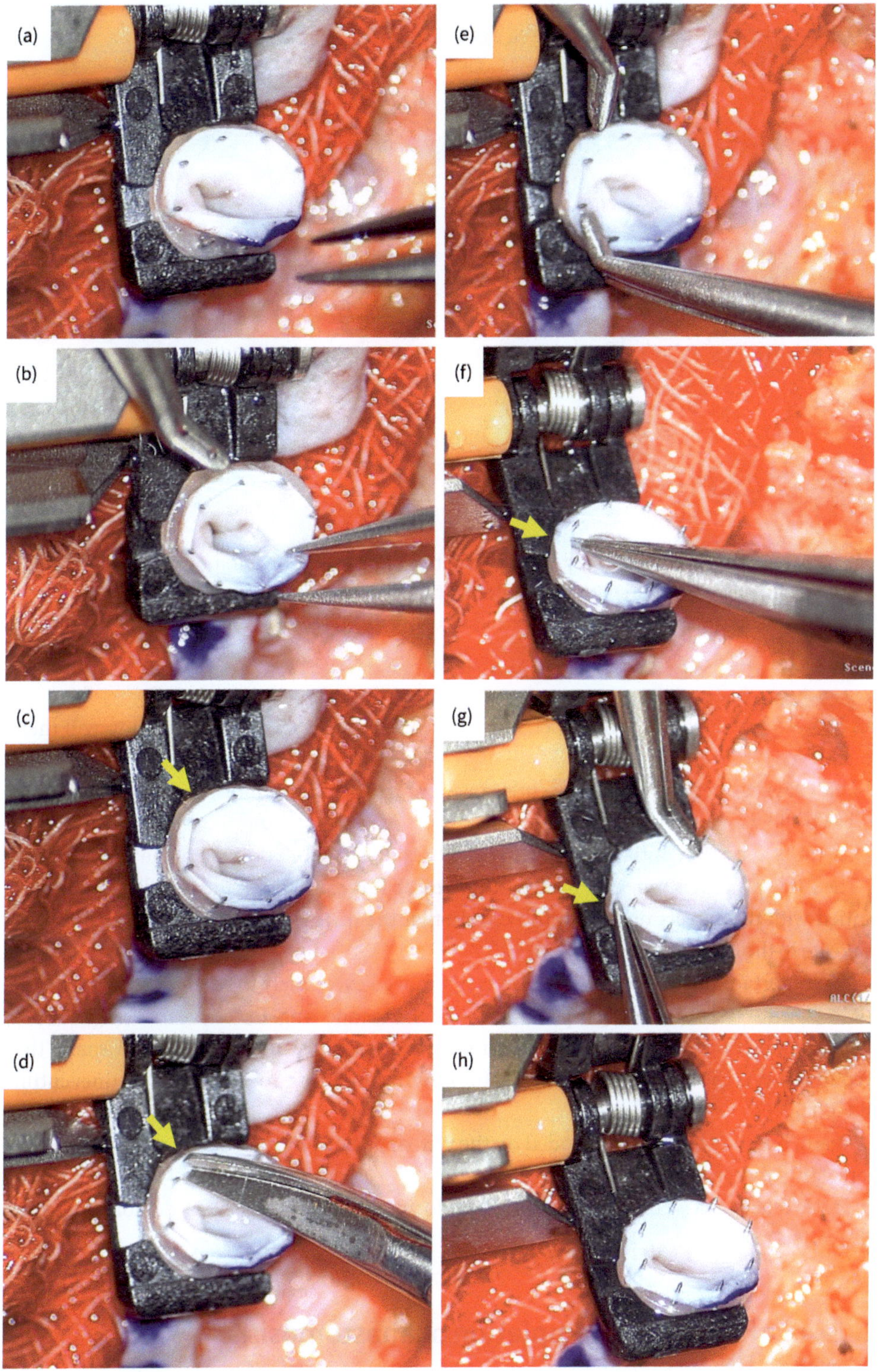
(a)
(b)
(c)
(d)
(e)
(f)
(g)
(h)

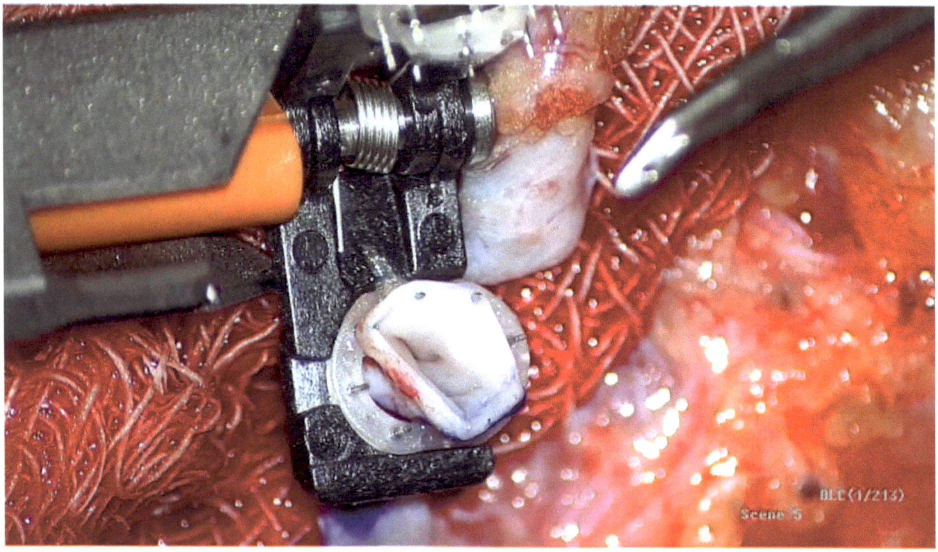

Video 9.4.1 Sequence of venous anastomosis with a microscopic anastomotic device (MACD). See this video online by searching for this book's title or ISBN at https://academic.oup.com/
Reproduced courtesy of Leandros Vassiliou, Manchester University NHS Foundation Trust, Manchester, UK.

can be performed with adventitia scissors to overcome the 'constriction'. Eversion will then be achieved (Figure 9.4.4).

Once this has been performed, gentle rinse and irrigation will moisturize the vessel edge and also allow for a final inspection.

Ensure that no adventitia tissue is impinged or trapped within the area of the ring.

The same process is repeated for the other vessel. It is crucial that the vessel is pulled and pinned with the correct orientation so ensure that the methylene blue dot is sitting exactly opposite to the complimentary vessel.

It is important that the coupler system is not moved excessively to reach the other system, but in contrast the other vessel is pulled through the second ring. Excessive movement of the coupler handler may stretch the already pinned vessel causing tears and damage. Usually, the second vessel is the vessel which is easier for pinning and this process should be uneventful and quick.

Again, once the vessel is suspended on the pin-ring gently irrigate and inspect the perfection of the vessel mounting.

The sequence of venous anastomosis performed with a MACD is demonstrated in Video 9.4.1.

Closure of frame and completion of anastomosis

Once both vessels have been mounted then the coupler frame is ready to close so that the rings are approximated together, and the pins inserted into their corresponding recipient holes of the opposite ring.

In cases of vascular mismatch when a larger vessel is pinned then there will be an excess of vascular edge tissue hanging out of the ring. It is not inappropriate to gently dissect these excess edges with microvascular curved or adventitia scissors.

The couplers knob is rotated clockwise, and the operator observes the frame closing (Figure 9.4.5). It is important at this point that the field remains clear, and no irrelevant tissue is entrapped within the anastomosis or within the closing frames that can cause the system to jump.

Once the rings have approximated to each other it is important to gently put pressure so that the ring system is properly locked. That is accomplished by clamping gently both sides of the frame, both the anterior and posterior with mosquito forceps.

Once this has been achieved and the rings are compressed against each other then the assistant holds the exposed part of the ring system gently with mosquito forceps. Usually, one or two teeth width of the mosquito forceps jaws are adequate the suspend the ring without pushing or pressing against the vessels.

As the knob continues to be rotated the rings will start releasing from the frame. It is important at this point that the assistant continues to stabilize the ring system until they are completely freed from the suspending frame.

The operator asks for a second pair of mosquito forceps and once the rings are released the handle is handed back to the scrub nurse, and with the other mosquito forceps the operator compresses the rings together both diametrically opposite where the assistant is holding the ring system and also on the posterior and anterior sides.

The whole anastomosis is then gently rotated, and appropriate approximation and compaction of the rings is confirmed. At this point the anastomosis is complete.

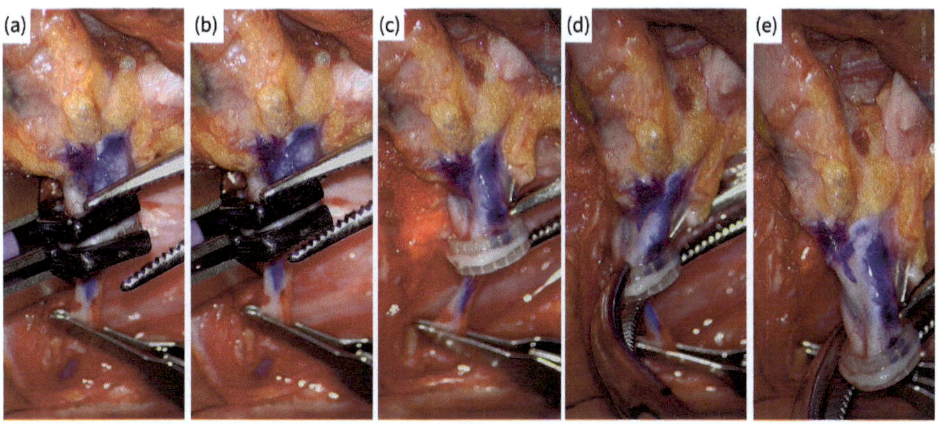

Figure 9.4.5 Closing the MACD a. The coupler frame has now closed, but note that the pins are not pushed against each other completely. Mosquito forceps are used for this purpose. b. The mosquito forceps first compress the frames, the anterior and posterior parts of the frame against each other. c. The mosquito forceps (one or a maximum of two teeth) are gently holding and immobilizing the rings while the coupler knob is rotated to release the rings from the frame. d. As soon as the operator releases the coupler rings from the frame, they take another mosquito forceps and holds the opposite side of the ring. While the assistant continues to immobilize the rings, the operator compresses the rings against each other in all other sites of the circle. e. Compression of the posterior side of the ring to allow a perfect lock of the couplers.

The next step is to release the vascular clamps and assess the patency and quality of the anastomosis. The pedicle side clamp is the first clamp to be released and by doing that all the accumulated blood in the venous system will flow through the anastomosis and will expand the vessels.

When the expansion, the shape of the anastomosis is deemed satisfactory and there are no areas of twists or constriction, then the vascular clamp distal to the anastomosis (recipient vein) is then released and the system is allowed to decompress, and the flow normalized.

The whole sequence is demonstrated in Figure 9.4.6 and Video 9.4.2.

An extremely challenging situation with potential detriment for the anastomosis may be encountered if the coupler frames become jammed and are unable to close (Video 9.4.3). This most often occurs due to the faulty installation of the single-use coupler frame system onto the handle. There is only one way to mount the frame correctly, and this is achieved by gently pushing the frame onto the receiver end of the handle until it clicks. However, if the frame is pushed forcefully the wrong way up, it may still click, offering false reassurance only to declare the problem later when the frame cannot close. It is highly recommended that the microvascular surgeon takes responsibility for mounting the frame themselves and not delegate the task to others.

Figure 9.4.6 Sequence of venous anastomosis using MACD. a. The vein is prepared. After adventitia dissection, a dilator is introduced to gently stretch the vessel edges. b. The coupler size is selected. As the picture shows, size '2.5' could be marginally smaller than the calibre of the vessel at rest after dilation. c. Size '3.0' is slightly larger and is preferred as it is predicted that the vessel can tolerate a little stretch. d. Passage of the vessel through the coupler ring. It is crucial at this point that the orientation is maintained, and the dots remain aligned to avoid inadvertent twisting of the vessel while it passes through the ring. e. Suspension of the vessel in the first two pins. f. The tip and whole of the hockey-stick is used to just pass the pin through the vessel wall. g. Further pinning is ensuing. h. Almost half of the pinning has occurred. Note that at this point, the vessel is under stretch and starts resisting full eversion. i. Gentle grasping of the vessel edge with the tips of the hockey stick. j. Gentle pushing of the tip of the pin only to maximize the vessel stretch as shown in the previous Figure 9.4.3. k. The last pin is now passed while the assistant is pinning the vessel area that displays the maximum resistance. l. Attempt to evert the vessel edges. m. As the vessel was marginally smaller than the coupler size, there is resistance in eversion. The restriction band is now cut. n. After the small edge venotomy, the vessel edges are slowly everted actively using forceps. o. The vessel frame is slowly released. Note that the assistant is holding the coupler rings with one or two teeth of mosquito forceps tips. p. The end result of the anastomosis after the release of the frame. The anastomosis is evenly expanded and running.

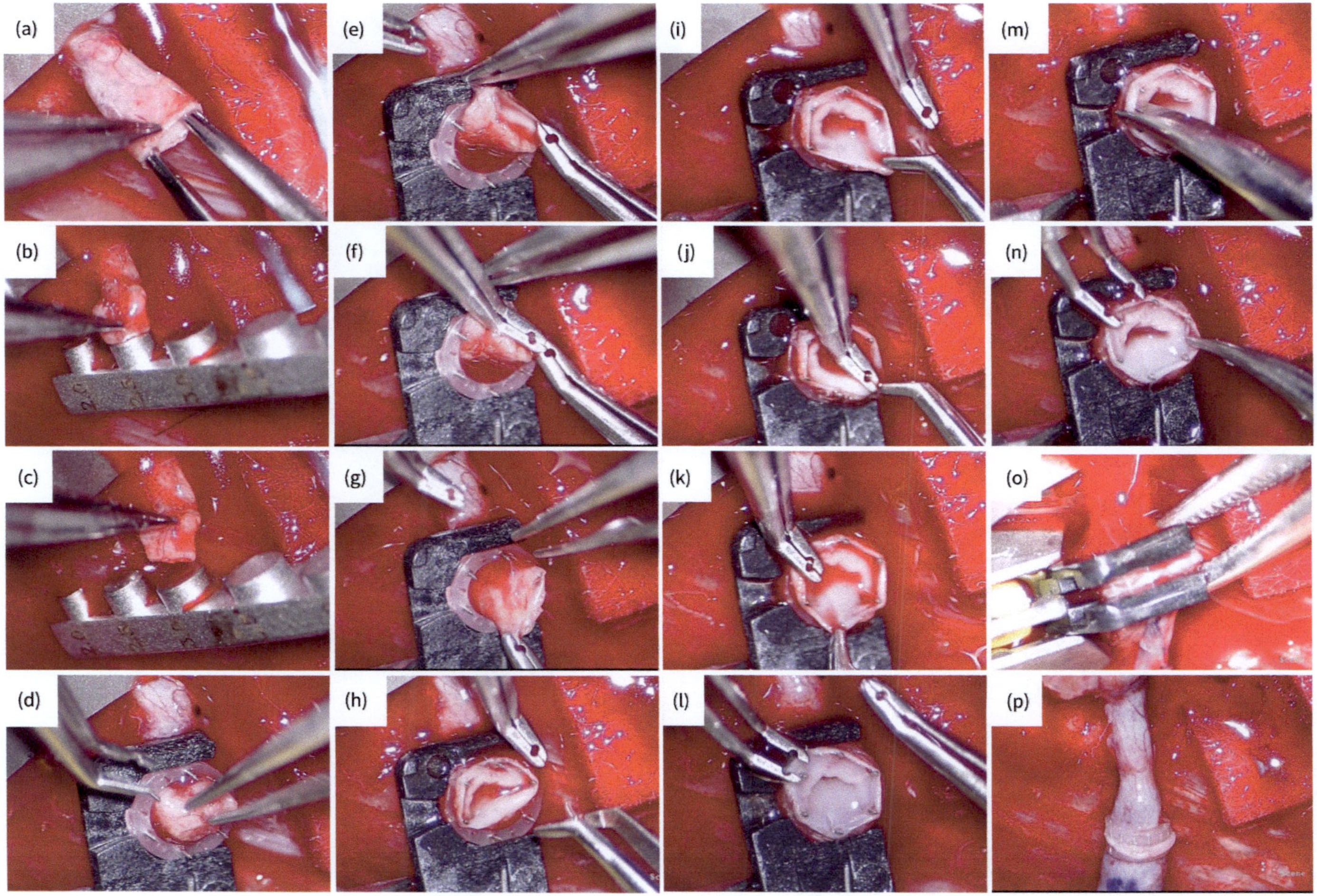

(a)
(b)
(c)
(d)
(e)
(f)
(g)
(h)
(i)
(j)
(k)
(l)
(m)
(n)
(o)
(p)

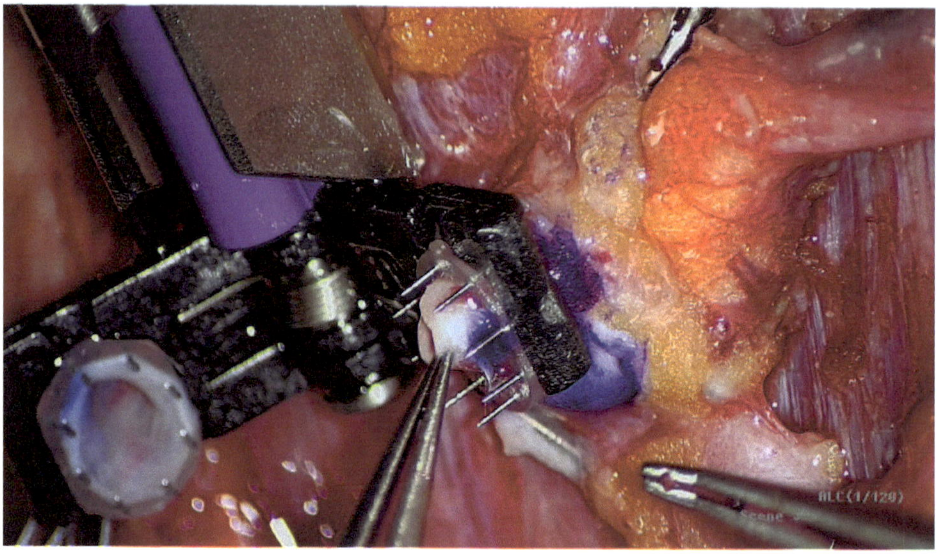

Video 9.4.2 Venous coupler closure.
See this video online by searching for this book's title or ISBN at https://academic.oup.com/
Reproduced courtesy of Leandros Vassiliou, Manchester University NHS Foundation Trust, Manchester, UK.

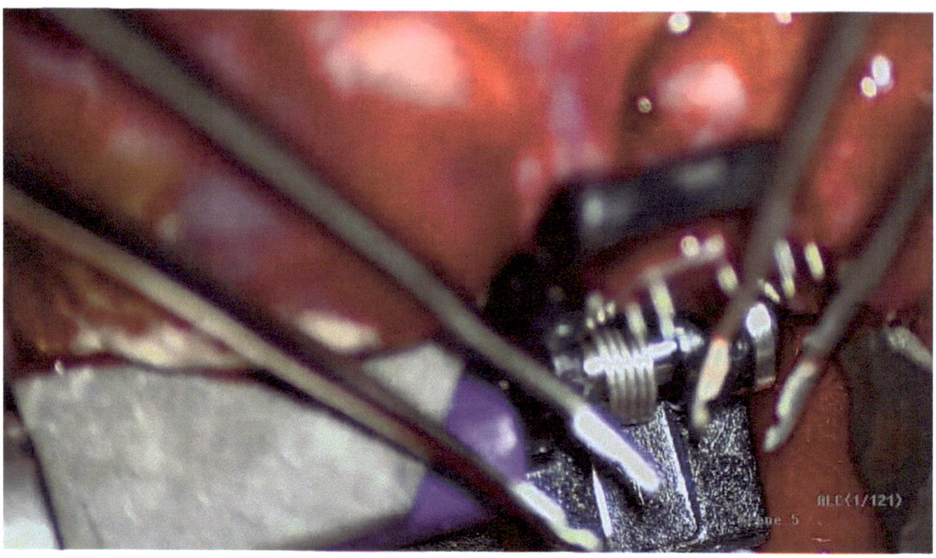

Video 9.4.3 Jammed microscopic anastomotic devices (MACD) complication.
See this video online by searching for this book's title or ISBN at https://academic.oup.com/
Reproduced courtesy of Leandros Vassiliou, Manchester University NHS Foundation Trust, Manchester, UK.

Further reading

Acland RD. *Practice Manual for Microvascular Surgery*. St Louis, MO: C.V. Mosby Company, 1989: p. 134.

DeLacure MD, Kuriakose MA, Spies AL. Clinical experience in end-to-side venous anastomoses with a microvascular anastomotic coupling device in head and neck reconstruction. Arch Otolaryngol Head Neck Surg. 1999 Aug;125(8):869–72. doi: 10.1001/archotol.125.8.869. PMID: 10448733.

Li MM, *et al.* Utilization of microvascular couplers in salvage arterial anastomosis in head and neck free flap surgery: case series and literature review. *Head Neck* 2020;42(8):E1–7.

Maruccia M, *et al.* Microvascular coupler device versus hand-sewn venous anastomosis: A systematic review of the literature and data meta-analysis. *Microsurgery* 2020;40(5):608–17.

Murugan MS, Mudigonda SK. End-to-side versus end-to-end venous anastomosis using couplers in mandibular reconstruction: a comparative study. *J Maxillofac Oral Surg* 2022;21(1):247–52.

Sullivan B, Zoppo M, Yao A, Henderson PW. Simple interrupted microvascular anastomosis: review of four sutures placement sequences. *J Reconstr Microsurg Open* 2020;5:e101–6.

Watanabe H, Ueda K, Ohkouchi M, Kajikawa A, Suzuki Y. Posterior-wall-first continuous suturing combined with conventional interrupted suturing for microvascular anastomosis. *J Reconstr Microsurg* 2006;22(8):617–23.

Wu GJ, Loewenstein SN, Mailey BA, Sasor S, Cook J, Hassanein AH. Unique complications of venous anastomotic couplers: a systematic review of the literature. *J Reconstr Microsurg* 2020;36(6):403–11.

Zhang T, Lubek J, Salama A, Caccamese J, Coletti D, Dyalram D, Ord R. Venous anastomoses using microvascular coupler in free flap head and neck reconstruction. *J Oral Maxillofac Surg* 2012;70(4):992–6.

10
Anastomosis initial assessment and final pedicle positioning

Andrew Goodall, Leandros Vassilios F. Vassiliou, Panayiotis Kyzas, and Nicholas Kalavrezos

10.1 Assessment of the anastomosis

Introduction

How the surgeon assesses the patency of the anastomosis depends on which vessel type has been anastomosed (different clinical signs are seen with arteries as compared to veins), and which technique has been used to complete the anastomosis (hand suturing versus use of anastomotic coupler).

Arterial anastomosis

Venous outflow

A definitive sign that the anastomosis is patent is to perform the arterial anastomosis first, and once all sutures are placed, release of the arterial clamp should result in visible blood exiting the vein, which is yet to be anastomosed. In our practice, this is our preferred method, and we recommend letting the flap run for a few minutes before performing the venous anastomosis (Figure 10.1.1).

Satisfactory venous outflow (volume and rate) is the most important indicator of a successful arterial anastomosis. It not only proves that the artery is running, but it also indicates that the whole circuit (microvascular circulation) of the flap is patent, functional, and the venous outflow system is uninhibited.

The first amount of blood that will come down from the vein will be dark in colour. This depends on the ischaemia time and also the flap type. This will improve and will soon resume to a bright red colour.

The surgeons should familiarize that the different flaps have different rate and volume of venous outflow. Of course, this depends on the blood pressure and upon release of the vascular clamp it is highly recommended that the main arterial pressure (MAP) will be maintained above 70 mmHg:

- The radial forearm free flap will produce a constant stream of blood from either the venae-comitantes (VCs), the cephalic, or the conjoined vein.

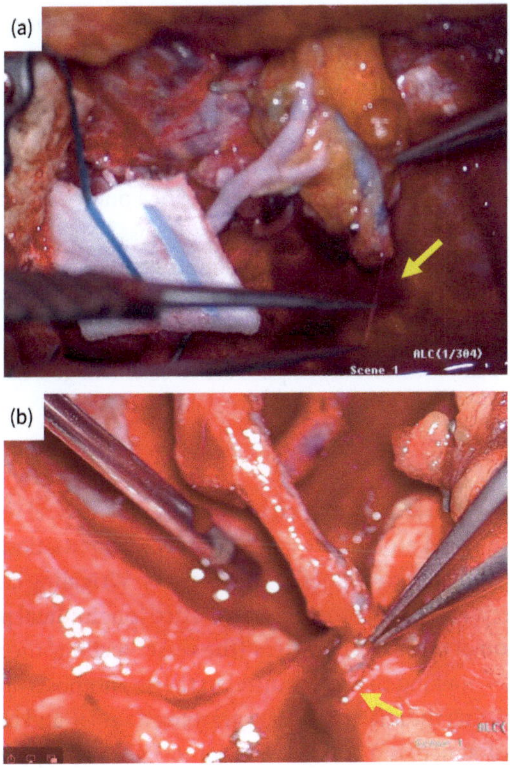

Figure 10.1.1 Venous outflow as an indicator of successful anastomosis.

- Low resistance flaps like the latissimus dorsi will demonstrate an impressive jet of blood that almost resembles arterial bleeding in terms of rate and speed. At this stage and depending on the average time for a venous anastomosis, a blood transfusion may be considered for these flaps, as an open vein may lead to a considerable amount of blood loss.
- Composite flaps such as the fibula or deep circumflex iliac artery (DCIA) are expected to bring down a good amount of volume and rate of blood from the veins.
- For fibula free flaps, it is anticipated that upon a successful arterial anastomosis almost instant venous outflow will confirm successful arterial microvascular surgery and also patent microcirculation.
- For bony flaps, if the venous outflow is not within a few seconds, and is not of satisfactory volume, that may signify a problem with the microcirculation, the anastomosis itself or the perfusion power of the recipient artery.

Shape of the anastomosis

Another sign of a healthy arterial anastomosis is the shape of the anastomosis. Upon release of the vascular clamp, the artery will start pulsating, and the anastomosis will fill up with the undercurrent of flowing blood.

The anastomosis should have a circumferential 360-degree expansion and it should look like a symmetrical funnel throughout or a symmetrical cylinder throughout. There should be no areas of inversion, areas where the vessel wall may look impinged.

Even if the venous is flowing any areas of asymmetry in the anastomosis must be closely examined as this may manifest with later thrombosis or failure.

Pulsatility

Arteries will demonstrate *expansile* pulsation (where the diameter of the vessel transiently expands with each heartbeat), but it is crucial to convince oneself that the pulsation is present *distal* to the anastomosis, representing blood flow across the anastomosis. This will seem obvious to say but proximal pulsation indicates blood flowing towards but not across the anastomosis (patency) and care should be taken to ensure that there is true distal pulsation.

It is important that the arterial pulsations are felt with two fingers gently holding the artery along the length of the pedicle as distally as possible to establish god quality and strength of pulsatility.

'Wriggling'

Another clinical sign visible in arteries is 'wriggling' of a curved vessel with each heartbeat as blood flows through the vessel around the curvature. As with pulsation of the artery, this is only valid when observed downstream of the anastomosis. Wriggling cannot be seen within a straight length of artery. False wriggling is a transmitted longitudinal pulsation that occurs when expansile pulsation of the proximal artery (the vessel 'feeding' the anastomosis) strikes the blocked anastomosis, making the artery distal to the anastomosis *appear to pulsate*. This can be stopped by stabilizing the anastomosis by grasping a suture and holding the vessel still (prevents the transmission across a blocked anastomosis). By grasping a suture at the site of and so stabilizing the anastomosis, false wriggling across a blocked anastomosis will be stopped, whereas true wriggling across a patent anastomosis will persist.

'Empty-and-refill' test

Acland first described the 'empty-and-refill test' in 1980 (see 'Further reading'). Using forceps, squeeze and occlude the artery proximal to the anastomosis (in the recipient artery site, for example, the facial artery). Using a second pair of forceps, squeeze gently, and occlude the pedicle artery immediately distal to the anastomosis. With this second pair of jeweller's forceps, hold the tips gently closed and run the forceps squeezing gently the artery towards a distal direction (downstream). This creates a segment of the (downstream) vessel that is empty of blood. Once the segment is empty (collapsed), release the first pair of forceps (proximal) and if the anastomosis is patent, the testing segment will refill with blood immediately.

Vasa vasorum

Another important indicator of a healthy anastomosis is perfusion of the vasa vasorum both of the artery and also the vein (Figure 10.1.2).

In the areas where the artery is stripped from the perivascular tissue, small lines of bright red vasa vasorum may be observed, indicating that the arterial perivascular tissues receive a blood supply. The rest of the pedicle perivascular tissue may demonstrate small punctate areas of bleeding. Again, these are areas of global pedicle perfusion.

Flap inspection

Finally, the ultimate sign of a successful anastomosis and flap perfusion is observation of the actual flap. If the flap has a skin paddle, then sufficient insufflation of the skin paddle,

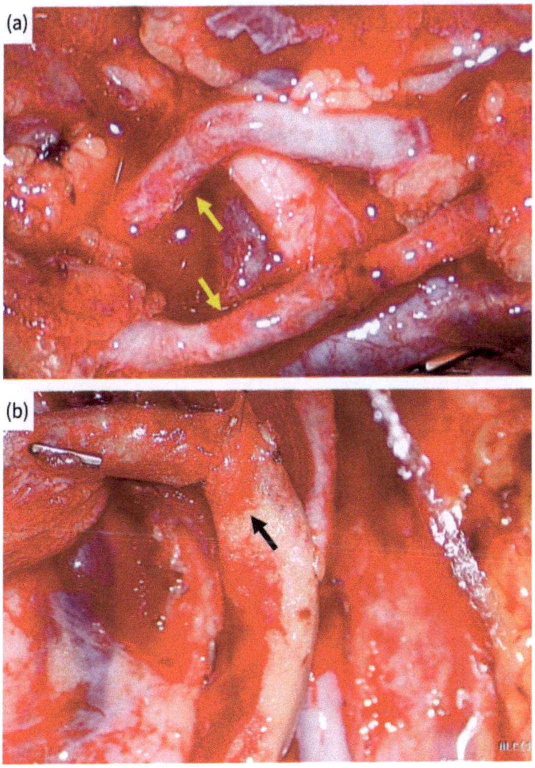

Figure 10.1.2 Perfusion of flap pedicle vasa vasorum as an indicator of successful anastomosis.

capillary refill, and healthy colour indicating blood inflow and healthy outflow is a key marker.

For composite flaps, bleeding from the bone edges is again a sign of reassurance

Adventitia bands

Once the artery is expanded, the whole length of the artery should be thoroughly checked. Occasionally, if the adventitia preparation or trimming is suboptimal, and especially if the adventitia preparation has not been performed with sharp dissection as described in Chapter 7, adventitia bands may constrict the area of artery (Figure 10.1.3).

These bands are advisable to be carefully divided, as otherwise they may constrict the blood vessel and induce a turbulent flow that may lead to thrombotic or thromboembolic complications.

Venous anastomosis

For hand-sewn venous anastomosis, the best advice is to get each suture right the first time, i.e. do not tie the suture unless you are confident that you have not caught the back wall. Any additional time this takes is well spent, as it avoids the lengthier problem of trying to correct a hastily bodged initial job.

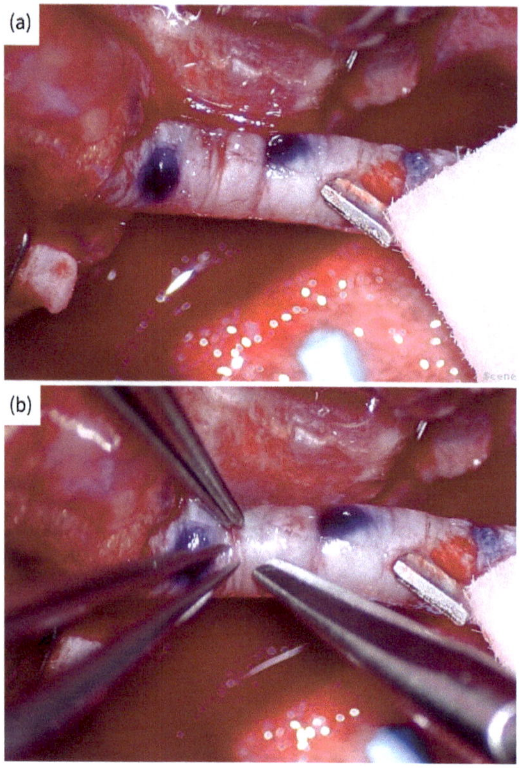

Figure 10.1.3 Adventitia bands and careful division.

Filling of the recipient vein

This is our preferred method for anastomosing the vein as it is simple, quick, and reliable. After squeezing the coupler with an artery forceps to ensure it is fully engaged and closed, the applicator is withdrawn, and the vascular clamps released. The empty and flaccid vessel should immediately fill with blood as soon as the clamp is released. If you release the distal venous clamp first, this will be backflow from the internal jugular vein. If you release the proximal clamp first, then filling and expansion of the vessel distal to the anastomosis is evidence of anastomotic patency.

Blood flow

If you study the completed anastomosis carefully it is sometimes possible to see blood flowing within the lumen of the vein. However, this is not always possible, and other means are necessary to confirm patency.

'Empty-and-refill test'

Another reliable test is the 'empty-and-refill test' described by Acland (see Further Reading) and in the section of the artery above. Using forceps, squeeze and occlude the vein distal to the anastomosis. Using a second pair of forceps, squeeze and occlude the vein immediately distal to the first, a section of vein downstream (i.e. further distal), and move the second forceps further distal. This will create a section of vein that is now emptied of blood. Release

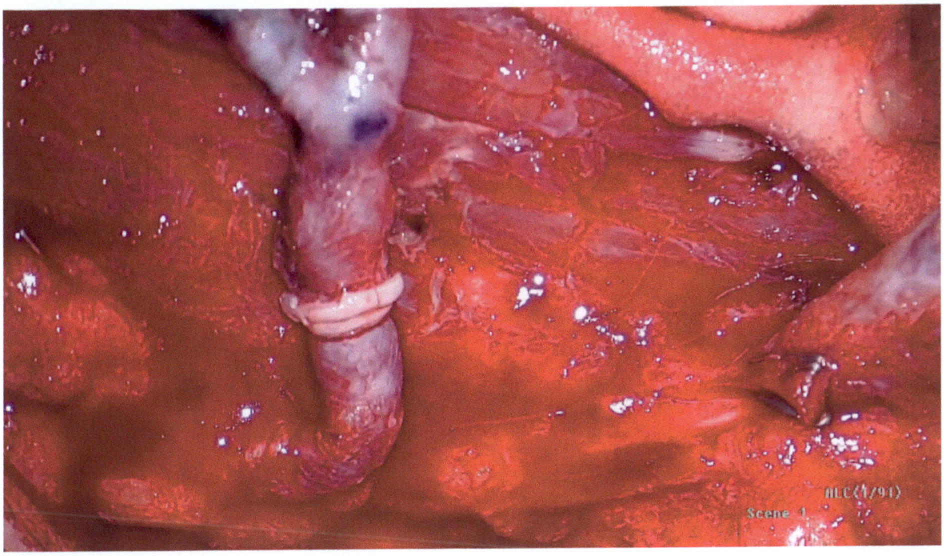

Video 10.1.1 Vein patency test via the empty and refill manoeuvre.
See this video online by searching for this book's title or ISBN at https://academic.oup.com/
Reproduced courtesy of Leandros Vassiliou, Manchester University NHS Foundation Trust, Manchester, UK.

the first pair of forceps (proximal) and if the anastomosis is patent, the vessel will refill with blood immediately (Videos 10.1.1 and 10.1.2). This method unfortunately carries a small risk of traumatizing the vein, which is to be avoided where possible, and the occlude/refill test should be used sparingly.

Obviously, this test can be used to assess patency in both hand-sewn and coupler device anastomoses.

Concerns regarding patency

Where confidence in this is low, use a curved instrument to gently lift the vessel distal to the anastomosis, lifting just until before the point that the vessel is almost occluded. The section of vessel that passes over the instrument will demonstrate alternating filling and collapsing with each beat of the heart (this is called the uplift test, and first described by Acland in 1980, see 'Further reading').

For a hand-sewn anastomosis, to prove patency, it is simple to remove a suture and observe for blood flowing across the anastomosis and escaping through the gap created by the removed suture. Having confirmed patency, it is easy to replace the suture without clamping the vessels off. The second surgeon irrigates the escaping blood briskly while the suture is reinserted and tied.

Where the anastomosis is found to be non-patent, this may be due to

- strictures
- twisting of the vessel, or
- because the suture has caught the backwall of the vessel leading to acute thrombosis.

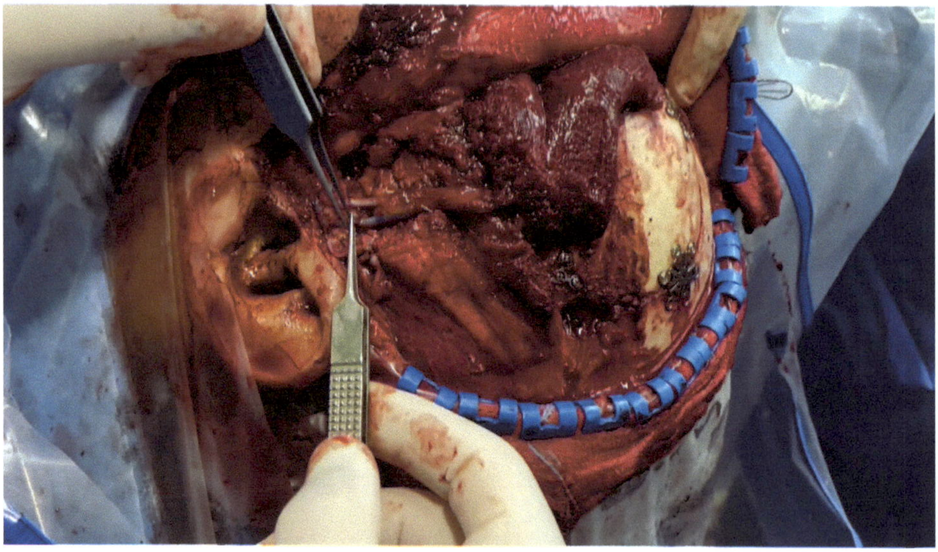

Video 10.1.2 Empty and refill test for anastomosis patency. In this case, an extended craniofacial resection for an adenoid cystic carcinoma of the lacrimal gland and reconstruction with a rectus abdominis flap anastomosed to the temporal vessels has been performed.
See this video online by searching for this book's title or ISBN at https://academic.oup.com/
Reproduced courtesy of Professor Julio Acero, and Dr Fernando Almeida, Ramon y Cajal University Hospital, Madrid, Spain.

A number of sutures will need to be removed to create a window of sufficient size to assess the suture line along the back wall of the vein. Any suture that is seen to be catching should be removed and replaced in a manner that ensures it does not catch the back wall.

Any thrombus within the vessel will need to be fastidiously irrigated away with heparin-saline solution. The sutures must now be expertly inserted. Ultimately the anastomosis may need to be repeated.

Once the failed anastomosis is divided and removed, the entire process will have to start again. Any trauma to the vessel risks promoting thrombi formation. This is likely to be less of a problem distal to the venous anastomosis if the flow through the flap is robust, as these microthrombi will be flushed away into the internal jugular vein rather than the microcirculation of the flap. However, best not to activate this pro-thrombotic effect, and avoid any trauma to the pedicle as best as is possible (see comment earlier regarding the empty-and- refill test).

Pedicle vein engorgement

If the pedicle veins are not soft, compressible, and relaxed, and start swelling up, and becoming firm and engorged, there is clearly an obstruction in the venous outflow.

The anastomosis has to be carefully inspected. Often the only alternative is to divide and remove the entire anastomosis and start again. Any trauma to the vessel risks promoting thrombi formation. This is likely to be less of a problem distal to the venous anastomosis if the flow through the flap is robust, as these microthrombi will be flushed away into the internal jugular vein rather than the microcirculation of the flap.

The recommended steps to confirm a healthy running anastomosis are summarized in Box 10.1.1.

Box 10.1.1 Recommended sequence for confirming anastomotic patency

Look for pulsation distal to the anastomosis. If this is not confidently assessed, gently raise the vessel until just before the point of vessel occlusion. Observe for the column of blood filling and the vessel transiently expanding with each heartbeat (the uplift test).

Assess for evidence of blood flow distal to the anastomosis around a length of curved vessel (wriggling sign). Beware of 'false wriggling'.

If the artery anastomosis was completed first, blood should be seen emerging from the cut edge of the pedicle vein. If there is no blood emerging the anastomosis is not patent or consider if the microcirculation within the flap itself has become thrombosed (isolate the flap and consider thrombolysis).

Once the arterial anastomosis is confirmed patent, turn your attention to the venous anastomosis. If hand sewing, securely tighten the knots on all but the final suture. Insert the final suture but do not yet tie the knot. Release the vascular clamps and blood can be seen passing across the anastomosis. Then tie the final knot. *This is not possible when using the coupler device, and instead you can use the empty-and-refill test.*

Consider the empty-and-refill test to test patency of the venous anastomosis. Use this sparingly as it can traumatize the vessels.

10.2 **Anastomotic leak**

Introduction

The best solution to deal with anastomotic leaks is to prevent them. Be mindful of the spacing requirements for a vessel when considering the position of each subsequent suture:

- Careful judgement
- Even placement of sutures
- Adequate number of sutures
- Optimum vessel wall apposition
- Judicious elimination of calibre and thickness mismatch

Placement of every suture should be viewed as a strategic 'mind game' to avoid drawbacks and failures once the clamp is released.

The principle is that sutures should be positioned to evert the cut vessel ends at the anastomosis. This also reduces the risk of debris entering the lumen and helps mitigate the risk of microthrombi formation. Once the clamp is removed, a low-flow leak between two adjacent sutures can be resolved by gently placing a soaked tonsil gauze swab or a neuro-patty on the anastomosis for a minute or two. This does not require drastic management with replacing or placing additional sutures and can be managed conservatively with time and patience.

But often careful troubleshooting may be required. Early recognition of an impending problem and steps taken to correct it along the way is a better approach than realizing after having (through the prism of tunnel vision) placed six sutures that were equally spaced but inappropriately located, when the vessel dimensions necessitated 8–10 sutures.

A substantial leak can be tricky to subsequently correct, and it is best to try to avoid finding oneself, having released the clamp, with widespread leak via large spaces between every suture. This may indicate that the spacing was improper at the time the suture was completed and is a point for reflection and future improvement.

To avoid tunnel vision, the second surgeon is well positioned to offer some advice as the first surgeon passes the suture needle. For a new partnership of microvascular surgeons, it may take time to develop the shared experiences and rapport to reach a 'surgical shorthand'.

Assessment and troubleshooting

There is always some degree of bleeding after the release of the vascular clamp an immediate blood flow through the anastomosis. A couple of minutes should be given for the flap to be perfused. During that time gentle anastomosis encasement between two neuro-patties and often changing the top neuro-patty with gentle application of low suction on top of it will be adequate.

It is important that the main neck drain has already been placed and its tube connected to the suction. This removes any blood from the dead space below the level of the anastomosis (space between the main neck vessels and the sternocleidomastoid muscle) and protects the field from flooding.

After a couple of minutes and under irrigation, careful inspection of the anastomosis both in the front wall and back wall is performed. If there is an obvious leak that will manifest with a stream of arterial blood leaking from at least one place.

As a rule of thumb, any bleeding that persists despite this period of pressure requires additional (and possibly repositioning existing) sutures. Any high flow bleeding once the clamp is removed usually immediately indicates the need for further sutures.

Application of an arrow or irrigation under high magnification will allow identification of its cause. Careful assessment and judgement need to be applied here as this anastomotic leak correction will be the point of perfection or compromise of the overall anastomosis. In other words, 'the make or break' of the anastomosis.

In brief there are three main causes of an anastomotic bleeding:

- Suture holes
- Suture gaps
- Telescoping/misapposition

Troubleshooting and technique

Addressing an anastomotic leak is an extremely delicate and demanding procedure and requires refines microsurgical skill and calmness. Maximum concentration and clear and detailed communication between the two microvascular surgeons is crucial.

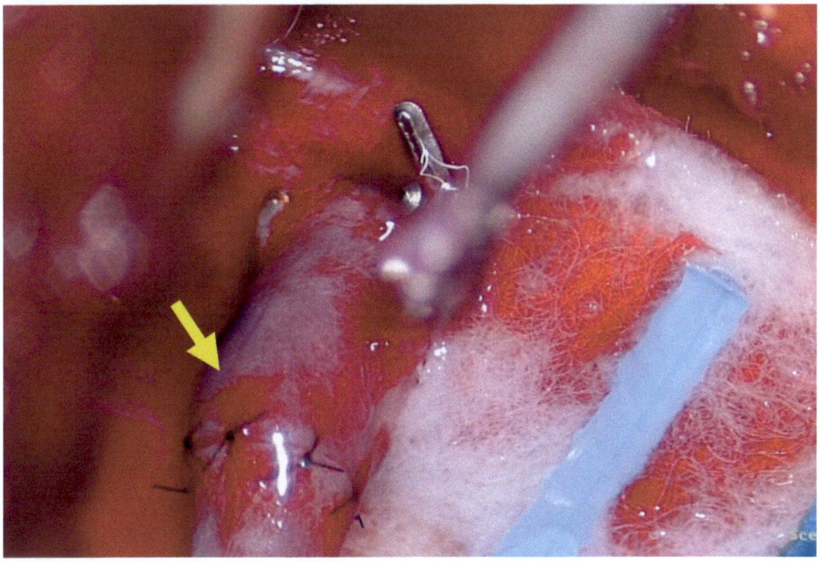

Figure 10.2.1 Suture hole leak.

Suture holes

Blood escaping through suture holes is very common when the needle had to pass twice during the anastomotic suturing or when the needle traversed the vessel wall not perpendicularly but through an oblique course through the vessel.

Stitch hole bleedings in the vast majority of cases will spontaneously cease to bleed.

An application of a neuro-patty with very gentle pressure with the suction on top of it, or serial application of arrows exactly on the point of the stitch hole bleeding may address the issue (Figure 10.2.1 and Video 10.2.1).

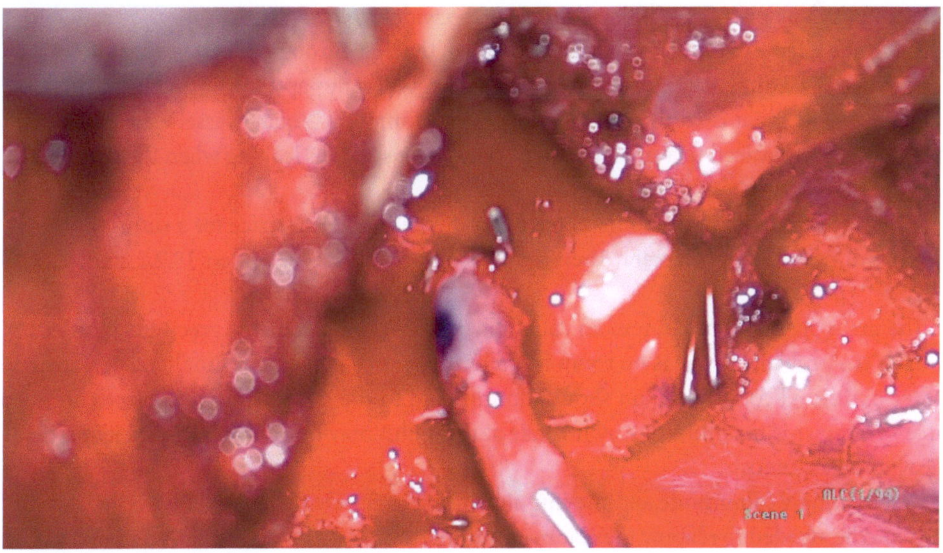

Video 10.2.1 Suture hole leak treated with an arrow.
See this video online by searching for this book's title or ISBN at https://academic.oup.com/
Reproduced courtesy of Leandros Vassiliou, Manchester University NHS Foundation Trust, Manchester, UK.

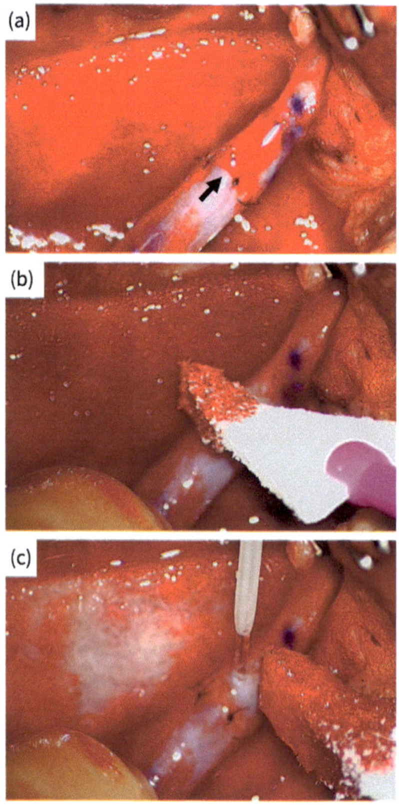

Figure 10.2.2 Anastomotic gap with optimum vessel wall apposition.

Suture gaps

Anastomotic leak may occur if the sutures are too widely spaced. A gap is most often identified after the release of the clamp and restoration of the flow through the vessel that allows the actual vessel wall dimensions to resume. The latter reveals any gaps.

Careful judgement is required at this stage. For example, adequate vessel wall apposition and alignment may lead to a small gap that spontaneously stops leaking when the vessel wall is correct (Figure 10.2.2).

If the gap is wider and the surgeon feels that there is adequate space for a suture, without overcrowding suture placement, then another suture is placed (Video 10.2.2 and Video 10.2.3).

The main operator should remain calm and control the movements precisely in order to address the problem. There is no room for failure, so every movement should be performed under optimized conditions and should not proceed to the next step unless every controllable parameter is maximized. Any mistake at this point may be detrimental and jeopardize the whole anastomosis.

Maintaining a calm mode and moving slowly and precisely is the key. It is very rare, and it should be avoided to reapply the clamp as the anastomosis is left to run now and every obliteration of blood flow may be predisposed to blood stasis and microthrombosis of the flap microcirculation.

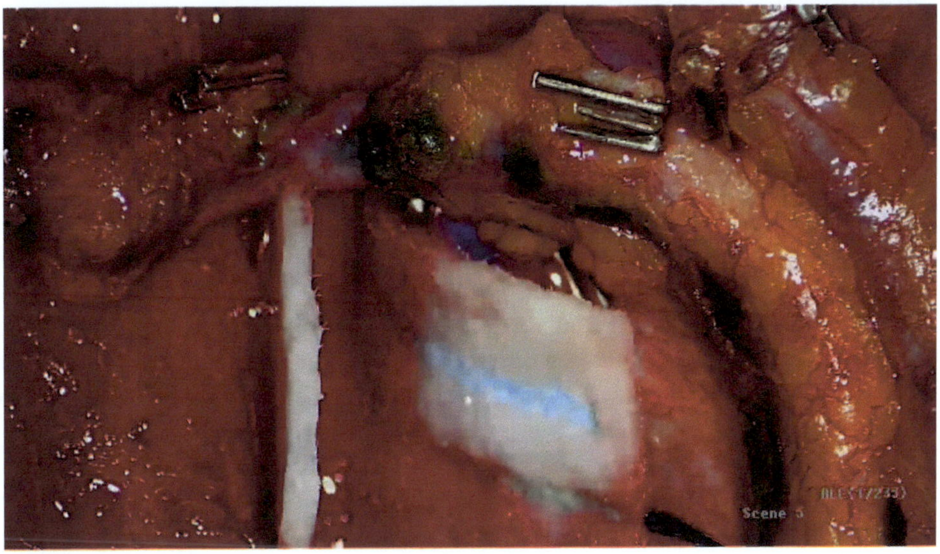

Video 10.2.2 Anastomotic leak due to suture gap requiring an extra stitch.
See this video online by searching for this book's title or ISBN at https://academic.oup.com/
Reproduced courtesy of Leandros Vassiliou, Manchester University NHS Foundation Trust, Manchester, UK.

A standard setting requires the assistant to hold one of the immediately nearby sutures next to the anastomotic leak with one hand holding the microvascular tulip forceps. The other hand holds the syringe with heparinized saline irrigation providing a steady stream of irrigation to allow visibility.

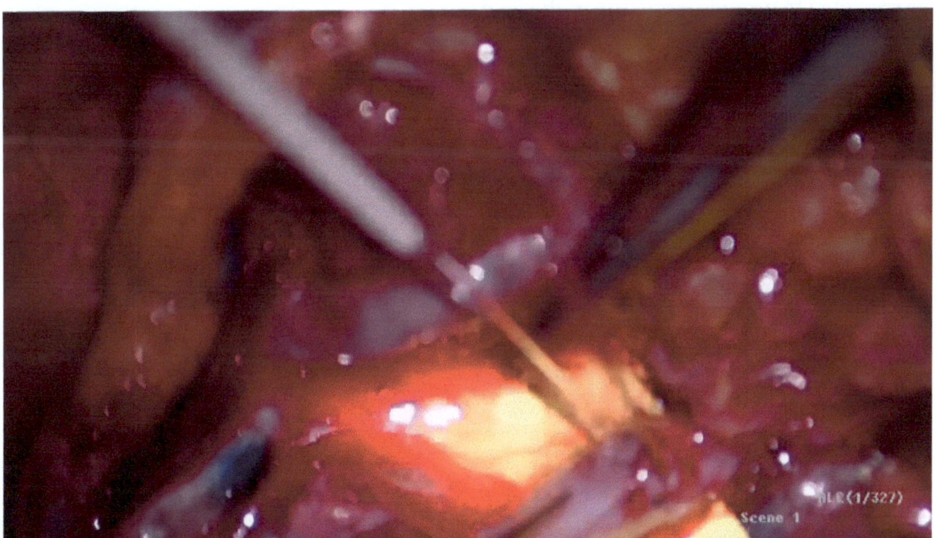

Video 10.2.3 Anastomotic leak due to suture gap requiring an extra stitch in a vertical anastomosis fashion.
See this video online by searching for this book's title or ISBN at https://academic.oup.com/
Reproduced courtesy of Leandros Vassiliou, Manchester University NHS Foundation Trust, Manchester, UK.

The main operator will hold the other stitch on the other side adjusting the tension to the optimum in order to provide adequate countertraction and stretching of the space between the two stitches to allow passage of the needle.

It is best to have anticipated the optimal spacing and ensured high quality, evenly spaced sutures of the utmost quality at each point. Irregularly spaced, poor-quality suture line with mismatching amounts of vessel wall captured in the sutures will affect lamellar flow through the vessel, increasing the risk of thrombi formation.

Where the additional suture needs to be placed at the vessel back wall, then the assistant may choose to pool the adventitia of the tissue instead from a distance of the anastomosis in order to control the whole artery and rotate it while gently may push the rotated vessel with the arrow held by the hand. If the manoeuvres are too difficult or demanding, then a second assistant may be required or alternatively the scrub nurse may be asked to irrigate while the assistant controls the vessel position.

The passage of the needle must be precise and perpendicular through the vessel wall and in this situation the tactile sensation and feedback is of paramount importance. The operator has to feel that the little 'give' signifying that the needle is through the full thickness of the arterial wall by also being extremely sensitive to avoid injuring the endothelial inner wall of the other side of the lumen.

In most vessels and under high magnification, the silhouette of the needle can be seen through the vessel wall, confirming the appropriate course when passing through the lumen.

Once the tip of the needle is felt to have passed through, then the needle is rotated to aim towards the exit point on the other side.

It is important to remember that during the passage of the needle due to the transient disruption of the anastomosis, the bleeding usually will increase (Figure 10.2.3). Appropriate visualization with constant irrigation is the key and, in this situation, if the assistant's both hands are occupied stabilizing the vessel, then a third person (second assistant) may need to be recruited to provide irrigation in the field.

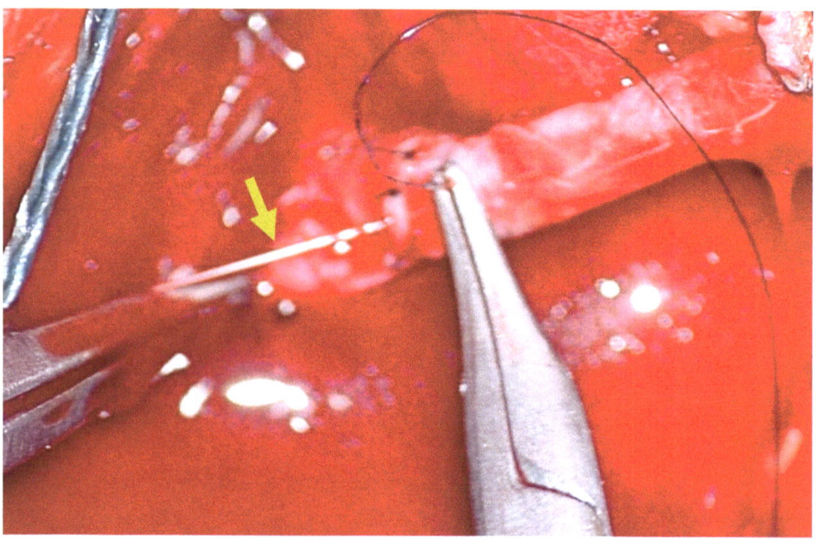

Figure 10.2.3 Extra suture on anastomotic gap.

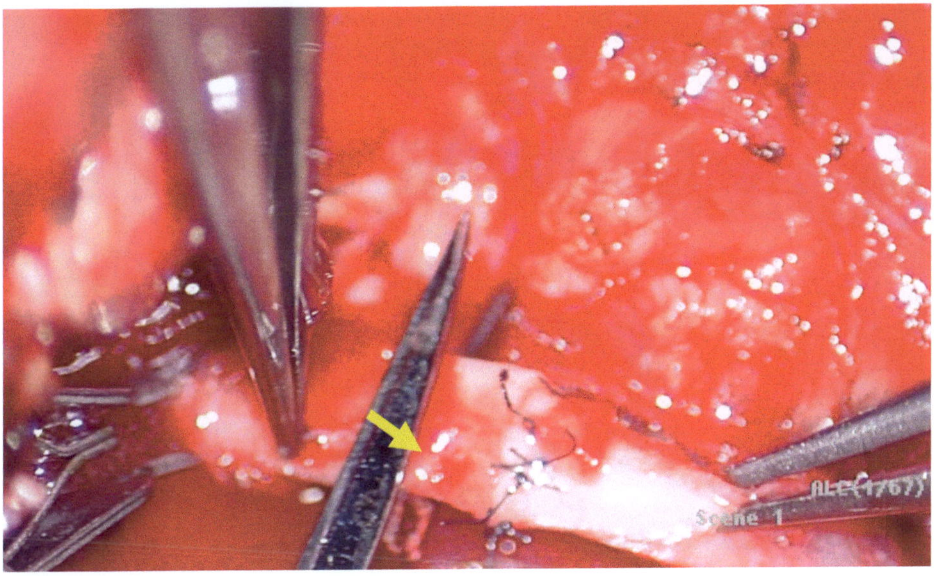

Figure 10.2.4 Vessel tear jeopardizing the whole anastomosis.

On tying the knot, a double square knot is important. Due to the underlying pressure of the blood flow, a single knot may become loose before it is locked with the reef knot; this may endanger the result. For anastomotic leaks when placing additional sutures, always use double knots.

In summary, it is important that any additional stitch on a running anastomosis is placed under extreme precision.

The surgeon and the operator must be well coordinated, and the suture must be inserted completely perpendicular to a relatively immobilized vessel. If additional help for irrigation is required, then the microvascular duet should not hesitate bringing in another assistant.

Careless or unsuccessful passage of the needle these extremely delicate circumstances can result in vessel wall tears that may jeopardize completely the whole anastomosis.

In that scenario, the anastomosis will have to be cut off and replaced back from the beginning (Figure 10.2.4). Clearly that will cause a significant amount of stress due to the added time and also contribute to the fatigue of the surgical team and this must be prevented by all means.

Telescoping/misapposition

The third cause of an anastomotic leak is a vessel wall misappositon. There might be an area of inversion or otherwise called telescoping or an area of eversion especially in cases of calibre mismatch.

Telescoping or otherwise the direction of inversion is crucial in decision making and selecting course of action.

Telescoping can be of two types:

- Type I: Recipient artery wall edge telescoped into the pedicle artery (narrow recipient artery, wider pedicle artery)

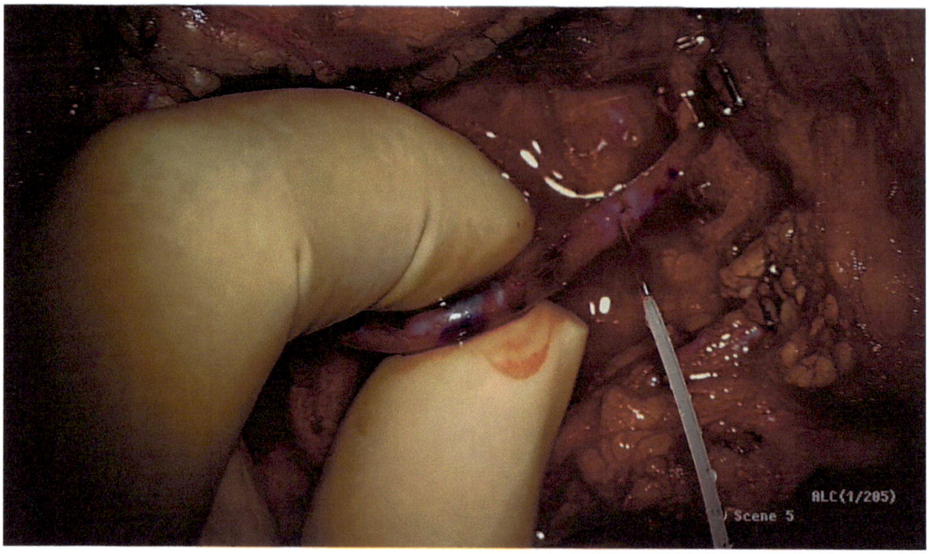

Video 10.2.4 Anastomotic leak, minimal misapposition treated with arrow pressure.
See this video online by searching for this book's title or ISBN at https://academic.oup.com/
Reproduced courtesy of Leandros Vassiliou, Manchester University NHS Foundation Trust, Manchester, UK.

- Type II: Pedicle artery wall edge telescoped into the recipient artery (narrow pedicle artery, wider recipient artery)

As the blood flows from the recipient to towards the pedicle artery, when the inversion is from the recipient to the pedicle artery and only a small one (Type I), the problem may not cause bleeding, and also the anastomosis is considered safe.

However, for type II telescoping when the donor (pedicle artery) is inverted into the recipient artery, there will be a brisk jet of bleeding. This will require correction even if there is a transient stop in bleeding. The reasons correction is indicated is that if postoperatively the patient's blood pressure increases or spikes bleeding will re-occur. Also, this vessel configuration in type II telescoping predisposes to turbulent blood flow and thrombosis.

For type II telescoping, correction is required as the anastomosis is not safe.

When planning the approach to correct the problem, it is best to try to avoid removing and repositioning sutures as each of these attempts cause unavoidable vessel wall trauma.

In some cases, using mild pressure with a series of arrows will help gently 'guide' the vessel edges to re-appose/re-align (Video 10.2.4).

Some cases will certainly require another suture, not for the closure of the gap, but for re-alignment or re-apposition of the vessel walls, especially the intima, to avoid turbulent flow and subsequent thrombosis.

There are two points to consider:

- For calibre and thickness mismatch and the needle is best first passed through the smaller or thinner vessel and a bigger bite is chosen (bigger distance of entry point to edge of vessel wall). A relatively smaller bite (small distance from edge of vessel wall to exit point) is preferred through the larger and thicker opposed vessel.

- On the contrary if the needle is passed through the larger thicker vessel first then a relatively smaller bite is preferred and once the needle is through the full thickness of the vessel wall then it aims towards the relatively larger bite on the other side.

This technique will help the smaller vessel lip to lie everted onto the full thickness edge of the larger vessels once the knot is placed. Precise targeting of the entry and exit points of the needle is important to eliminate any thickness or calibre mismatch at this stage.

Once the needle is through then a double loop is created and a flat square knot is pulled. It is highly important that for anastomotic leaks a double knot is created as a single knot with the underlying blood flow pressure may become loose, destabilizing the anastomosis and effectively fail.

Once the square knot is placed with adequate (adjust the tension of the knot) in order to not strangulate the anastomosis but not be too loose either. A second locking knot in a reef manor is placed. Following that the anastomosis is secured with a third knot and effectively if the whole sequence has been efficient, the leak will stop, and the anastomosis will continue to run without leaks.

10.3 Pedicle suspension and neck positioning

Introduction

During the first one or two days postoperatively the pedicle is not completely fixed even if the platysma flap is repaired and the neck wound closed over suction drains.

During the first phase of wound healing (haemostasis), the blood clot forms fibrin that acts as natural 'glue' and 'cements' all structures including the pedicle and all its components into the embedding neck tissue planes. However, the process, even without complications (collections, seromas, haematomas) may take three to five days before the pedicle is considered stable and hence positionally safe.

There is hence potential for movement that may cause alteration of the blood flow, kinking of the pedicle, and even stasis and thrombosis.

Once the two anastomoses are inspected and the microsurgeons are pleased with the end result, care must be given to suspending the pedicle in order to establish equilibrium in the blood flow and the microcirculation of the flap.

Pedicle course and configuration

The optimum course and configuration of the pedicle needs to be determined. This will need to have gentle curvature, with no acute angles or areas where the vessels are kinked.

The provisional course of the pedicle is set once the flap is inset and the pedicled dropped through the tunnel into the neck to reach the recipient vessels. Having secured the flap *in situ* (do not prolong ischaemic time by completing all sutures needed to make the flap watertight, instead only place enough to ensure the flap is secured against falling away from the tissues. The remaining sutures needed to become watertight can be finished once the microvascular anastomoses have been completed) draw the pedicle across the neck tissues, creating a path from its emergence through the submandibular tunnel to the chosen anastomotic vessels. This path should ensure the vessels are allowed to sit passively and avoid any tight turns or twist, which may kink or otherwise impede luminal blood flow.

Having identified our arterial and venous vessels at the distal end of the pedicle, a trial and error of different paths that the pedicle can trace from the submandibular tunnel to the available anastomotic vessel choices is performed. The optimum choice is the one that allows the most natural path where the pedicle sits passively with favourable ergonomics: we avoid any acute twists or curves and avoid the pedicle passing over structures where it can become compressed (hence we divide the digastric muscle) (Figure 10.3.1).

The summary of steps to ensure the anastomosis is accomplished is a satisfactory fashion are highlighted in Box 10.3.1.

Forward thinking regarding the patient's positioning once they leave the theatre has to be given. It is important to bear in mind that the anastomosis is assessed with the patient lying supine, flat, and with the neck rotated against the side of the anastomosis. The operator has to visualize what are the potential movements of the pedicle will be once the patient's upper body is raised by 30° and 45° degrees and when the patient is sat upright.

In cases with long pedicles such as the radial forearm, once the patient assumes a more vertical position, due to gravity, a sag may incur, from forming a 'U' shaped curvature into an acute 'V' angle (Figure 10.3.2).

Having established the preferred optimal path, the pedicle can be tacked in place with a few well-placed 5/0 or 6/0 round body Prolene plication sutures through the fat attached to the vessel adventitia and the muscle in the anterior triangle.

We recommend the suspension/plication is performed using in 1 to maximum 3 points of the pedicle. The sutures placed are only for suspension, therefore the knot should not be too tight as this can cause constriction or compression of the vessel and compromise the blood flow.

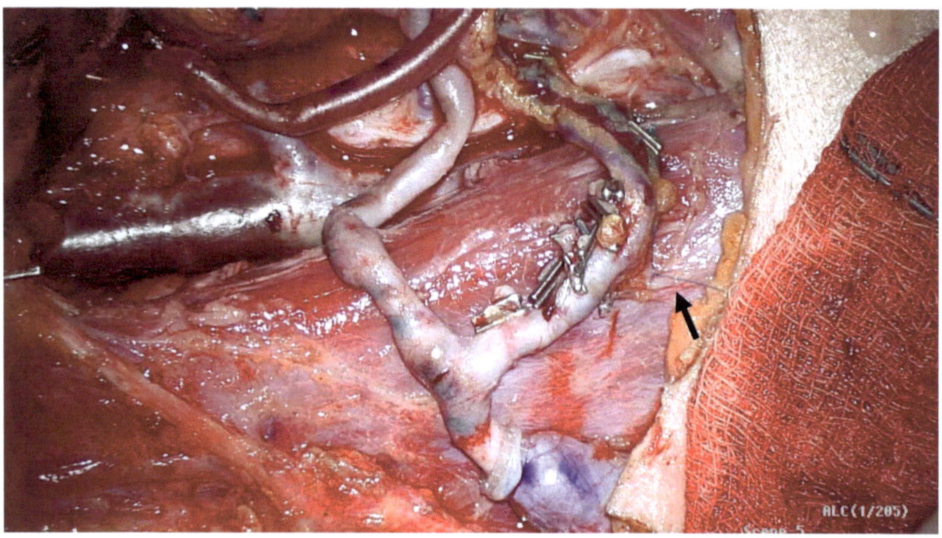

Figure 10.3.1 Pedicle suspension. Note the Prolene stitch (arrow) placed to prevent migration of the pedicle vein that may cause blood flow complications.

Box 10.3.1 Recommended sequence for securing optimal patency

- Place the free flap into its desired position and bring the pedicle into the neck.
- Time economy is important during insetting the flap. Appropriate meticulous inset is of paramount importance; however, if it is expected to take time, place the strategic sutures, continue with the anastomosis and return post-anastomosis to complete the detailed work. Spend no more than 15 minutes insetting a composite free flap—fix the bone with one or two screws and place sufficient sutures to prevent the flap falling or moving are required—the remaining screws and sutures needed to make the reconstruction watertight can be placed after the anastomoses are completed.
- Determine the optimal path for the pedicle to pass across the neck tissues to the chosen anastomotic vessels. Tack the pedicle along the chosen path with a few 5/0 or 6/0 Prolene round-bodied needle sutures.
- Complete the handsewn artery (see later detailed description of how to plan for and execute optimal suture configuration for anastomotic patency while avoiding anastomotic leak) and release the arterial clamp. Watch for blood egress from the (yet to be anastomosed) flap's outlet vein(s), and other signs of arterial patency (pulsation, wriggling, etc.,).
- Apply venous clamps, irrigate the lumen of any residual blood with heparin-saline solution, and complete the venous anastomosis using your chosen method (coupler device versus handsewn). Release the venous clamps and check for clinical signs of patency.
- If satisfied that the anastomoses are both patent, the anastomosis is not leaking, and the pedicle has been suspended to maintain a favourable path for the pedicle, you can return to completing the free flap inset. Apply all the additional sutures required to ensure the flap is secure and mucosa/flap junction is watertight. This process usually takes 15 minutes or so, after which recheck the pedicle and the microvascular anastomoses. The preceding 15 minutes completing the flap inset was adequate time for any technical issues with the anastomoses to manifest and declare themselves.
- With the correct correlation of choices chosen to this point (flap choice, preparing of vascular tunnel, sacrifice of digastric, pedicle length, pedicle path and suspension, anastomotic branch choices from external carotid and tributary branches of the external or internal jugular vein) the anastomoses should still be patent and attention can be turned to closing the neck.

The needle is usually passed from an area of perivascular tissue or abundant adventitia and fixed on a stable point such as a muscle belly in the neck (Figure 10.3.3).

Stabilization of the pedicle with sutures is an inexpensive, simple, and safe technique. Some microvascular surgeons are using various haemostatic or coagulation factors (see Further Reading), such as fibrin glue to achieve that, however this may induce thrombogenic effects or make any subsequent access for exploration of the anastomosis if a complication is incurred difficult. We advise against the use of those agents.

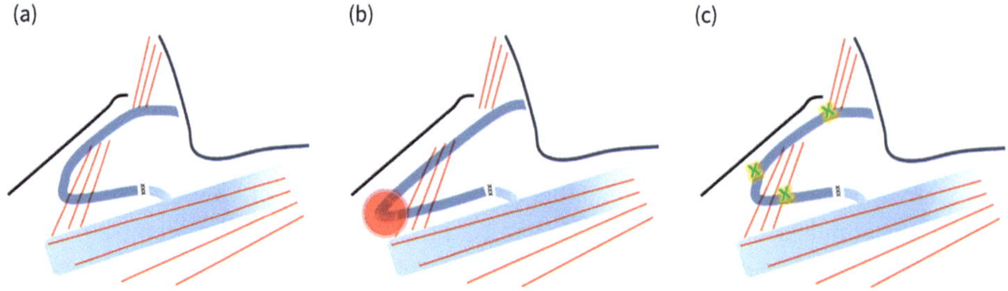

Figure 10.3.2 Schematic presentation of the reasons and technique of pedicle suspension a. Note the 'natural' course of a long pedicle (vein) with an anastomosis (end-to-end) to the common facial vein of the IJV. b. Without suspension and due to gravity, the pedicle 'sags' resulting in an acute angle (kinking) which predisposes to turbulent flow and thrombosis. c. Demonstration of 3-point pedicle fixation using sutures to suspend the pedicle and immobilize it, maintaining the most optimal configuration for patent blood flow.

Sternocleidomastoid (SCM) gutter

Another useful tip for accommodating suspension of the pedicle vessels, as well as avoidance of compression is strategic myotomes, especially of the sternocleidomastoid muscle (SCM).

Remember that the vein lacks muscle and is very thin-walled and has the propensity to collapse upon itself if it is forced to take an unfavourable path. Any collapse will impact blood flow and risks thrombus formation and microvascular failure. The artery is relatively protected against this collapse, being a high-pressure system and with vessel walls containing smooth muscle making the vessels more robust and able to tolerate tighter angulations or a twisting course.

When the venous anastomosis is on the external jugular vein, then creation of a gutter by a limited myotomy on the antero-lateral border of the SCM, creating a small 'nest' where

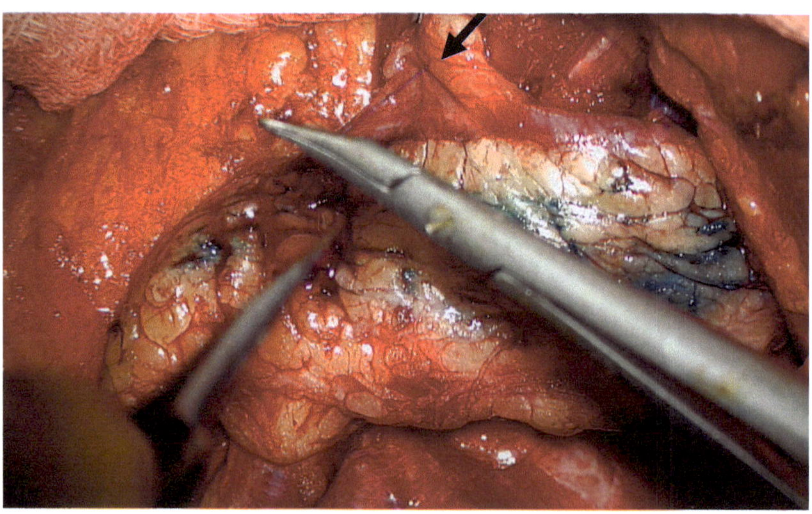

Figure 10.3.3 Pedicle suspension. Note the suspension of the perivascular tissue onto the underlying muscle.

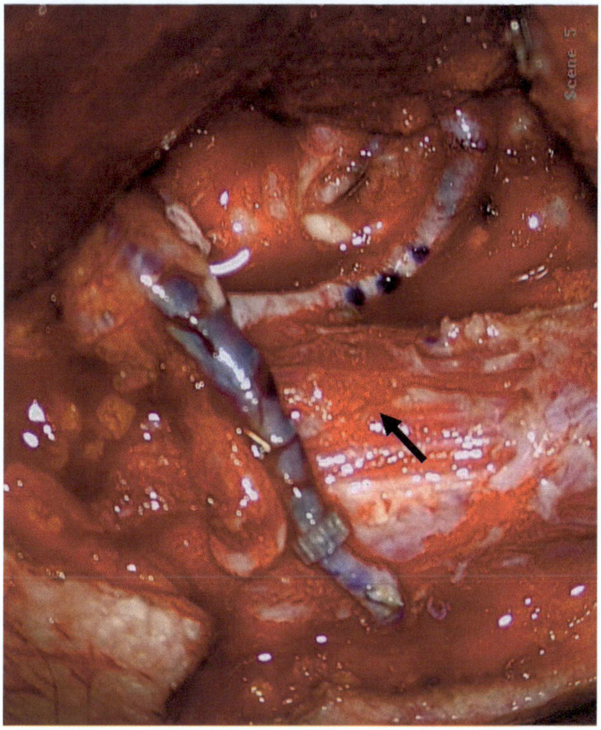

Figure 10.3.4 Sternocleidomastoid muscle myotomy to create a gutter to host the vessel.

the vessel can rest, supported and also without any external compression (Figure 10.3.4 and Video 10.3.1).

The gutter also prevents the vein from downwards (caudal) movement when the patient's neck is raised postoperatively by acting as a 'step' to support it. Vein movement in the postoperative period can be dangerous as if kink occurs acute obstruction can be detrimental.

Similarly, for veins anastomosed to the internal jugular vein a SCM, a myotomy on the inner medial or anterior border may again avoid any compression or kinking by the bulk of the SCM over the fresh venous anastomosis and may create a pocket or a pouch where the vein is running uninhibited.

Postoperative positioning of the head and neck

Once the anastomoses have been checked and they are flowing fine and the pedicle stabilized in the optimum configuration of choice, the ideal position of the neck needs to be assessed.

In most cases slight rotation to the direction opposite the anastomosis side is the normal.

However, it is not unusual especially for shorter pedicles of midface flaps that a neutral position, or a mild rotation towards the ipsilateral site to avoid stretching of the vessels is preferred.

A careful assessment is made and once a decision is made the optimum position is clearly communicated to the anaesthetic and surgical team as well as the theatre team.

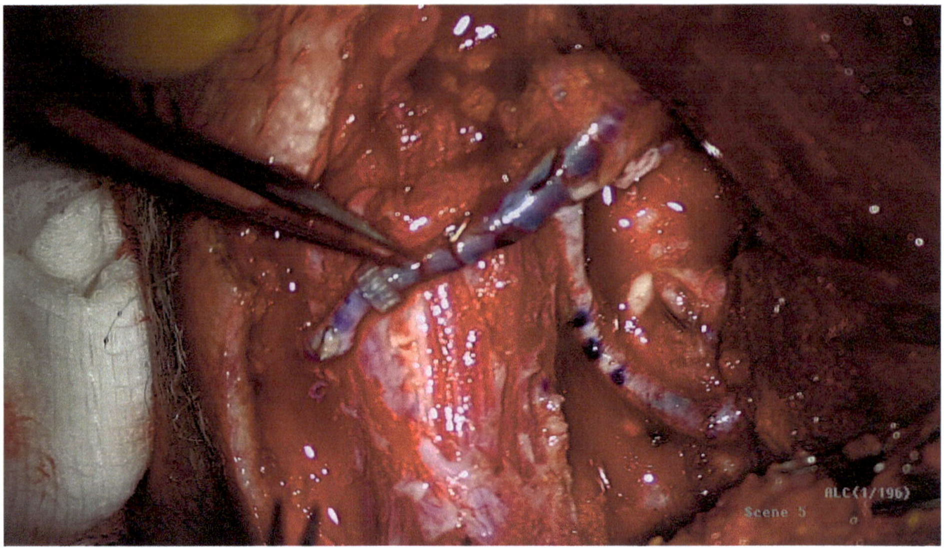

Video 10.3.1 Sternocleidomastoid (SCM) gutter for vein.
See this video online by searching for this book's title or ISBN at https://academic.oup.com/
Reproduced courtesy of Leandros Vassiliou, Manchester University NHS Foundation Trust, Manchester, UK.

This is important because any change from this position has to be carefully undertaken and after the patient's transfer to the bed the correct neck position needs to be re-established as soon as possible.

The correct (optimum) position has to be documented in the postoperative notes and clearly communicated to the recovery team and the intensive care unit team that will receive the patient in the immediate postoperative period.

It is strongly recommended that upon transfer of the patient to the intensive care a senior member of the surgical team attends the handover process, confirms correct positioning of the patient's neck and ensures the message and the relevant instructions are passed on to the critical care team.

Further reading

Acland RD. *Practice Manual for Microvascular Surgery*. St Louis, MO: C.V. Mosby Company, 1989: p. 134.

Isogai N, Ueda Y, Kurozumi N, Kamiishi H. Wound healing at the site of microvascular anastomosis: fibrin-stabilizing factor XIII administration and its effects. *Microsurgery* 1990;11(1):40–6.

Kamiji T, Maeda M, Matsumoto K, Nishioka K. Microvascular anastomosis using polyethylene glycol 4000 and fibrin glue. *Br J Plast Surg* 1989;42(1):54–8.

Kim JT, Kim YH, Kim SW. Effect of fibrin sealant in positioning and stabilizing microvascular pedicle: a comparative study. *Microsurgery* 2017;37(5):406–9.

Liang X, Liu S, Fang Z, Sun G, Guo Z. Prevention of vascular anastomotic stenosis with 2-octylcyanoacrylate. *J Craniofac Surg* 2019;30(1):74–80.

11
Troubleshooting
Recognition

Fu-Chan Wei, Gonzalo Mallarino, Nidal Al Deek, Leandros Vassilios F. Vassiliou, Panayiotis Kyzas, and Nicholas Kalavrezos

11.1 Troubleshooting: Recognition of flap compromise

Introduction

The evolution of microsurgery has allowed consistent and favourable outcomes for a diverse group of pathologies. Undeniably, a large percentage of the growing success in microsurgical procedures, derives from the capacity to timely identify and intervene in adverse situations that might compromise flap viability.

Adequate planning and accurate execution of a microsurgical procedure will decrease the rate of complications; prompt recognition of a problem, and precise identification of its cause, will increase the salvage success after flap re-exploration.

The present chapter aims to provide a guide on how to identify the signs of a failing flap, and the thought process behind detecting the cause of the impending failure. The focus is the particulars of head and neck reconstruction.

Early recognition of flap compromise must prompt return to theatre for exploration and revision. The earlier the problem is detected, the higher the chances for successful flap salvage.

Signs of flap compromise

Any newly vascularized flap has to be viewed as a 'closed-loop' tissue-block system with an arterial input and a venous output. This forms a circuit with the endpoint being the perfusion of the tissue block with oxygenated blood.

There should be an equilibrium between the volume of blood that is pumped in by the arterial segment and the blood that is drained out by the venous outflow. Any disturbance of this flow balance will produce haemodynamic consequences that will manifest at the microvascular (tissue microcirculation) and '*macro*'-vascular level (flap larger vessels and pedicle).

For at least the first week of flap recovery and integration the blood flow within the tissue closed loop is dependent on the principal anastomosed vessels. Progressively, during the process of integration, the flap will connect with the surrounding tissues via new blood vessel formation (neoangiogenesis) that will create collateral channels of blood inflow and outflow (thus achieving peripheral blood supply).

In order to better understand problems related to the vascular pedicle of the flap and how to better troubleshoot and recognize the underlying cause, we will classify the potential flap perfusion issues into:

1 Primarily arterial failure.
2 Primarily venous failure.

In a state of healthy recovery where there is adequate perfusion and balanced blood inflow and outflow if the flap contains a skin paddle, the latter will be expected to appear and feel healthy as any part of the patient's body.

The main parameters are colour, temperature, texture, capillary refill, and for flaps whose vascular pedicle is within reach (i.e. fasciocutaneous radial forearm free flap), an acoustic Doppler signal.

Primarily arterial failure

In the event of acute arterial obstruction/failure, the flap tissue will appear pale, flaccid, and will feel cold. There will be an absence of capillary refill, and on needle prick test or a small incision there will be no bleeding or there will be stagnant venous blood.

If the problem is recognized early, there is a chance of potential flap salvage by immediate return to theatre and revision of both anastomoses (arterial and venous—the venous anastomosis is revised to allow flashing of the flap with heparinized saline and/or alteplase in order to clean the system from debris, clots, and free radicals that can potentially damage the microcirculation). Of course, a full troubleshooting process to identify the cause that led to arterial failure has to be undertaken as discussed in the relevant chapters.

Primarily venous failure

As most of the flaps are inset intraorally with the anastomosis in the neck, venous failure often manifests first with neck swelling. This is because if there is a blockage at the point of the venous anastomosis, the blood outflow will first stop at the point of the anastomosis, and the congestion will start developing retrograde from the level of the anastomosis and backwards to the flap. This is an extremely important point as early venous failure may manifest as an increasing neck haematoma (the 'chicken and egg' dilemma).

Manifestations of venous congestion at the level of the skin paddle such as early bruising (Figure 11.1.1) may be a relatively late phenomenon in the process of venous congestion as this usually occurs at a lower level (anastomosis).

This is where lack of experience on a fresh anastomosis and a newly appearing neck swelling will lead to the false impression that there is a haematoma in the neck triggering removal of sutures and drainage. Whereas, in reality, that early neck swelling signifies the first signs of venous congestion and should trigger a return to theatre and revision of the anastomosis instead.

If the venous failure remains undetected, the progressive venous outflow obstruction with a working arterial anastomosis will further lead to progressive tissue firm engorgement, change of the tissue colour and hue from light blue to deep purple, brisk capillary refill, and bleeding at late stages.

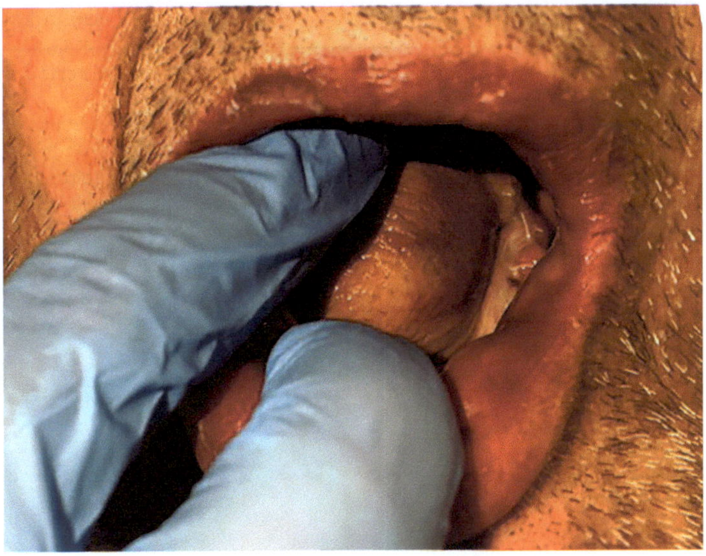

Figure 11.1.1 Clinical picture of early venous failure on a radial forearm free flap.

As mentioned earlier—venous congestion manifests first in the neck and that is clinically visible initially with fullness of the neck, progressively obvious swelling, and later on, if the artery continues to pump blood against an obstructed outflow, with haemorrhage. Exploration of the neck at a late stage will confirm a thrombosed venous anastomosis.

In the event of venous failure and assuming that there is an acute blockage of the venous outflow with a strong working arterial anastomosis that is still pumping blood into the flap tissue, the presentation can be spectacular with fast progressing venous engorgement that manifests with rapid tissue swelling and discoloration, brisk capillary refill that quickly develops into bleeding.

The speed of the clinical evolution depends on the blood rate and volume that the artery is pumping into the tissue. This complication can quickly progress into significant and even massive flap engorgement in the mouth and neck, and development of haemorrhage as the blood is constantly pumped into the flap with no outflow passage through the vein. The trapped blood is under significant and increasing pressure, which effectively decompresses by opening of the vascular channels from the original incisions.

In summary, venous failure due to its often dramatic presentation is far easier to recognize, whereas arterial failure is far more subtle. Unless trained staff members are monitoring the flap and have relevant background experience, the problem is usually identified when it is too late to salvage the flap (unless other monitoring methods are applied).

11.2 **Methods for early detection of flap compromise**

Introduction

This subchapter discusses the available methods, both non-invasive and invasive, that are currently in practice or have been developed.

The summary of the techniques can be found in Table 11.2.1.

Table 11.2.1 Clinical signs of flap compromise

	Intraoperative to early postoperative period (<7 days)	Late postoperative period (7 days or more)
ARTERIAL	**Skin flaps:** - *Colour:* Pale. - *Temperature:* Cold. - *Turgor:* Decreased. - *Capillary refill:* Slow (>5 sec) or absent. - *Bleeding:* Slow or absent.	- *Colour:* Patchy with pale areas. - *Temperature:* Decreased. - *Turgor:* Oedematous. - *Capillary Refill:* Slow (>5 sec) or absent. - *Bleeding:* Slow.
	Intestinal Flaps: - Loss of peristaltic movements. - Pale mucosa. - Decrease in mucous production.	
	Muscle flaps: - No bleeding is observed. - Darker/dim colour. - No contractions. - Flap's surface becomes pasty.	- Turbulent and/or purulent discharge, clinical signs of infection.
VENOUS	**Skin flaps:** - *Colour:* Blue/dark. - *Temperature:* Normal. - *Turgor:* Increased. - *Capillary refill:* Fast (<2 sec). - *Bleeding:* Brisk, dark.	**Skin flaps:** - *Colour:* Dusky, blueish. - *Temperature:* Normal—decreased. - *Turgor:* Oedematous. - *Capillary Refill: Fast* (<2 sec). - *Bleeding:* dark.
	Intestinal flaps: - Dark-looking mucosa. - Engorged or swollen vessels. - Edematous mucosa	**Intestinal flaps:** Very low tolerance to congestion; look for signs of infection.
	Muscle flaps: - Dark-looking fibres. - Excessive bleeding from muscle (dark blood). - Weak responsiveness.	**Muscle flaps:** Look for infection signs.
BOTH	The flap is less full, pale and bluish (patchy appearance), slow to no puncture bleeding (when blood comes out, it is usually dark and uncontinuous). Often, there is wound breakdown due to areas of malperfusion, full/partial thickness ischaemia zones, turbulent discharge due to wound dehiscence and purulent exudates secondary to infection.	

Clinical observation

Intraoperatively

An invaluable predictor of the anastomosis prognosis is the intraoperative assessment of the quality of the anastomosis. It is imperative that upon completion of both arterial and venous anastomoses that a series of validation checks is performed to establish patency and successful flap perfusion:

- Quick and satisfactory flow and volume of venous output as soon as the arterial clamps are released is a powerful prognosticator.

- Perfusion and refill of the arterial vasa vasorum is another indicator of healthy anastomosis.
- Strong pulsation along the arterial pedicle indicates unimpaired flow to the distal end of the artery.
- Sustainable venous outflow (full veins) with no reduction in flow until the neck is closed indicates a good patent anastomotic circuit.
- Intraoperatively, there are some factors that can produce transitory changes, such as hypotension, transient vasospasm, or intraflap blood-flow redistribution; those need to be addressed fully before considering other more severe causes of vascular compromise.

If any of these parameters change while the patient is still on the operating table, the anastomoses need a thorough comprehensive re-assessment and a troubleshooting process needs to be instigated immediately. Often the anastomoses need to be revised, but it is better done at that time rather than a return to theatre with ischaemia anytime later on.

Postoperatively

Flap viability needs to be constantly evaluated during every stage of the surgical procedure, until the patient is transferred to the intensive care unit (ICU), where ideally a routine check on flap status will be conducted by trained staff. Well-developed skills for clinical flap assessment should be instinctive for reconstructive microsurgeons.

Most units have established flap observation protocols and relevant charts where the recordings can be documented. Hourly flap observations are recommended for the first 72 hours. The frequency of flap monitoring may decrease to 2–4 hourly for the fourth and fifth postoperative day to twice per day from the fifth postoperative day onwards. This is based on studies shown that the likelihood of microvascular complications arises mainly in the first 72 postoperative hours as demonstrated by Devine et al. (see 'Further reading').

Flaps containing a skin paddle are more easily monitored. Flap colour, capillary refill, skin turgor, and temperature are some of the clinical parameters that reflect a flap's vascular status (Table 11.2.2).

Even though some specific parameters of what is considered normal have been established, during the postoperative period, it's important to bear in mind that each patient should be held against their own standards, and that a slight deterioration (even within the range of normality) needs to be considered as a herald of early vascular compromise until proven otherwise. Neoangiogenesis usually takes place during the first week after flap transfer, this can alleviate the repercussions of vascular compromise during the late postoperative period and result in a viable flap. For this reason, the signs of arterial and/or venous insufficiency, might be less clear as they are intraoperatively or during the first few days after surgery, and will have a different manifestation.

Additionally, due to the functional demands in head and neck reconstruction, flap underperfusion and ischaemia can result in wound breakdown and cause fistulas to appear. An accurate track on the drainage in order to identify a sudden change in wound discharge, can help to identify wound dehiscence secondary to focal ischaemia.

Monitoring of flaps composed of tissue different to skin requires special observation. Intestinal flaps suffering from ischaemia will undergo similar changes in flap colour when undergoing venous or arterial ischaemia; additional signs like decrease or absence of mucous

Table 11.2.2 Detailed overview of the free flap monitoring methods

	Strengths	Limitations	Applicability/suitability in elderly patients
Clinical examination	Non-invasive Low cost Quick assessment	Limited use in buried flaps without skin island Dependence on a light source Lack of standardization Expertise and experience required	Challenging due to interindividual skin/flap appearance and lacking standardized protocols
Handheld Doppler (acoustic Doppler sonography)	Non-invasive Simple to use Low cost Quick assessment	Typically not applicable for buried flaps Lack of quantitative measurement Non-continuous Expertise and experience required	No definitive conclusions; age may be considered a potential confounder
Implantable Doppler	Simple to use Easy handling and simple setup Use in buried flaps Continuous	Invasive Expensive Implantable probe needs to be removed (possible port of entry for infectious agents)	Might be beneficial, future large-scale studies are needed
Flow coupler	Simple to use Easy handling and simple setup Use in buried flaps Continuous	Invasive Implantable probe needs to be removed, (possible port of entry for infectious agents)	Might be beneficial, future large-scale studies are needed
Colour duplex ultrasonography	Non-invasive Use in buried flaps Quantifications of vessel inflow and outflow	Expertise and experience required Expensive Non-continuous	Lack of robust data regarding postoperative free flap monitoring
Laser Doppler flowmetry	Non-invasive continuous Arterial and venous occlusion differentiation	Expensive Lack of quantitative measure User training and experience required	Blood flow parameters may differ among elderly patients; standardized norm values are lacking

Near-infrared spectroscopy	Non-invasive continuous real-time measurement Simple to use Remote monitoring possible	Expensive Regional oxygen saturation might be influenced by internal and external variables Patient mobility can influence signal quality Requires skin island and taping of large probe that can limit clinical assessment of flap	Might be beneficial, future large-scale studies are needed
Hyperspectral imaging	Non-invasive Quick assessment Ability to differentiate arterial and venous occlusion	Noncontinuous Expensive Sensitivity to small movement Lack of large-scale validation studies Reliance on ambient lighting	Resting posture might be problematic in elderly patients (e.g. due to tremor and restlessness)
Oxygen partial pressure measurement	Continuous	Invasive Single-point measurement	Might be beneficial, future large-scale studies are needed
Thermal imaging	Noninvasive	Unclear, future studies are needed	Future large-scale studies are needed

Adapted from Knoedler S, Hoch CC, Huelsboemer L, Knoedler L, Stögner VA, Pomahac B, Kauke-Navarro M, Colen D. Postoperative free flap monitoring in reconstructive surgery-man or machine? Front Surg. 2023 Feb 22;10:1130566 under a Creative Commons CC-BY-4.0 license.

production, and reduction in peristaltic movements should be noted as early vascular compromise.

Muscle flaps will develop a pale and later 'mottled' appearance (Figure 11.2.1) and will have reduced bleeding in the presence of arterial insufficiency. If venous compromise occurs, bruising, engorgement of the underlying muscle before the skin paddle and bleeding will ensue.

In the event of flaps located deep within the oral cavity, or highly pigmented skin phenotypes and patients' darker skin complexity, or musculocutaneous flaps where the arterial function cannot be monitored with Doppler, monitoring of the aforementioned parameters might be difficult. In this scenario, performing a needle pin prick or a superficial incision will provide a direct visualization of the vascular status at the dermis, and will not increase the risk of infection or heal inadequately.

Clinical monitoring of buried flaps is more challenging. Intraoperatively, it's possible to detect vascular changes in the muscle, periosteum, or bowels; however, during the postoperative period, it might be difficult (or even impossible) to determine vascular impairment based on clinical signs, and gross manifestations, such as purulent discharge will become apparent when it's too late to act. A study conducted by Yuen and colleagues (see Further Reading) describing a monitoring protocol for 55 buried flaps used in head and neck reconstruction, determined that assessing flap viability through an exteriorization of a flap's component, was superior to other methods of monitoring, and resulted in a 100% successful re-exploration rate.

Clinical observation combined with acoustic Doppler is considered the gold standard in flap monitoring to date. However, and taking this a step further, we recommend that the best practice lies in serial flap observations. A 'snapshot' recording of the flap clinical status may not always reveal a problem or detect an evolving complication especially in complex

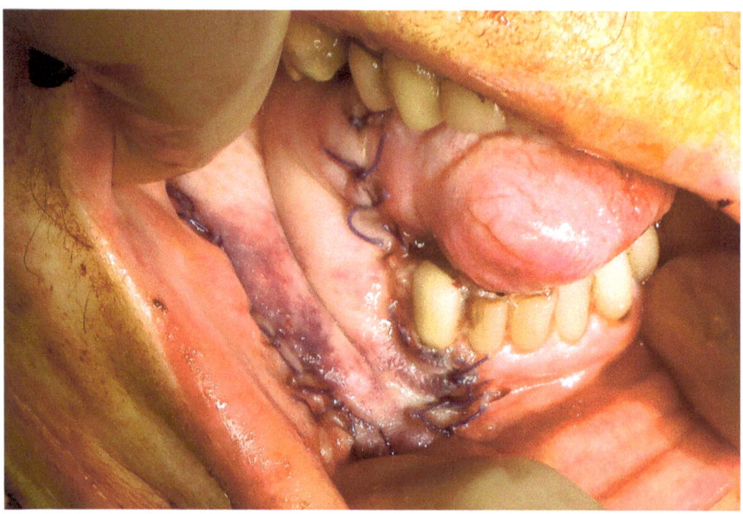

Figure 11.2.1 Late recognition of arterial failure in myocutaneous free flap (latissimus dorsi). Note the 'deflated' pale skin with areas of mottling due to progressive ischaemia.

reconstructions or flaps difficult to monitor. Serial observations and a high index of suspicion are keys for early recognition and detection of a compromise. Subtle changes, a swelling in the neck or a small area of discoloration are of significant value if monitored over short time and proved to evolve.

Handheld Doppler

This is acoustic Doppler sonography based on a small portable Doppler device with a probe that can be applied on the flap and can pick up arterial pulsations. This method works on perforator flaps and flaps with pedicles, but it can be difficult to apply for monitoring of musculocutaneous flaps such as latissimus dorsi due to the absence of an underlying arterial vessel.

The principle of its function is that the probe picks ultrasonic waves from the pulsatile blood and translates those bio signals into acoustic feedback (see Salgado et al. in 'Further reading').

The handheld Doppler only monitors the arterial part of the flap and is not applicable for monitoring the venous outflow.

The method is quite economic, as the portable Doppler devices are not considered expensive.

Implantable Doppler

This method was introduced by Swartz et al. in 1988 (see Swartz et al. in 'Further reading') and is also based on Doppler science. Rather than a portable probe, there is a small-sized piezoelectric crystal applied on the anastomosis (both the arterial and the venous) and embedded in a silicone sheath gently tied around the vessels.

The connecting wires transmit a single inner acoustic Doppler device. This method offers constant monitoring of both the arterial and the venous anastomosis.

The downside of this is that there are a quite high false-positive signals (see Ferguson and Yu in 'Further reading') due to dislocation of the probes or disconnection of the delicate wiring.

Flow coupler

A flow coupler Doppler monitors a combined vascular anastomosis coupler as described in the MACD chapter with an implantable ultrasonic micro-Doppler probe. This can provide similar information as an acoustic implant Doppler (see Zhang et al. and Troob et al. in 'Further reading'). However, it is only applicable to the venous anastomosis as coupler devices are not applied to arteries.

Although the method is regarded as very sensitive, there are still reports of a relatively high false-positive rate.

Colour duplex ultrasonography

This is based on more advanced duplex ultrasonography (see Ensat et al. in 'Further reading') and a device that is designed to provide visualization of the ultrasonic waves translating blood flow and blood velocity.

The principle is very similar to acoustic Doppler sonography. However, the yield and quality of information are more advanced. The device monitors the actual microvascular anastomosis, and the blood flow can be assessed by a viewing monitor.

This is applicable for the monitoring of buried flaps that are not approachable to direct clinical inspection.

The equipment is very expensive.

Laser Doppler

The Doppler shift from laser light backscattered by red cells can be used to assess circulation at a capillary level. Jones et al. were the first to describe the use of laser Doppler flowmetry (LDF) for free flap monitoring in 1982, and ever since it's a practice that has been refined and gained a wide acceptance since it's a non-invasive and safe method for continuous flap assessment. The most basic configuration of LDF consists of a probe placed in the flap intraoperatively, which is usually connected to a helium-neon laser through an optical fibre. With the assistance of specialized software, the signals of blood flow are amplified, and transduced to a monitor, where tissue perfusion can be observed as an oscillating curve (as described by Jones et al., Frerichs et al., and Oberg in 'Further reading').

Clinical experience shows that flow values can vary greatly between patients and the tissue type being monitored. For this reason, in order for LDF to be accurately interpreted, it's necessary to establish the baseline measurements intraoperatively. Yushino et al. (see 'Further reading') described the use of LDF for monitoring of 37 flaps used for head and neck reconstruction, at different time-points in order to describe the patterns in which LDF is able to predict vascular collapse; instead of using absolute parameters, baseline perfusion was defined as 100% before flap elevation. Even though a slight decrease was noted after microvascular anastomosis, flaps with an uneventful evolution usually showed a pattern of increasing flow during the first postoperative day, which reached 100% of flow during the second or third postoperative day. In contrast, when a flap presented with vascular compromise, an abrupt collapse 50% or more of blood flow was observed, usually preceding clinical manifestations. Heller et al. (see 'Further reading') developed a protocol combining clinical observation and objective measurement of flow using LDF; whenever a deterioration of 50% of the baseline measurement, or a drop of 0.4 LDF units was observed for more than 30 minutes, clinical observation was increased and additional measurements (e.g. suture release, optimization of haemodynamic parameters and the patient's position) were set in place. A salvage rate of 88% was reported with the use of the combined protocol, and LDF was able to predict vascular compromise before clinical manifestations in 94% of the cases. A wide body of evidence is available (Pafitanis et al. in 'Further reading'), describing the use of LDF for the postoperative monitoring, specifically of free flaps used for head and neck reconstruction. Yoshino et al. used adhesive LDF probes in order to monitor intraoral flaps in a series of 38 flaps, obtaining a similar success rate. Hellner et al. (see 'Further reading') described the use of LDF monitoring in 28 cases for head and neck reconstruction, which included flaps where clinical observation can be difficult, such as buried muscular flaps and intestinal flaps, reporting a positive predictive value of 85%. Yuen and collaborators (see 'Further reading') described the use of LDF in diverse clinical settings, including a protocol for buried flaps for hypopharyngeal reconstruction, that combines clinical observation with LDF monitoring in an exteriorized flap component in 55 consecutive cases, were a salvage rate of 100% was obtained. Limitations of LDF include the fact that the probe only takes account 1 mm of tissue, which can lead to false-negative in cases of partial flap ischaemia. Moreover, some studies suggest that LDF is able to predict vascular collapse before clinical signs when it's caused by arterial occlusion; however, when venous thrombosis occurs, the deterioration of flow parameters can occur over a long period of time, which makes clinical observation a more reliable tool (see Yuen and Feng in 'Further reading'). Additionally, there is a rate of around 4% of erroneous readings due to artefacts like partial detachment of the probe or vibration. Lastly, the high cost of both the equipment and probes (which can be around 15.000 and 120 USD, respectively) has also hindered the way LDF has been fostered as a postoperative monitoring technique (see Yuen and Feng in 'Further reading').

Indocyanine green near-infrared video angiography

Indocyanine green near-infrared video angiography (ICG-NIR-VA), is a safe, non-invasive method to assess flap perfusion in real time, which has been shown to determine areas of flap hypoperfusion, even before clinical signs arise. ICG is a molecule that binds to plasmatic proteins and is confined exclusively to the vascular space, which makes it ideal for assessing perfusion. There is a small but documented risk of anaphylaxis. The molecule has a half-life time of 3–5 minutes.

With the aid of near-infrared video, it is possible to assess the perfusion of a flap in real time by objectively characterizing the flap's fluorescence as reported by Hembt et al. and Sahovaler et al. (see 'Further reading'). ICG-NIR-VA can aid during flap harvest and inset by identifying and selectively excluding segments with poor perfusion and has been found to decrease complications that arise from tissue necrosis, and partial or total flap loss. In a study conducted by Kneser et al. that described the impact of using ICG-NIR-VA during flap harvest in 88 free flaps for different indications, ICG-NIR-VA was found to have a sensitivity of 100% for detecting underperfused areas, with a negative predictive value of 100% (Bigdeli et al. in 'Further reading'). Additionally, when the poorly perfused areas were resected, a 38.6% decrease in complications (i.e. fistula formation) rate was observed. This method can be used after flap anastomosis as well. Hembt et al. (see 'Further reading') described the use of ICG-NIR-VA in a series of 506 DIEP flaps for breast reconstruction after the anastomosis was concluded. When compared with cases where it wasn't used, ICG-NIR-VA significantly decreased fat necrosis. Use of ICG-NIR-VA for determining acute vascular compromise during the postoperative period is yet to be fully developed, especially considering that it's not possible to differentiate venous from arterial compromise based on fluorescent parameters. Bettega et al. (see 'Further reading') published a pilot study where 20 patients undergoing head and neck reconstructions with free flaps, were monitored using sequential injections of ICG with hourly monitoring and perfusion assessment with the assistance of a NIR camera.

Even though deterioration of perfusion parameters based on fluorescence (curve slope and amplitude) allowed to detect flap failure in some cases; the high rate of false positives due to variation of such parameters over time, and the difficult logistics behind periodical use of indocyanine green, would seem to preclude ICG-NIR-VA from being an efficient postoperative method of flap monitoring, especially in the head and neck. An additional downside of this method is the fact that it is not possible to visualize deep tissue, as the penetration of ICG-NIT-VA is limited to 5–8 mm of tissue.

Hyperspectral imaging

This method is based on spectrometric tissue analysis (see Karim et al. in 'Further reading'). It is a non-invasive method. The target tissue is illuminated by a halogen light source and the remitted light is analysed in a spectrum of 380–1,000 nanometers (from visual wavelength to infrared software). Algorithms process the data into colour-coded images. Different levels of haemoglobin, oxygenation, and saturation produce different-coloured signals warning the operator about the level and quality of flap profusion.

The method, although scientifically astute, has not been validated by large-scale studies (see Schulz et al. in 'Further reading').

The device is able to detect early vascular compromise of the flap and can discriminate between material blockage and venous congestion.

One downside of the method is the reliance on specific light conditions and the cost of the equipment.

Metabolic monitoring

When deprived of oxygen, cells will access the glycogen deposits in order to produce adenosine triphosphate (ATP) molecules. This leads to the production of high levels of lactic acid. These metabolic changes occurring within the extracellular space can be tracked as well, in order to assess response to ischaemia (Jyraenki et al. in 'Further reading').

Microdialysis (MD) for monitoring brain tissue was initially described by Delgado et al. in 1972 and was later adapted for the surveillance of flaps and peripheral tissues by Ungerstedt and colleagues (see 'Further reading'). By placing a double-lumen catheter with a dialysis membrane perfusing Ringer's lactate, the collected dialysate is analysed at bedside during the postoperative period, in order to provide continuous monitoring of flaps. Edsander-Nord et al. (see 'Further reading') reported the results of postoperative flap monitoring in 22 free and pedicled TRAM flaps, and compared concentration levels of glucose, lactate, glycerol, and the glucose/pyruvate ratio, between zone II and III, and were able to describe the metabolic response to different types of ischaemia during the postoperative period. One of the main conclusions drawn by this study is that even though absolute values can be used as parameters in order to define alert levels, baseline concentrations of the different metabolites should ideally be defined by analysing tissue near the donor area. Nielsen and collaborators (see 'Further reading') described the first protocol adapting MD for monitoring of free flaps after head and neck tumour ablations. 78 flaps were monitored, and whenever glucose levels dropped by more than 1 mmol/L or lactate levels increased >10 mmol/L, nurses alerted the surgeon in order to decide if flap re-exploration was required. In this study, MD was reported to have a false-positive and false-negative rate of 25.5% and 0%, respectively. Birkenfeld et al. (see 'Further reading') tested a similar protocol comparing the outcomes on 96 flaps used for head and neck reconstruction that were monitored by clinical observation exclusively vs. MD. Interestingly the results were less favourable, reporting a false-negative rate of 10% in the MD group. After measuring the concentrations of different metabolites in 34 buried flaps used for mandible reconstruction with bony flaps, Dakpe et al. (see 'Further reading') concluded that deterioration in the metabolic parameters during the first postoperative days, was able to predict complications such as impaired wound healing and flap failure. However, due to the relatively low sample this correlation was not statistically significant. Disadvantages of DM include the possibility of catheter dislodgement and false readings due to the presence of hematomas between the probe and the monitored tissue. Additionally, care must be taken when interpreting the readings based on absolute results, since there are factors that can greatly change these parameters, such as previous conditions or the particular metabolic profile that each tissue has (Kwasnicki et al. in 'Further reading').

Other methods for monitoring metabolic factors in free flaps include the capillary measurement of glucose and lactate (see Karakawa et al. and Setala et al. in 'Further reading'). The use of capillary glucose by Hara et al. (see 'Further reading') found a specificity and sensitivity of 88% and 82%, respectively, for detecting venous compromise during the early postoperative period. Heunalt and colleagues (see 'Further reading') noted an increase in the performance of capillary measurements when lactate was included in the protocol. Glucose level <3.85 mmol/dL and lactate levels >6.4 mmol/dL, had a sensitivity of 98.5% and specificity of 99.5% for detecting vascular compromise in free flaps.

Other methods—oxygen partial pressure monitoring

Direct measurement by diverse methods of tissue partial oxygen pressure (pti O_2) has also been used as a method to determine flap viability and to timely predict complications. Use of the Licox® microcatheter for monitoring of free flaps was first described by Wechselberger and colleagues in 17 TRAM flaps, and later by Kamolz et al. (see 'Further reading'), who published one of the largest series on the subject on 60 cases, where a decrease of 10 mmHg in pti O_2 had 100% of positive-predictive value for detecting vascular compromise. Monitoring with pti O_2 for head and neck reconstructions with similar results.

Overall, the different technologies described for flap monitoring stand out as a useful supplement for clinical observation (which remains the gold standard for determining vascular compromise), especially aiding untrained staff. On a broader context, the actual impact of such ancillary methods for flap monitoring has on enhancing postoperative care, decreasing length of ICU stay, or increasing the success rate in reinterventions, is yet to be proven, particularly in the context of head and neck reconstruction.

Other methods—thermal imaging

Thermal imaging is a relatively novel non-invasive method for flap monitoring. Its operating principle is based on measuring tissue temperature, which is directly correlated to blood flow converting it to visual images (see Frohwitter et al. and Rabani et al. in 'Further reading').

The method is contactless and hence infection control risks encountered in other methods such as the use of handheld probes in multiple patients are omitted.

11.3 Causes for flap failure in head and neck reconstruction

Introduction

Undoubtedly, a significant portion of free flap failures is attributed to technical aspects of the microvascular anastomosis, especially for the less experienced microvascular surgeon. But there is a much wider amplitude of factors that can affect the viability of the flap and those could be systemic physiological factors, local factors as previous neck treatments, and more complex technical procedures that increase the risk of thrombogenesis.

It is important that the vascularized flap is seen as a 'system' or better said as an 'organ' whose perfusion and viability are directly depended to the host's (patient's organism) physiological condition.

Postoperative parameters and physiological factors

Even in the context of patients in ideal conditions, undergoing perfectly executed reconstructions that are well-designed for the patient's needs; an inadequate perioperative management that doesn't take into consideration the special requirements these complex reconstructions have, will eventually end up causing flap loss and other devastating consequences. There are multiple factors with the potential to limit a flap's circulation that need to be addressed by the team in charge of delivering the anaesthesia. Central hypothermia can lead to vascular constriction, which can in turn cause spasm of donor or recipient vessels (see Hagau et al. in 'Further reading'). Inadequate management of hemodynamic parameters can compromise a flap's vitality as well (see Kass et al. in 'Further reading'). After studying the effects of intraoperative hypotension for 445 free flaps for head and neck reconstruction; Kass et al. (see 'Further reading') concluded that consistent hypotension and large-volume fluid administration (particularly >7 litres of crystalloids), led to higher rates of flap failure. Very similar results were found by Ettinger and colleagues (see 'Further reading'), which concluded that administration of more than 7 litres of crystalloids had a correlation with higher risk of flap loss (O.R 1.2) and other clinical complications. Use of vasopressors represents a good solution for avoiding hypotension without having to appeal to liberal fluid administration. In a meta-analysis that pooled the outcomes of 8,653 flaps conducted by Goh et al. (see 'Further reading') studying the impact that perioperative vasopressors have on flap loss after head and neck reconstruction, it was reported that use of vasopressors was a protective factor against pedicle thrombosis in head and neck reconstruction (O.R 0.7). Kim and collaborators (see 'Further reading') developed a goal-directed hemodynamic therapy protocol that was found to decrease the risk of flap failure by maintaining a mean arterial pressure >65 mmHg. This protocol was found to have a reduction of 10.5% of flap loss in a comparative study that included 62 patients undergoing head and neck reconstructions. After undergoing free tissue transfer, patients are usually at high risk of developing postoperative agitation and other types of delirium, with the potential to cause traction of the vessels or to cause bleeding and hematoma in the wounded.

Although no studies can be found that objectively measure this correlation, there are many available protocols describing different types of sedation schemes in this specific population (see Yang et al. and Yamagata et al. in 'Further reading'). Prolonged anaesthesia and operative times also have a clear correlation with the development of flap failure and other major clinical complications. A study analysing this correlation in 1.305 free flaps (see Kim et al. in 'Further reading'), showed that flap failure could increase by up to 23% with prolonged operative times, and increase the risk of requiring blood transfusion, and other medical comorbidities as well. Additional elements of the perioperative care of patients undergoing head and neck reconstructions, which can cause injury to the pedicle and result in flap failure include drain displacement, inadequate position, and transportation of the patient resulting in pedicle strain, and direct injury to the pedicle when replacing wound dressings.

Counting on a trained staff is fundamental for avoiding these types of adverse events. Additionally, efficient communication between the surgical team and the postoperative care staff is needed, specifically regarding the exact location of the anastomosis and perforators, as well as additional particularities that a patient might have.

Technical factors during flap harvest

Finding the cause of vascular compromise is just as important as timely identification of flap failure signs. Human error plays the most important role in free flap failure and unfavourable microsurgical reconstructions. More specifically, technical errors during flap harvest, inset, and microvascular anastomosis, are estimated to be the cause of 5.5–28.3% of complications of head and neck reconstructions (see Wei et al. in 'Further reading'), although in our view this figure is a gross underestimation. Perforator injury is an under-reported complication that can occur at multiple moments during free tissue transfer. Miyamoto and collaborators (see 'Further reading') reported a total incidence of 1.5% of this complication after retrospectively analysing 476 perforator-based flaps used for head and neck reconstruction. The flap with the highest percentage of perforator injury the deep inferior epigastric perforator (DIEP) flap (4.3%) followed by the fibula flap (2.0%), and by the anterolateral thigh (ALT) flap (0.9%). Contrary to what might be expected, most of the injuries occurred during flap tailoring rather than when the flap was being harvested (71%), especially when osteotomies were performed for mandibular reconstruction.

ALT flaps harvested as musculocutaneous flaps had a higher incidence of perforator injury than when perforator skeletonization was performed. A study (see Celik et al. in 'Further reading') analysing unfavourable outcomes in 672 ALT flaps, concluded that lack of skills to properly identify a sizeable perforator could account for 1% of the causes for flap failure. Additional errors, such as unfavourable geometry during flap inset causing pedicle and/or perforator kinking and errors during anastomosis, need to be addressed urgently in order to avoid catastrophic consequences (see Chang et al. in 'Further reading').

Infection

Surgical site infections have been reported to be as high as 41% after microsurgical reconstruction of the head and neck, caused mainly by MRSA, *P. Aeuroginosa*, *K. Pneumoniae*, and other enterobacteria (Karakida et al. in 'Further reading'). Given the anatomic continuity that microvascular anastomosis have with the aerodigestive tract, infection, and fistulas represent an additional threat to flap viability and cause late flap failure. In a systematic review pooling patients with late flap loss (>7 days) in head and neck reconstruction, Forner et al. (see 'Further reading') established that fistula and abscess formation, was the cause for flap loss in 42% of the cases.

Previous radiotherapy

Reconstruction of defects compromising the head and neck, includes specific challenges that can potentially compromise a flap's viability. Radiotherapy (RT) at the recipient site has been associated with a higher risk of flap failure. A meta-analysis conducted by Mijiti et al. (see 'Further reading') that pooled over 12,668 free flaps used for of head and concluded that preoperative RT had a higher risk for flap failure with an O.R of 1.92. The additional risk that RT portrays, is dose dependent. Benatar and collaborators (see 'Further reading') described the impact that RT dose has by studying the outcomes on 429 cases of free flaps for head and neck reconstruction. Patients that received irradiation doses >60 Gy, had a statistically significant increase in the risk of free flap failure, hematoma formation, and overall complications.

The negative effect of RT comes from impaired endothelial function and has an impact on head and neck reconstruction at many different levels, since irradiated recipient vessels have a lower quality, and can represent an additional challenge that requires the development of specific skills and experience for handling these types of vessels (see Smith et al. in 'Further reading'). An experimental study conducted by Watson (see 'Further reading') showed that anastomosis patency can decrease from 94% to 54% when anastomosis is attempted within an irradiated field. Higher doses of radiation and prolonged time elapse since radiation until, surgery increased the risk of thrombosis at the anastomosis site. Additionally, irradiated tissues have extremely low capacity to generate nutrient exchange with transferred flaps, prolonging the period in which a free flap will depend on its vascular pedicle, and decreasing the capacity of a flap to react to unfavourable situations.

Shultze-Mosgau (see 'Further reading') objectively compared the vascularization patterns on the interface of 217 free flaps and the recipient beds. It was found that that RT had a correlation with a decrease in capillary angiogenesis, increased precapillary fibrosis, and an increased risk of flap failure. These findings were more marked at higher doses of irradiation.

Harvesting of recipient vessels is an additional cause for flap complications in heavily irradiated necks; ionizing radiation causes a steep decrease in arterial vasa vasorum and constricts the smooth muscle, which make the irradiated vessels more prone to rupture.

Osteoradionecrosis (ORN) is a condition in which bone turnover is affected by fibrosis and hypovascularization due to the endothelial damage caused by RT, that often requires resection of the affected tissue and reconstruction with free tissue transfer. In the context of ORN, the risk of flap failure is even higher than the one faced in irradiated wound beds (Lee et al. in 'Further reading').

Previous surgery

A study conducted by Ishimaru et al. (see 'Further reading') that included 1,791 free flaps for head and neck reconstruction, in which recurrent and primary cases were paired according to intraoperative factors (use of vein grafts, number of veins used, and surgeon's experience), showed that total flap loss increased from 3.5 to 5.5% in recurrent cases when compared with primary cases. When facing flap failure, other factors known to favour the circumstances that cause vascular compromise should be kept in mind as well; especially considering the overall high prevalence in patients suffering from head and neck malignancies, such as malnutrition, smoking history, advanced age, and presence of other comorbidities.

Coagulopathy

The relationship between a hypercoagulable state and macrovascular thrombosis (e.g. deep venous thrombosis or pulmonary thromboembolism) has been studied at large. The use of different tools in order to assess the risk of macrovascular thrombosis, such as the Caprini score, to properly select the need for a perioperative anticoagulation scheme. This association has been described with thrombosis at the anastomosis site (microvascular thrombosis) as well (see Pannucci et al. in 'Further reading'). One of the largest studies (see Wang et al. in 'Further reading') found on the subject where 58 patients with hereditary conditions such as Factor V Leiden mutation, protein C deficiency, and antiphospholipid syndrome among others, found that pedicle thrombosis rate increased from 4.2% to 20.7% in patients suffering from hereditary conditions, and recommended consulting to hematology in order to determine a proper thromboprophylaxis regimen.

Patients who receive anticoagulants should be carefully managed according to the respective guidelines. Dual oral anticoagulants (DOACs) should be discontinued at appropriate timings and replaced by appropriate regimes of low-molecular-weight heparin (LMWH). They should be recommenced when the risk of bleeding is overcome. Patients on direct oral anticoagulants (DOACs) should be carefully monitored. If the underlying condition is atrial fibrillation (AF), then there is a high risk in free flap reconstruction. Paroxysmal AF is considered low risk; however, careful consideration of the reconstructive plan is required.

Hemoglobinopathies can predispose to coagulopathy, such as in sickle cell trait (see Platt et al. in 'Further reading'). Abnormal erythrocytes in extreme circumstances such as major surgery may precipitate thrombosis even if the anastomosis is technically sound. In such patients every effort must be made perioperatively to maintain normal physiological parameters and avoid at any cost prolonged tissue ischaemia, hypoxia, or dehydration.

Vein grafts

Use of vein grafts (VG) in head and neck reconstruction has shown to increase a risk for pedicle thrombosis as well. In a study evaluating the outcome of 3,240 free flaps used for head and neck reconstruction, Maricevich et al. (see 'Further reading') established that the interposition of VG increased the risk of pedicle thrombosis from 1.1% to 6.4%.

Haemorrhage

Carotid blowout syndrome (CBS) is a relatively rare but potentially fatal complication in surgeries involving the neck, where rupture of a vessel in the carotid system can cause life-threatening haemorrhages (see Suarez et al. in 'Further reading'). Risk of CBS is higher in patients undergoing surgical interventions that require artery manipulation, infection, and previous irradiation. For this reason, complex reconstructions in the cervicofacial area after tumour ablation represent a perfect scenario for this complication to arise (see Lu et al. in 'Further reading'). Postoperative CBS should be suspected whenever massive bleeding occurs and requires immediate intervention.

Further reading

Al Deek NF, Wei F-C, Kao H-K. Free tissue transfer to head and neck: lessons learned from unfavorable results-experience per subsite. *Clin Plast Surg* 2016;43(4):621–30.

Benatar MJ, *et al.* Impact of preoperative radiotherapy on head and neck free flap reconstruction: a report on 429 cases. *J Plast Reconstr Aesthetic Surg* 2013;66(4):478–82.

Bigdeli AK, Thomas B, Falkner F, Gazyakan E, Hirche C, Kneser U. The impact of indocyanine-green fluorescence angiography on intraoperative decision-making and postoperative outcome in free flap surgery. *J Reconstr Microsurg* 2020;36(8):556–66.

Birkenfeld F, Naujokat H, Helmers A-K, Purcz N, Möller B, Wiltfang J. Microdialysis in postoperative monitoring of microvascular free flaps: experiences with a decision algorithm. *J Cranio-Maxillo-Fac Surg* 2019;47(8):1306–9.

Celik N, *et al.* Technique and strategy in anterolateral thigh perforator flap surgery, based on an analysis of 15 complete and partial failures in 439 cases. *Plast Reconstr Surg* 2002;109(7):2211–16.

Chang EI, Hanasono MM, Butler CE. Management of unfavorable outcomes in head and neck free flap reconstruction: experience-based lessons from the MD Anderson Cancer Center. *Clin Plast Surg* 2016;43(4):653–67.

Chen H-C, Tan B-K, Cheng M-H, Chang C-H, Tang Y. Behavior of free jejunal flaps after early disruption of blood supply. *Ann Thorac Surg* 2002;73(3):987–9.

Chorath K, et al. Enhanced recovery after surgery for head and neck free flap reconstruction: a systematic review and meta-analysis. *Oral Oncol* 2021;113:105117.

Dakpé S, *et al.* Intraosseous microdialysis for bone free flap monitoring in head and neck reconstructive surgery: a prospective pilot study. *Microsurgery* 2020;40(3):315–23.

Devine JC, Potter LA, Magennis P, Brown JS, Vaughan ED. Flap monitoring after head and neck reconstruction: evaluating an observation protocol. *J Wound Care* 2001;10(1):525–9.

Dort JC, et al. Optimal perioperative care in major head and neck cancer surgery with free flap reconstruction: a consensus review and recommendations from the Enhanced Recovery After Surgery Society. *JAMA Otolaryngol—Head Neck Surg* 2017;143(3):292–303.

Edsander-Nord A, Röjdmark J, Wickman M. Metabolism in pedicled and free TRAM flaps: a comparison using the microdialysis technique. *Plast Reconstr Surg* 2002;109(2):664–73.

Ensat F, *et al.* The efficacy of color duplex sonography in preoperative assessment of anterolateral thigh flap. *Microsurgery* 2012;32(8):605–10.

Ettinger KS, et al. Higher perioperative fluid administration is associated with increased rates of complications following head and neck microvascular reconstruction with fibular free flaps. *Microsurgery* 2017;37(2):128–36.

Ferguson REH Jr, Yu P. Techniques of monitoring buried fasciocutaneous free flaps. *Plast Reconstr Surg* 2009;123(2):525–32.

Forner D, Williams BA, Makki FM, Trites JR, Taylor SM, Hart RD. Late free flap failure in head and neck reconstruction: a systematic review. *Ear Nose Throat J* 2018;97(7):213–16.

Frerichs KU, Feuerstein GZ. Laser-Doppler flowmetry. A review of its application for measuring cerebral and spinal cord blood flow. *Mol Chem Neuropathol* 1990;12(1):55–70.

Frohwitter G, Nobis CP, Weber M, Oetter N, Rau A, Kesting MR, Lutz R. Thermal imaging in a clinically non-assessable free flap reconstruction of the face. *Plast Reconstr Surg Glob Open* 2021;9(2):e3440.

Goh CSL, Ng MJM, Song DH, Ooi ASH. Perioperative vasopressor use in free flap surgery: a systematic review and meta-analysis. *J Reconstr Microsurg* 2019;35(7):529–40.

Hagau N, Longrois D. Anesthesia for free vascularized tissue transfer. *Microsurgery* 2009;29(2):161–7.
Hand WR, *et al.* Intraoperative goal-directed hemodynamic management in free tissue transfer for head and neck cancer. *Head Neck* 2016;38 Suppl 1:E1974–80.
Hara H, *et al.* Blood glucose measurement for flap monitoring to salvage flaps from venous thrombosis. *J Plast Reconstr Aesthetic Surg* 2012;65(5):616–19.
Heller L, Levin LS, Klitzman B. Laser Doppler flowmeter monitoring of free-tissue transfers: blood flow in normal and complicated cases. *Plast Reconstr Surg* 2001;107(7):1739–45.
Hellner D, Schmelzle R. Laser Doppler monitoring of free microvascular flaps in maxillofacial surgery. *J Craniomaxillofac Surg* 1993;21(1):25–9.
Hembd AS, Yan J, Zhu H, Haddock NT, Teotia SS. Intraoperative assessment of DIEP flap breast reconstruction using indocyanine green angiography: reduction of fat necrosis, resection volumes, and postoperative surveillance. *Plast Reconstr Surg* 2020;146(1):1e–10e.
Henault B, Pluvy I, Pauchot J, Sinna R, Labruère-Chazal C, Zwetyenga N. Capillary measurement of lactate and glucose for free flap monitoring. *Ann Chir Plast Esthet* 2014;59(1):15–21.
Hitier M, Cracowski J-L, Hamou C, Righini C, Bettega G. Indocyanine green fluorescence angiography for free flap monitoring: a pilot study. *J Craniomaxillofac Surg* 2016;44(11):1833–41.
Lorenzetti F, Giordano S, Suominen E, Asko-Seljavaara S, Suominen S. Intraoperative hemodynamic evaluation of the radial and ulnar arteries during free radial forearm flap procedure. *J Reconstr Microsurg* 2010;26(2):73–7.
Ishimaru M, Ono S, Suzuki S, Matsui H, Fushimi K, Yasunaga H. Risk factors for free flap failure in 2,846 patients with head and neck cancer: a national database study in Japan. *J Oral Maxillofac Surg* 2016;74(6):1265–70.
Jones BM, Mayou BJ. The laser Doppler flowmeter for microvascular monitoring: a preliminary report. *Br J Plast Surg* 1982;35(2):147–9.
Jyränki J, Suominen S, Vuola J, Bäck L. Microdialysis in clinical practice: monitoring intraoral free flaps. *Ann Plast Surg* 2006;56(4):387–93.
Kamolz LP, Giovanoli P, Haslik W, Koller R, Frey M. Continuous free-flap monitoring with tissue-oxygen measurements: three-year experience. *J Reconstr Microsurg* 2002;18(6):487–91.
Karakawa R, Yoshimatsu H, Narushima M, Iida T. Ratio of blood glucose level change measurement for flap monitoring. *Plast Reconstr Surg Glob Open* 2018;6(7):e1851.
Karakida K, *et al.* Analysis of risk factors for surgical-site infections in 276 oral cancer surgeries with microvascular free-flap reconstructions at a single university hospital. *J Infect Chemother Off J Jpn Soc Chemother* 2010;16(5):334–9.
Karim S, Qadir A, Farooq U, Shakir M, Laghari AA. Hyperspectral imaging: a review and trends towards medical imaging. *Curr Med Imaging* 2022;19(5):417–27.
Kass JL, *et al.* Intraoperative hypotension and flap loss in free tissue transfer surgery of the head and neck. *Head Neck* 2018;40(11):2334–9.
Kim BD, Ver Halen JP, Grant DW, Kim JYS. Anesthesia duration as an independent risk factor for postoperative complications in free flap surgery: a review of 1,305 surgical cases. *J Reconstr Microsurg* 2014;30(4):217–26.
Kim HJ, *et al.* Effect of goal-directed haemodynamic therapy in free flap reconstruction for head and neck cancer. *Acta Anaesthesiol Scand* 2018;62(7):903–14.
Knoedler S, *et al.* Postoperative free flap monitoring in reconstructive surgery-man or machine? *Front Surg* 2023;10:1130566.
Kwasnicki RM, Noakes AJ, Banhidy N, Hettiaratchy S. Quantifying the limitations of clinical and technology-based flap monitoring strategies using a systematic thematic analysis. *Plast Reconstr Surg Glob Open* 2021;9(7):e3663.
Lee M, Chin RY, Eslick GD, Sritharan N, Paramaesvaran S. Outcomes of microvascular free flap reconstruction for mandibular osteoradionecrosis: a systematic review. *J Craniomaxillofac Surg* 2015;43(10):2026–33.
Lindeborg MM, *et al.* Predictive factors for prolonged operative time in head and neck patients undergoing free flap reconstruction. *Am J Otolaryngol* 2020;41(2):102392.
Lu H-J, *et al.* Predisposing factors, management, and prognostic evaluation of acute carotid blowout syndrome. *J Vasc Surg* 2013;58(5):1226–35.

Luu Q, Farwell DG. Advances in free flap monitoring: have we gone too far? *Curr Opin Otolaryngol Head Neck Surg* 2009;17(4):267–9.

Maricevich M, Lin LO, Liu J, Chang EI, Hanasono MM. Interposition vein grafting in head and neck free flap reconstruction. *Plast Reconstr Surg* 2018;142(4):1025–34.

Mijiti A, Kuerbantayi N, Zhang ZQ, Su MY, Zhang XH, Huojia M. Influence of preoperative radiotherapy on head and neck free-flap reconstruction: systematic review and meta-analysis. *Head Neck* 2020;42(8):2165–80.

Miyamoto S, Sakuraba M, Nagamatsu S. Inadvertent injury of critical perforator vessels during perforator flap surgery. *J Reconstr Microsurg* 2012;28(2):95–8.

Mücke T, *et al.* A comparative analysis using flowmeter, laser-Doppler |spectrophotometry, and indocyanine green-videoangiography for detection of vascular stenosis in free flaps. *Sci Rep* 2020;10(1):939.

Nielsen HT, Gutberg N, Birke-Sorensen H. Monitoring of intraoral free flaps with microdialysis. *Br J Oral Maxillofac Surg* 2011;49(7):521–6.

Oberg PA. Laser-Doppler flowmetry. *Crit Rev Biomed Eng* 1990;18(2):125–63.

Pafitanis G, Raveendran M, Myers S, Ghanem AM. Flowmetry evolution in microvascular surgery: a systematic review. *J Plast Reconstr Aesthetic Surg* 2017;70(9):1242–51.

Pannucci CJ, Kovach SJ, Cuker A. Microsurgery and the hypercoagulable state: a hematologist's perspective. *Plast Reconstr Surg* 2015;136(4):545e–52e.

Platt AJ, Robertson A, Batchelor AG. Successful free flap transfer and salvage in sickle cell trait. *Br J Plast Surg* 2000;53(8):707–8.

Rabbani MJ, Bhatti AZ, Shahzad A. Flap monitoring using thermal imaging camera: a contactless method. *J Coll Physicians Surg Pak* 2021;31(6):703–6.

Ritschl LM, Schmidt LH, Fichter AM, Hapfelmeier A, Wolff K-D, Mücke T. Multimodal analysis using flowmeter analysis, laser-Doppler spectrophotometry, and indocyanine green videoangiography for the detection of venous compromise in flaps in rats. *J Craniomaxillofac Surg* 2018;46(6):905–15.

Sahovaler A, *et al.* Applications of intraoperative angiography in head and neck reconstruction. *Acta Otorhinolaryngol Ital* 2021;41(3):215–20.

Salgado CJ, Moran SL, Mardini S. Flap monitoring and patient management. *Plast Reconstr Surg* 2009;124(6 Suppl):e295–e302.

Schulz T, Marotz J, Stukenberg A, Reumuth G, Houschyar KS, Siemers F. Hyperspektralimaging zum postoperativen Lappenmonitoring von lokoregionären Lappenplastiken [Hyperspectral imaging for postoperative flap monitoring of pedicled flaps]. *Handchir Mikrochir Plast Chir* 2020;52(4):316–24. German.

Schultze-Mosgau S, *et al.* Vascularization in the transition area between free grafted soft tissues and pre-irradiated graft bed tissues following preoperative radiotherapy in the head and neck region. *Head Neck* 2002;24(1):42–51.

Setälä LP, Korvenoja EM-L, Härmä MA, Alhava EM, Uusaro AV, Tenhunen JJ. Glucose, lactate, and pyruvate response in an experimental model of microvascular flap ischemia and reperfusion: a microdialysis study. *Microsurgery* 2004;24(3):223–31.

Smit JM, Zeebregts CJ, Acosta R, Werker PMN. Advancements in free flap monitoring in the last decade: a critical review. *Plast Reconstr Surg* 2010;125(1):177–85.

Smith DJ. Effects of gamma radiation on isolated surviving arteries and their vasa vasorum. Am J Physiol 1961;201:901–4.

Suárez C, *et al.* Carotid blowout syndrome: modern trends in management. *Cancer Manag Res* 2018;10:5617–28.

Swartz WM, Jones NF, Cherup L, Klein A. Direct monitoring of microvascular anastomoses with the 20-MHz ultrasonic Doppler probe: an experimental and clinical study. *Plast Reconstr Surg* 1988;81(2):149–61.

Troob SH, *et al.* Venous flow coupler in head and neck free flap reconstruction. *Otolaryngol Head Neck Surg* 2021;164(3):574–9.

Tsuzuki K, Yanai A, Bandoh Y. A contrivance for monitoring skin flaps with a Doppler flowmeter. *J Reconstr Microsurg* 1990;6(4):363–6.

Ungerstedt U. Microdialysis--principles and applications for studies in animals and man. *J Intern Med* 1991;230(4):365–73.
Wang TY, *et al.* Free tissue transfer in the hypercoagulable patient: a review of 58 flaps. *Plast Reconstr Surg* 2012;129(2):443–53.
Watson JS. Experimental microvascular anastomoses in radiated vessels: a study of the patency rate and the histopathology of healing. *Plast Reconstr Surg* 1979;63(4):525–33.
Wechselberger G, Rumer A, Schoeller T, Schwabegger A, Ninkovic M, Anderl H. Free-flap monitoring with tissue-oxygen measurement. *J Reconstr Microsurg* 1997;13(2):125–30.
Wei F-C, Al Deek NF, Cheng M-H, Lin C-H. The triangle of unfavorable outcomes after microsurgical head and neck reconstruction: planning, design, and execution. *Clin Plast Surg* 2016;43(4):615–20.
Yamagata K, Onizawa K, Yusa H, Wakatsuki T, Yanagawa T, Yoshida H. Risk factors for postoperative delirium in patients undergoing head and neck cancer surgery. *Int J Oral Maxillofac Surg* 2005;34(1):33–6.
Yang X, Li Z, Gao C, Liu R. Effect of dexmedetomidine on preventing agitation and delirium after microvascular free flap surgery: a randomized, double-blind, control study. *J Oral Maxillofac Surg* 2015;73(6):1065–72.
Yoshino K, Nara S, Endo M, Kamata N. Intraoral free flap monitoring with a laser Doppler flowmeter. *Microsurgery* 1996;17(6):337–40.
Yuen JC, Feng Z. Distinguishing laser Doppler flowmetric responses between arterial and venous obstructions in flaps. *J Reconstr Microsurg* 2000;16(8):629–35.
Yuen JC, Feng Z. Reduced cost of extremity free flap monitoring. *Ann Plast Surg* 1998;41(1):36–40.
Yuen JC. Enabling remote monitoring using free apps and smart devices for a free-flap adjunct monitor. *Plast Reconstr Surg Glob Open* 2017;5(9):e1507.
Yuen JC. Techniques of external monitoring of buried free flaps. *Ann Plast Surg* 2005;55(5):460–5.
Zhang T, Dyalram-Silverberg D, Bui T, Caccamese JF Jr, Lubek JE. Analysis of an implantable venous anastomotic flow coupler: experience in head and neck free flap reconstruction. *Int J Oral Maxillofac Surg* 2012;41(6):751–5.

12
Troubleshooting
Immediate/early management

Leandros Vassilios F. Vassiliou, Panayiotis Kyzas, and Nicholas Kalavrezos

12.1 **Arterial failure: Immediate management**

Introduction

The first and foremost step in managing a compromised flap is the recognition that there is a problem with the microcirculation as discussed in the previous chapter (see Chapter 11).

As discussed in the previous chapter, compromise of the arterial supply to a free flap (arterial insufficiency), is relatively rare, and potentially catastrophic/detrimental to the survival of the flap.

Flap arterial insufficiency is more difficult to recognize and more difficult to salvage than venous compromise. Given the potentially catastrophic consequences of prolonged ischaemia, the ultimate step when the flap is salvageable is early/immediate return to the operating theatre for exploration and salvage.

Recognition

While most fasciocutaneous flaps are easy to monitor in cases of muscle only flaps, composite flaps or flaps with myocutaneous skin paddle an anterior failure may be difficult to timely recognize. Often when recognition takes place the flap is no longer salvageable. With arterial failure the top problem is time critical.

Fasciocutaneous

If there is an arterial circulatory problem the flap would initially usually look pale/yellow, lacking capillary refill and turgor. The flap will look empty.

Musculocutaneous/Muscle

Within half an hour of cut-off arterial blood supply, the skin component of a free flap will start look mottled, with bruising at the periphery/edges, which gradually moves towards the centre of the flap. This is due to stagnant blood in the capillaries/microcirculation, of a previously perfused flap that now lacks arterial supply.

Muscle flaps can be particularly difficult to judge—colour change with loss of a beefy red appearance is the most common finding, alongside with loss of the bright glistening superficial muscle layer. If one can tease the muscle fibres apart, then there is significant concern for arterial insufficiency.

Critical considerations

The problem has to be recognized early when there is a salvageability prospect for the flap and immediate action needs to take place.

For fasciocutaneous flaps an acute change in the clinical appearance, where the flap looks pale, empty (deflated), lacking capillary fill, and turgor may be adequate to establish the problem. Needle pinprick or a small incision through the skin paddle will confirm the problem.

There are two crucial questions that need to be answered at this critical moment:

1. Is the flap salvageable?

Free flaps can have the prospect of successful salvage if reperfusion takes place within 2 hours, within the maximum 3 hours after the onset of ischaemia/arterial occlusion. For bone flaps, the window is far more narrow as microthrombi lodge in the Harvesian channels and it is almost impossible to restore patency of the microcirculation.

2. Can the patient tolerate another general anaesthetic (GA)?

A comprehensive, thorough, and holistic assessment of the patient's fitness for another GA and a projection of how this is likely to impact their further recovery needs to take place, in conjunction with anaesthetic and intensive care specialist input.

- Flaps sometimes fail because the patient's general physiological status is compromised. Pneumonia, cardiovascular events, hypotension, sepsis may affect the flap perfusion and lead to ischaemia and a clinical picture of arterial failure. The problem is systemic and not of microvascular nature. In these scenarios taking the patient back to theatre is the wrong decision. This will likely put the patient at risk of further deterioration and will not achieve much in terms of salvaging the flap.
- Similarly, if the problem is deemed microvascular in its origin however the patient is unfit for surgery due to postoperative systemic complications, decision to follow an expectant course of management with systemic support and optimization of the patient and a delayed intervention (debridement) may be wise.
- Finally, if the flap problem is recognized early, the flap is deemed salvageable and the patient likely to tolerate a return to theatre then provision and mobilization of all relevant teams needs to take place for immediate action.

If the flap is considered salvageable and the patient fit to return to theatre, then the team has to work fast and efficiently.

- **Alert the operating theatre and anaesthetic teams.** When the suspicion of a flap compromise is raised, any member of the surgical team must alert theatres to be prepared for an impending (immediate) return to theatre. This allows time for the consultant on-call for microvascular flap salvage to attend, assess the situation, and to discuss the case with the attending anaesthetist and theatre nurse leader.

- The patient is booked as Category 1 (immediate within less than an hour) transferred to theatre (see Box 12.1.1 and National Confidential Enquiry into Patient Outcome and Death https://www.ncepod.org.uk/classification.html in 'Further reading').
- The airway is managed, the tracheostomy cuff is inflated, and oxygen therapy commenced.
- Blood is sent to the lab and also crossmatched for potential transfusion.
- Intravenous fluids are administered and the patient kept warm.
- Broad spectrum antibiotics are commenced if not been administered already.
- An initial treatment with low-molecular-weight heparin is commenced.
- Once the patient is transferred to the operating theatre, central venous and arterial lines are inserted. These are for administration of fluids, blood transfusion, and inotropic support (central line) and for cardiovascular monitoring.
- Arrangements are made for postoperative admission to the intensive care unit.

Troubleshooting and management algorithm

A situation of acute arterial failure can be stressful and complex. It is useful to organize our thought process and management in a stepwise algorithm. A useful guide is the *ABCDE resuscitation approach:*

The patient's general status and clinical appearance should be taken into account.

Box 12.1.1 National confidential enquiry into patient outcome and death, classification of intervention, December 2004

Category 1—IMMEDIATE—Immediate life, limb, or organ-saving intervention—resuscitation simultaneous with intervention. Normally within minutes of decision to operate.

Category 2—URGENT—Intervention for acute onset or clinical deterioration of potentially life-threatening conditions, for those conditions that may threaten the survival of limb or organ, for fixation of many fractures and for relief of pain or other distressing symptoms. Normally within hours of decision to operate.

Category 3—EXPEDITED—Patient requiring early treatment where the condition is not an immediate threat to life, limb, or organ survival. Normally within days of decision to operate.

Category 4—ELECTIVE—Intervention planned or booked in advance of routine admission to hospital. Timing to suit patient, hospital, and staff.

Reproduced from https://www.ncepod.org.uk/classification.html

A—Airway
B—Breathing
C—Circulation
D—Disability
E—Exposure

This sequence is run simultaneously in order to identify causes underlying the arterial compromise and also to manage the patient in the safest possible way. The general management resembles the sepsis protocol. The steps in detail are explained in the next paragraphs.

A—Airway

Most of the arterial failures would occur in the first five days postoperatively. During this time the patient's almost always still have a tracheostomy although they may be in a different stage of respirating weaning.

Once an arterial failure is identified and the possibility of return to theatre is evident, the cuff has to be inflated and the patient has to start oxygen therapy.

If the tracheostomy tube has been recently removed and there are still rescue stitches in place (see Chapter 3), then consideration has to be given for replacing the tracheostomy. This is in conjunction with the anaesthetic team or the intensive care unit team.

B—Breathing

Head and neck cancer patients often during the first week of their recovery may develop hospital acquired pneumonia, lung atelectasis or an exacerbation of their chronic obstructive pulmonary disorder (COPD). That may lead to a physiological decline and inability to tolerate general anaesthetic.

In a compromised flap it is prudent that the management is proactive and hence optimization of the respiratory function, oxygen therapy, and physiotherapy are important.

In the event of an active chest infection therefore a decision has to be made regarding the risks of another general anaesthetic and the impact on the overall recovery.

In our opinion, if the flap has less chance to be salvaged and the patient is respiratorily compromised, consideration for a later delayed intervention may be given.

C—Circulation

An early arterial flap failure may be a result of the following:

- Hypovolaemia can lead to hypertension and is not uncommon in patients having had major head and neck surgery. An immediate bolus fluid challenge must be attempted.
- Cardiovascular factors such as postoperative hypotension
  Atrial fibrillation and concomitant thrombus formation (stasis) or thromboembolic episode. The atrial fibrillation could be of a new onset, paroxysmal, or exacerbation of a

known one. Consideration of pharmacological management of atrial fibrillation should be discussed with the attending anaesthetist.

- An electrocardiograph (ECG) is important to assess and explore the possibility of a cardiac event such as atrial fibrillation, arrhythmia, or a perioperative myocardial infarction (MI). This should be discussed with the anaesthetist/attending intensivist and/or cardiology if required.
- Exacerbation or deterioration of heart failure. In that case, the findings of hypovolemia/hypotension are relative and in the context of cardiogenic shock rather than hypovolemic shock.

On the other hand, an arterial occlusion and a delayed flap failure may cause sepsis which will in many cases lead to hypertension.

Management with broad-spectrum IV antibiotics is usually considered.

It is prudent to check the recent Hb levels, haematocrit, and obtain another one as quickly as possible, such as a blood gas sample to rule out the possibility of occult bleed.

Blood transfusion should be considered and an urgent sample for crossmatch should be sent to the blood bank.

Central venous and arterial lines inserted, as mentioned earlier.

Initiate treatment with a therapeutic dose of low molecular weight heparin (LMWH). LMWH is an anticoagulant that binds to anti-thrombin, a serine protease inhibitor, and creates a conformational change. This change accelerates its inhibition of activated factor X in the conversion of prothrombin to thrombin. Thus, thrombin cannot convert fibrinogen to fibrin strands and cause clot formation. In simple terms, LMWH stops the propagation of an existing blood clot and reduces the chance of another blood clot formation. It is not a thrombolytic agent (it doesn't dissolve clots). Therefore, it cannot remove the mechanical obstacle of a clot formed distally to the arterial anastomosis. Its use is to ensure the protection of the flap microcirculation, which, if compromised, will render a flap beyond any salvage. It is a way of 'buying time' until surgical salvage occurs.

D—Disability

If the patient is sedated, then they may be not able to provide informed consent. The possibility of return to theatre should have been discussed during the initial consultation pre-operatively.

A consent form 4 is filled out for the patient's best interest in case the surgical team feels that an urgent return to theatre and exploration of the flap may lead to successful salvage. Communication with the family is prudent.

The nasogastric (NG) feeding must stop; however, the anaesthetic team may run a rapid sequence induction if the patient has not been starved.

E—Exposure

Apart from a compromised flap, a thorough examination of the neck is performed. Local or mechanical factors may lead to acute arterial failure.

At the first 2–3 days postoperatively, the pedicle is still technically mobile until its position is fixed with the clotted blood and an initial healing tissue. A wrong head position may lead to an acute kink and occlusion.

It is not uncommon that external compressions such as a tracheostomy ties may cause pressure on the pedicle and compromise the arterial flow leading to thrombosis. The optimum head position must be known to all members of the team, checked constantly by the attending nursing staff and be clearly written on the handover sheet.

If for any reason the head position is altered and there is a suspicion that this could have contributed to the clinical picture of arterial occlusion, then the optimum position must be reinstated. This, however, must not change the endpoint of the salvage plan which is surgical re-exploration.

It would be uncommon for an arterial anastomosis to be so sensitive to position of the neck and if there is an established clinical picture of arterial failure, anastomosis should be revisited.

Often neck collections, haematomas, or infections may compromise the arterial anastomosis. It is important to check the contents of the neck bottles.

The possibility of chyle leak must be explored as well. In such scenario a cloudy milky fluid will be seen in the neck drain bottles, or the neck skin will appear erythematous and indurated with possible offensive discharge from the wound. Chyle is extremely toxic and causes immediate vessel spasm.

Once the patient is safely transferred to theatre for exploration and salvage then the next steps of troubleshooting and mitigation take place as is discussed in Chapter 13.

Delayed/Expectant management

If the patient is not fit to return to theatre or if the problem isn't recognized early enough to ensure flap salvageability then a decision for delayed intervention may be taken.

A) Delayed intervention
B) Debridement and wound healing under primary or secondary intention
C) Debridement and regional flap

In that case the patient is covered for antibiotics and optimized until fit for return to theatre. It is important to properly gauge the correct timing to debride the non-vital flap.

In cases where a small radial forearm flap has been used then debridement can be partially performed under local anaesthetic in the outpatient's department, depending on the size and the site of the flap.

In the scenario of late intervention, the question that needs to be answered 'is how is the defect going to be reconstructed?' For T1 and T2 intraoral tumours, a few days postoperatively some granulation tissue may have started appearing and upon debridement of the flap the defect may be amenable for secondary healing or partial primary healing. That may not necessarily result in the most aesthetic closure.

For example, a lateral mandibulectomy defect with a failed fibula flap may be closed primarily by suturing the buccal mucosa onto the remaining floor of mouth and tongue maintaining the plate for continuity of the jaw and better function. If the defect is too large or if there is a communication with the neck such as in floor of mouth defects, then in order to avoid oro-cutaneous fistulas provision for a flap like the original may be required.

The surgeon will have to determine whether the original flap will be performed at the time of debridement or at a different stage depending on the patient's status. A thorough anaesthetic assessment and comprehensive conversation between the surgeon and the anaesthetic team needs to take place.

12.2 **Venous failure: Immediate management**

Introduction

Venous insufficiency is the most common cause for return to theatre for free flap salvage but is not the leading cause of flap failure. A free flap fails when the artery indefinitely stops perfusing the flap, and all efforts of reperfusion fail. It is therefore clear that an established and continuing venous obstruction will inevitably lead to arterial insufficiency within a matter of hours. This is due to microcirculation thrombi that propagate backwards, leading to mechanical obstruction of the arterial flow and eventually thrombosis of the arterial anastomosis. At this stage, salvage of the flap is impossible. The window of opportunity to salvage a venously compromised flap varies between composite and soft tissue only flaps, composite flaps progress to arterial insufficiency much quicker. The sooner a venously compromised flap is explored surgically, the higher the chance of salvage. Generally, these cases need to return to theatre within 1–2 hours as a maximum.

Recognition

Recognition of early signs of venous insufficiency is vital for early intervention.

A venous compromise in most cases can be first recognized by changes in the neck. As the level of the obstruction is usually the site of the anastomosis in the neck, it is important to understand that the venous stasis and congestion will first manifest at the pedicle location.

As the flap veins become congested and engorged while the artery is still pumping blood against an obstructed outflow the neck will start swelling.

The neck swelling is first localized around the site of the venous anastomosis and then gradually expands as the whole pedicle tenses and swells up. The problem will quickly move backwards to reach the flap site. This is where, in fasciocutaneous flaps, skin paddle changes start to emerge.

Early recognition and intervention are key. If recognition and immediate action are not taken, then the flap intraorally will start swelling. A very full, pink flap, with obvious brisk capillary refill, that might look perfect in the eyes of an inexperienced junior doctor or nurse, is the cardinal sign of early venous insufficiency.

Serial frequent clinical assessment, with comparison of the initial postoperative stage will highlight the transition from a pale pink healthy skin flap to a pink hyperaemic skin paddle indicating venous congestion. If this is left without intervention, the flap will become swollen and engorged, the colour will change from pink to purple to blue/black, and the artery will eventually stop perfusing the flap.

If the artery is still pumping blood, then bleeding will ensue from all the obliterated channels of the microcirculation. Small tributaries in the pedicle veins will open up due to increasing pressure, and quickly the clinical picture may evolve to a dramatic picture of intraoral and neck bleeding.

It is well recognized that a neck hematoma can lead to venous thrombosis due to mass effect/compression. What is not appreciated, however, is the fact that venous insufficiency (from any cause other than neck haematoma) will lead to a tense neck haematoma.

This is because at the early stages of venous drainage compromise, blood escapes from the raw undersurface of the flap in the neck, to decompress the microcirculation. This forms a neck haematoma, and the microvascular reconstruction enters a futile circle of venous insufficiency—neck haematoma—further venous compression.

In late stages of venous failure, the phenomenon resembles the 'chicken and egg' paradox; it is difficult to determine whether bleeding and haematoma led to venous compression and failure or venous anastomosis obstruction caused blood congestion in the flap and bleeding due to mounting pressure from the working artery.

Experienced surgeons often don't really need to look at an intraoral flap to confirm venous insufficiency; the look and feel of the neck is enough to realize the underlying problem, even if the intraoral skin paddle hasn't changed colour (yet).

Types of venous failure based on clinical presentation

There are two main types of venous compromise depending on the clinical presentation and the 'acuteness' of how the problem evolves:

Type A: Acute and/or hyperacute
Type B: Slow, pervasive, and non-critical

Type A: Acute or hyperacute

This is met when the pedicle vein is acutely obstructed at the arterial anastomosis. A strong artery pumping blood against obstructed venous outflow will lead to massive pedicle and flap engorgement. The sequence is: progressive neck swelling—flap swelling and rapid development of blue/purple hue—bleeding—and possible blowout.

The events may develop relatively slowly in the 'acute' type or rapidly, and dramatically in the 'hyperacute' form, potentially resulting in a life-threatening emergency.

For this type of complication, the two questions mentioned in the arterial failure chapter (Chapter 12.1), namely,

1. *Is the flap salvageable?*
2. *Can the patient tolerate another GA?*

do not apply. The patient needs to be transferred urgently (Category 1) to the theatre for decompression.

The management algorithm is similar to the arterial insufficiency one. The management will follow the A, B, C, D approach that was described in the arterial failure paragraph (see Chapter 12.1).

Airway

It is important to secure the airway. If a tracheostomy tube is still present, then it must be ensured that it is secure and the cuff is inflated.

If the patient has been decannulated, then a tracheostomy tube is re-inserted (using the rescue sutures and appropriate kit) and the cuff is inflated. It is important to know that in its very dramatic presentation, venous failure can cause quickly massive neck swelling and obstruction of the upper airway, rendering the tracheostomy wound the only possible way to access the airway. Tracheostomy re-insertion must take place as soon as possible before the neck swells up, rendering any decannulation attempt extremely difficult.

Alert the operating theatre and anaesthetic teams

As stated in Chapter 12.1 the first action is to inform theatres about the impending return. It is important to note, that blood loss can be significant in venous insufficiency and blood transfusion is the norm in these cases.

Local decompression

It is important when the presentation is acute or hyperacute to release mounting venous pressure by opening the neck and, if possible, cutting the venous anastomosis in order to allow decompression of the venous system.

The following manoeuvres must be considered in preparation to return to theatre.

Evaluate and address systemic and mechanical factors

Venous insufficiency almost always signifies thrombosis at, before, or after the venous anastomosis. If the cause is external pressure (by a neck collection, i.e. hematoma) then there is usually a window of opportunity to prevent this mechanical venous obstruction from becoming an established thrombosis by removing the mechanical factor. This is achieved by opening and decompressing the neck at the bedside, while preparations for neck exploration in theatre are ongoing. We utilize marking sutures in the neck, indicative of where the venous anastomosis is, so that emergency neck decompression can take place without damaging the underlying pedicle/anastomosis. Opening the neck at the bedside allows direct inspection of the underlying venous anastomosis. If that is found thrombosed, we advocate releasing it with scissors, above the anastomosis, to allow flap decompression/decongestion (venous anastomosis transection). Obviously, this is easier done when the recipient vein is the external jugular vein, as if the recipient vein is the internal jugular vein the venous transection manoeuvre carries a significant risk of bleeding. In our practice, we use the external jugular vein as the recipient vessel.

Other mechanical factors as discussed earlier (neck position, external compression) must be looked at and addressed, but in our experience these attempts will not resolve an established venous insufficiency problem. The patient should be optimized from a circulatory point of view in preparation to return to theatre.

Initiate treatment with a therapeutic dose of LMWH

Low-molecular-weight heparin (LMWH) should be considered in venous insufficiency except the occasion that the sole reason of venous compromise is external pressure to neck hematoma due to bleeding. In that case, the use of anticoagulation should be carefully balanced to the risk of further bleed. This requires identifying the cause of neck bleed in theatre. For example, bleeding from a named vessel that is identified and controlled during neck exploration/salvage, doesn't indicate an increased bleeding tendency ('medical' bleed), therefore LMWH can be safely used. On the other hand, generalized oozing from multiple areas in the neck, is suggestive of an underlying coagulopathy; in that case, LMWH must be temporarily withheld until this is investigated further.

Salvage of the flap in the hyperacute form is most of the times impossible due to the extensive damage to the microcirculation. In most cases after this has been validated the flap is taken down and closure of the defect is achieved either with primary or secondary intention if possible (for relatively small defects) or with locoregional flaps.

Chepeha et al. (see 'Further reading') have tried to categorize flap venous compromise depending on the presumed (based on clinical evaluation) 'site' of the venous obstruction:

- flap microcirculation,
- cutaneous perforators in composite (osseocutaneous) flaps,
- diffuse (global) venous thrombosis

This is a useful approach as it can direct management decision-making on potential salvageability and next steps.

For acute types of venous congestion, once decompression is achieved, an attempt for salvage can be made as discussed in Chapter 14.

Type B: Slow, pervasive, and non-critical

The clinical presentation is less acute and impressive. The neck is usually soft or mildly swollen and the skin paddle initially hyperaemic with fast capillary refill or slowly assuming a darker hue or purplish colour.

The troubleshooting possibilities are the following:

- Partial venous obstruction.
- Single venous obstruction in flaps with two or more venous anastomoses.
- Combined arterial and venous failure (as the flap does not develop significant congestion, hindering towards weakness of the artery).

For this type of complication, we will again refer to the two main questions mentioned in the arterial failure chapter (Chapter 12.1):

1. *Is the flap salvageable?*
2. *Can the patient tolerate another GA?*

If the flap is deemed salvageable and an exploration worth doing, then the patient is immediately transferred to theatre and the troubleshooting commences as described in Chapter 14, otherwise an expectant plan may be set in place or consideration for leech therapy.

Expectant/delayed management

For delayed and slow venous failure, sometimes an expectant approach can be considered, especially if the patient is unlikely to tolerate a general anaesthetic or if the microvascular surgeon feels that exploration of the venous anastomosis would not yield any benefits.

The patient is managed with systemic support covered with antibiotics. Often, a delayed venous anastomosis with an otherwise functional arterial anastomosis may still result in partial take of the flap and the cost will only be the loss of some of the superficial skin paddle layers that will either slough or require a degree of debridement.

For delayed cases, there is still some time when the flap develops collateral vascular bridges with the surrounding tissue.

Leech therapy

Leech therapy has been described and utilized in venous insufficiency (Figure 12.2.1). In our opinion, it doesn't address the underlying microsurgery problem; however, it is a valid approach for Type B venous compromise, especially when the patient is not fit enough for return to theatre.

Leech therapy aims to decompress venous congestion until the flap develops collateral draining venous channels in its integration bed.

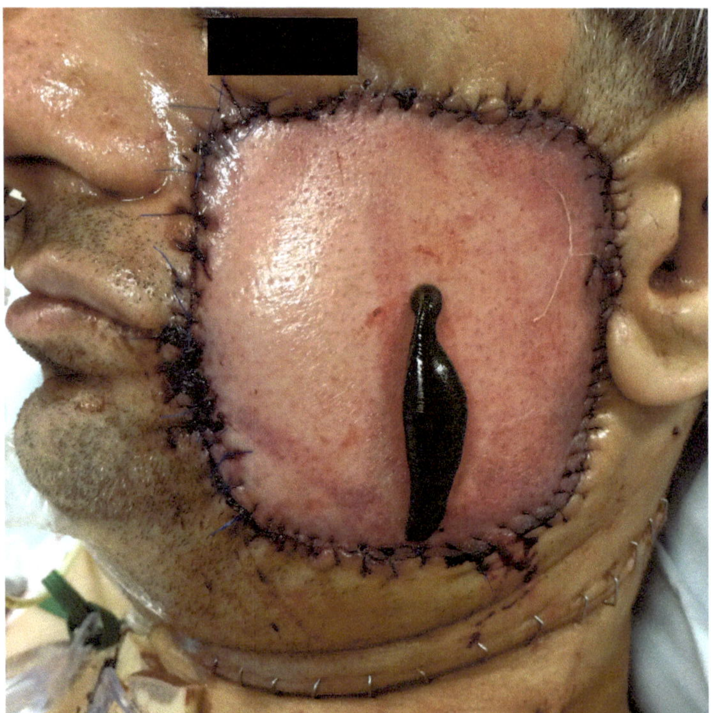

Figure 12.2.1 Initiation of leech treatment in a venous congested (Type B) latissimus dorsi flap used for reconstruction of cheek through-en-through defect.

The species used in *Hirudo medicinalis*. Leeches carry *Aeromonas hydrophila* in their gut, which can be transmitted through their bite and cause gastroenteritis, hence antimicrobial prophylaxis is required. This will be guided by local protocols; however, the bacterium is usually sensitive to tetracyclines, sulfonamides, trimethoprim/sulphamethoxazole, or ciprofloxacin. *Aeromonas hydrophila* is usually resistant to penicillin.

Contraindications for leech therapy are the following:

- Cardiovascular instability
- Previous exposure to leeches (risk of hypersensitivity reaction)
- Immunosuppression
- Type A venous compromise (see earlier in this chapter)
- Arterial compromise
- Patient's refusal of leech therapy or blood transfusion

Standard protocols for leech therapy will include the following:

- Admission to the intensive care unit for monitoring, 1:1 nursing, and cardiovascular support
- Consider insertion of central venous and arterial lines
- Anticoagulation with LMWH with or without aspirin (75 mg OD)
- Antimicrobial cover as discussed earlier
- Blood transfusion when haemoglobin <8 gr/dL
- Use of three leeches per hour
- Avoid application of ointment, Doppler gel on the skin paddle to encourage leech attachment
- Hourly cleaning of flap with heparinized saline
- Minimum possible benzodiazepines/narcotics to avoid reduced leech activity
- For intraoral leech therapy (rare) patients must be sedated the airway is maintained via a tracheostomy tube with the cuff inflated and the oropharynx is obliterated with a throat pack, to protect the aerodigestive track against leech migration
- After completion of leech treatment, leeches are detached and immersed in 70% ethanol solution

Further reading

Chalian AA, Anderson TD, Weinstein GS, Weber RS. Internal jugular vein versus external jugular vein anastomosis: implications for successful free tissue transfer. *Head Neck* 2001;23:475–8.

Chepeha DB, Nussenbaum B, Bradford CR, Teknos TN. Leech therapy for patients with surgically unsalvageable venous obstruction after revascularized free tissue transfer. *Arch Otolaryngol Head Neck Surg* 2002;128(8):960–5.

Herlin C, Bertheuil N, Bekara F, Boissiere F, Sinna R, Chaput B. Leech therapy in flap salvage: Systematic review and practical recommendations. *Ann Chir Plast Esthet* 2017;62(2):e1–13.

Hidalgo DA, Disa JJ, Cordeiro PG, Hu Q. A review of 716 consecutive free flaps for oncologic surgical defects: refinement in donor-site selection and technique. *Plast Reconstr Surg* 1998;102:722–32.

Hidalgo DA, Jones CS. The role of emergent exploration in free-tissue transfer: a review of 150 consecutive cases. *Plast Reconstr Surg*1990;86:492–8.

Kerrigan CL, Wizman PH, Jortdal VE, Sampalis J. Global flap ischemia: a comparison of arterial versus venous etiology. *Plast Reconstr Surg*1994;93:1485–95.
Kroll SS, *et al.* Anticoagulants and hematomas in free flap surgery. *Plast Reconstr Surg* 1995;96:643–7.
Lineaweaver WC, *et al. Aeromonas hydrophila* infections following use of medicinal leeches in replantation and flap surgery. *Ann Plast Surg* 1992;29:238–44.
Nakajima T How soon do venous drainage channels develop at the periphery of a free flap? A study in rats. *Br J Plast Surg* 1978;31:300–8.
National Confidential Enquiry into Patient Outcome and Death. The NCEPOD Classification of Intervention. 2024. Available at: https://www.ncepod.org.uk/classification.html
Urken ML, *et al.* Microvascular free flaps in head and neck reconstruction: report of 200 cases and review of complications. *Arch Otolaryngol Head Neck Surg* 1994;120:633–40.

13 Troubleshooting and cause-directed management

Artery

Leandros Vassilios F. Vassiliou, Panayiotis Kyzas, and Nicholas Kalavrezos

13.1 Troubleshooting in arterial compromise

Introduction

Rarely and despite the microsurgeon's best ability, free flaps fail. It is important for the operator to follow a calm systematic approach in troubleshooting the situation and identify the underlying cause in order to successfully salvage the flap if this can be possible.

The causes of the failure are predominantly either:

- an arterial anastomosis failure, or
- a venous anastomosis failure as will be discussed in this and the next Chapter 14.

Broadly, any free flap arterial compromise can be categorized in two types based on the acuteness of the presentation the speed of its evolution (Figure 13.1.1).

A thorough and comprehensive troubleshooting process will define which steps need to be further undertaken in order to rescue the flap.

In summary and as it will be further discussed in this chapter the prevailing classification or stratification includes (Figure 13.1.2):

1. TECHNICAL: Arterial anastomosis revision only required—Primary and Technical cause.
2. REGIONAL: Arterial anastomosis revision only required—Secondary with Underlying cause.
3. COMPLEX-TECHNICAL: Arterial and venous anastomosis revision required, or arterial and venous anastomosis revision and flap re-inset. The latter represents the most complex situation of free flap salvage and most commonly encountered in cases of erroneous inset and free flap pedicle contortion (twist).
4. COMPLEX-PHYSIOLOGICAL: This is an entirely different category as the aetiology of the flap failure is ischaemia due to physiological reasons, such as weak cardiovascular stamina (Figure 13.1.3).

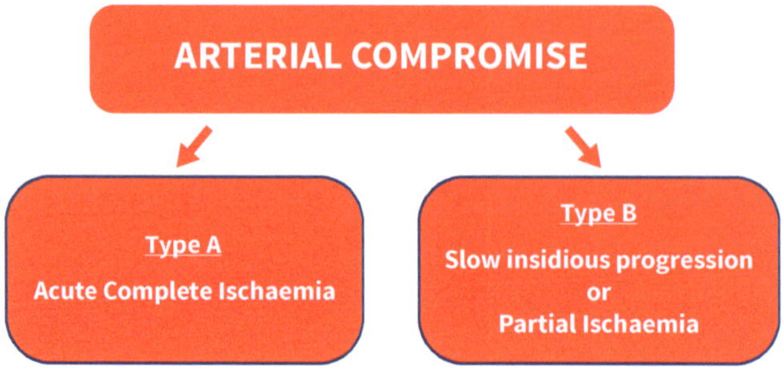

Figure 13.1.1 Broad categorization of free flap arterial compromise. Type A refers to acute and complete ischaemia manifesting with all the typical signs of arterial failure as described in Chapter 11. Type B refers to a less profound change of the free flap. Perfusion assessment based on clinical criteria can be perplexing. The free flap can display signs of partial or slow progressive hypoperfusion. Careful clinical judgement is required for initial troubleshooting. A comprehensive assessment of the patient's clinical status and physiology is mandatory prior to definitive decision-making.

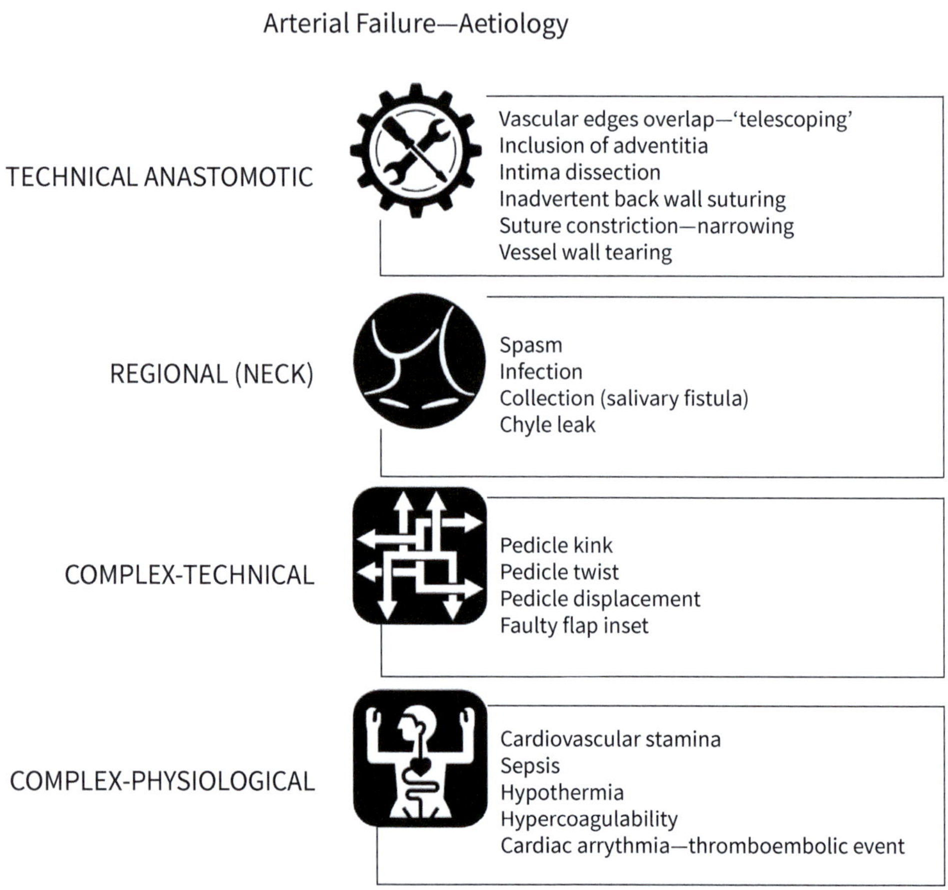

Figure 13.1.2 Summary of flap arterial failure aetiology.

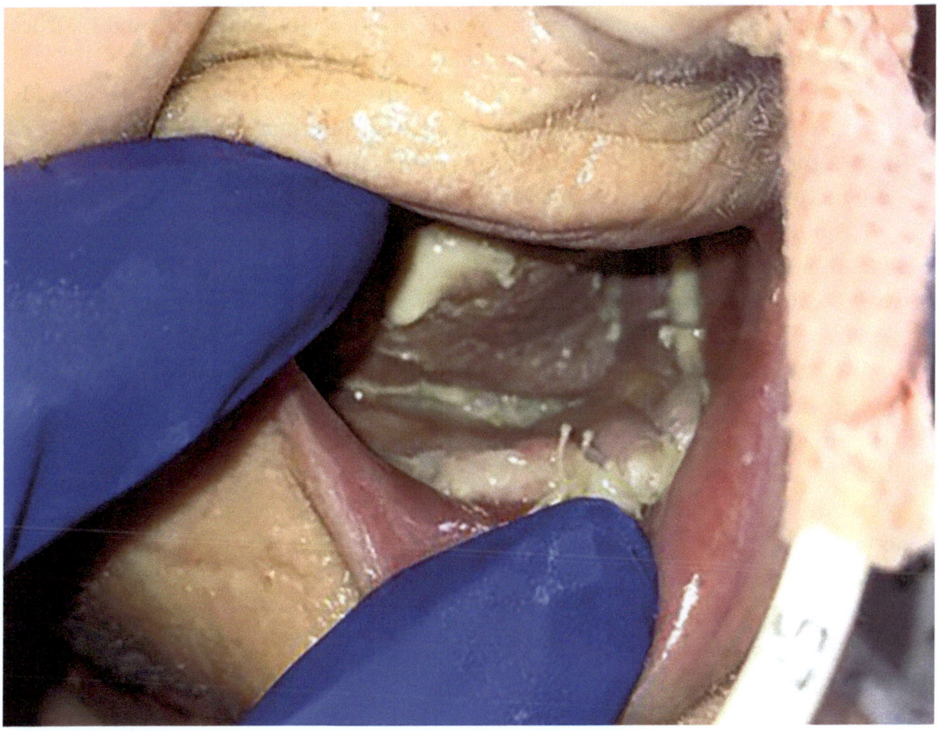

Figure 13.1.3 Clinical presentation of Type B arterial compromise of a radial forearm free flap used for the reconstruction of a floor of mouth defect. The flap did not display signs of complete arterial failure (bleeding was evident on the needle prick test). There were signs of ischaemia and hypoperfusion. However, due to the patient's frailty, a decision against exploration was made. The patient was managed medically and optimized. The end result was a partial take of the free flap with only partial loss of the superficial layer.

Other classifications of microvascular related troubleshooting simply divide the causes in 'microvascular' related ones, implying that the issue is based on the anastomosis (technical), and 'macrovascular' ones when the root cause stems from conditions in the neck or the patient's physiology (regional and complex, based on the proposed classification in this textbook). We prefer the categorization into technical–regional–complex as this is more analytical, helps define the cause more precisely and provides guidance towards the appropriate action plan.

Troubleshooting

The troubleshooting exercise starts with the recognition that there is a free flap compromise.

A comprehensive assessment of the free flap, the regional condition of the tissues i.e. the neck and the patient's overall clinical status needs to take place:

- The overall clinical picture and the vitals of the patient need to be carefully assessed. Is the patient septic? Is the patient hypotensive? Is the patient hypovolaemic?

- The appearance of the flap needs to be carefully assessed as in Chapters 11 and 12. Does the flap demonstrate features of predominantly arterial or venous failure?
- The condition of the neck needs to be carefully assessed. Is the neck swollen? Is there any palpable collection? Are there signs of bleeding or a haematoma? Are there signs of a collection? Are there signs of infection? This needs to be assessed in conjunction with blood tests including C-reactive protein (CRP) levels and white cell count.
- Check the contents in the drains and drain bottles to obtain a preliminary idea why of what the nature of the collection is in the neck. Is there blood in the drain bottles and what is the volume? Sometimes bleeding in the neck can cause excessive drainage in the drain bottles. Is there turbulent or white debris elements in the drain fluid? This could be consistent with an infection in the neck or chyle leak.
- Is there any malodourous smell suggestive of acute infection?
- Blood tests are important in providing a preliminary cause for a potential free flap compromise. The CRP levels, white count levels, and haemoglobin will guide the surgeon to formulate an initial impression of what the underlying of the free flap compromise might be.

Operative management

Further to what has been discussed in Chapter 12 regarding the early recognition of a free flap compromise, and if the overall comprehensive evaluation of the patient and the potential free flap compromise falls within the **Type A** failure which means that the free flap is deemed salvageable.

The aim is to revascularize the flap by successfully revisiting the anastomosis. In order to achieve this the underlying cause of failure i.e. troubleshooting must be undertaken and addressed in order to reverse the cause of the compromise and prevent further damage.

Once the steps in Chapter 12 have been completed and the patient is back in the operating theatre and on the table, the troubleshooting and addressing the complication starts by carefully opening the neck. At this stage photographic documentation may assist for future learning and reflective practice.

Neck contents assessment

The contents in the neck wound have to be carefully evaluated.

- Is there blood suggestive of a haematoma or acute bleeding?
- Is there pus suggestive an acute infection? In that case a pus sample needs to be sent to the microbiology laboratory for Gram staining and also microbiology cultures and sensitivities. The patient is commence immediately placed on broad spectrum antimicrobial therapy.
- Saliva could be suggestive of salivary collection from a defective flap inset and oro-cervical fistulation and salivary leakage.
- 'Milky' white fluid suggests chyle leak especially when addressing a left sided free flap and dissection. Management of chyle leak is further addressed in Chapter 13.3.

Once the contents of the neck have been assessed and addressed with further investigations being sent, the neck is carefully irrigated, and further assessment follows:

Vessels (anastomosis assessment)

The next step is to assess the vessels (arterial and venous anastomosis) condition.

The artery must be carefully assessed under the microscope. Is the artery empty but the anastomosis appears patent? Is there a thrombus in the anastomosis? Is the donor artery post anastomosis site narrowed and thrombosed suggestive of a spasm as the original event prior to the compromise.

Is there evidence of a thrombosed artery or vein? Is there evidence or a clinical picture of (empty) veins suggestive poor profusion due to arterial compromise first.

Technical common pitfalls involve:

- Inadvertent suturing of the back wall.
- Inadequate calibre mismatch between the donor and recipient vessels.
- Anastomotic gaps or strictures due to uneven distribution of sutures predisposing in unequal expansion of the anastomosis with localized narrowing and turbulent flow.
- Inclusion of adventitia.
- Intima dissection—especially atherosclerotic vessels.

This topic is further discussed in Chapter 13.2.

Pedicle condition assessment

The pedicle condition needs to be assessed. Is the pedicle in the original position and suspension as at the closure of the original operation? Are there any signs of kinking or malposition predisposing for arterial compromise? Are there any signs of congestion suggestive of predominantly venous congestion leading to arterial failure due to pumping against a blocked microcirculation.

- Acute angulation or kinking of the pedicle leading to increased workload for the artery to profuse the flap and eventually resulting in thrombosis due to decompensation.
- Twisting of the pedicle leading to turbulent flow, and increased perfusion resistance.

This topic is further discussed in Chapter 13.4.

From this assessment onwards the operating surgeon must have already completed an evaluation and will have a working diagnosis of what the situation is with the anastomoses and also what the underlying cause of the compromise might have been in order to further address this.

Poor arterial flow from the recipient artery due to inappropriate vessel selection or patient factors such as physiological compromise and poor cardiovascular output (hypotension).

13.2 Technical causes: Primary arterial compromise

Introduction

Returning to the operating theatre for exploration of a flap with signs of arterial insufficiency is a daunting task. The chances of a successful salvage are significantly smaller compared to venous insufficiency (Chapter 14). Identifying a technical cause is not always possible and when it is, the critical time point for salvage might have already passed. Nevertheless, the attending surgical team must employ a systematic approach, aiming to identify and rectify the underlying failure cause whenever possible.

An analysis of 14 cases showed technical errors in four. These consisted of

- inadvertent back wall sutures in one case and
- three cases of intimal overlap due to the wrong correction of thickness mismatch.

The rest of the histological studies of thrombosed arterial anastomosis have suggested that possible causes would be pre-existing or accentuated intima hyperplasia, and also medial layer smooth muscle necrosis due to compression within the suture cycle.

This highlights the importance, as described in Chapter 8, of the sutures only being tied to the point to achieve a good apposition of the vessel edges, and not so tight to result in tissue necrosis and swelling at the site of the anastomosis predisposing to obstructed patency and thrombosis.

The rest of the arterial anastomosis failures were attributed to arterial spasm, secondary to other causes, as further described.

The most common causes of technical anastomotic errors and as illustrated in Figure 13.2.1 are the following:

- Vascular edges overlap—'telescoping'
- Inclusion of Adventitia
- Intima dissection
- Inadvertent back wall suturing
- Suture constriction—narrowing
- Vessel wall tearing

Management

The theatre scrub team, equipment and anaesthesia must follow the same steps as the original surgery (set up, instrumentation, cardiovascular optimization, positioning). This has been previously described in Chapters 1, 3, and 11).

It is important for every team member to realize the time-critical nature of the exploration/salvage procedure, and it is the responsibility of the attending surgeon to emphasize this.

With the patient anaesthetised, prepped, draped, and positioned, the first step is to carefully open-up the neck, with care and diligence to avoid damage to the external jugular vein and venous anastomosis. Following that, the neck is gently but thoroughly washed with warm normal saline and heparinized saline, and the vascular pedicle is inspected.

In reality, in almost every case of arterial insufficiency, the first encounter of the exploring microvascular surgeon is a lifeless pulseless vascular pedicle. Therefore, the forward plan is threefold: Revision of the arterial anastomosis, identification, and rectification of the causal factor (s) and revision of the venous anastomosis.

To facilitate a standardized salvage technique, we have divided our approach into steps:

Step 1

The first step is to set up the microscope as previously described (Chapter 4). A 3A vascular clamp is placed on the recipient artery (usually the facial) and the arterial anastomosis is divided distally (on the donor vessel site). At that point, the 3A clamp is released. The presence of good arterial flow at the anastomosis is suggestive (but not definitive) of a good technical arterial anastomosis suturing, and points towards a more distal cause (distal pedicle twist or kink, thrombi or emboli in the arterioles, tunnel issues). Lack of flow through the anastomosis indicates either a technical issue at the anastomosis site or another issue that has been established for a prolonged period, with the thrombus propagating proximally towards the anastomosis.

The very rare exception (and a fortunate finding) is when the artery is still functional and patent but there is reduced flow due to vasospasm. This becomes evident if there is pulsation distally to the anastomosis, which indicates a functioning artery and a possible cause of arterial spasm. In that case, the anaesthetic team is asked to increase and maintain a high mean arterial pressure (MAP) (usually over 75–80 mmHg), and the pedicle is irrigated with papaverine and heparinized saline. It is then allowed to rest while the surgeon assesses all other potential causes for compromise (orientation, tunnel, haematoma, chyle leak). If vasospasm is the case, the flap picks up within minutes and this becomes apparent both from the clinical inspection of the intraoral skin component and by formally assessing venous drainage with the milking test (see Chapter 10). Unfortunately, the scenario just described is very rare, and in our experience, this is almost never the case. We can record only one case in over 1,000 free flap cases in which reversible vasospasm with patent anastomosis was the cause of arterial insufficiency, and it was reversed without the need of anastomosis revision.

Step 2

Every effort should be made to try and identify the cause of the arterial insufficiency. Any neck hematoma must be evacuated, and the cause must be identified and controlled (Chapter 13.3). The presence of chyle leak, if not already known, must be addressed and sealed (see Chapter 13 for a more detailed description).

If a technical error is identified, then the operator can proceed to Step 3.

In more complex cases when the cause is not deemed to be technical at the level of the anastomosis but an inset or tunnel problem is suspected, as discussed in Chapter 13.4. For the venous anastomosis(es) may need to be divided (proximal to the sutures or couplers), and the vascular pedicle is laid loose in the neck. It is then traced all the way up to the intraoral component of the flap and the tunnel patency is checked for adequacy. In composite oropharyngeal resections/reconstructions where a lip split approach has been utilized, this must be opened-up to ensure appropriate orientation of all the components of the pedicle. Any pedicle suspension sutures must be released. Essentially, the steps are the same as at the primary surgery, with the difference of working against the clock, handling tissues that have entered the stage of the inflammatory reaction of the healing process—not pleasant.

Step 3

Once the cause of the problem has been identified, the artery must be flushed with copious amounts of warm heparinized saline under the microscope. This allows the surgeon to feel any intraluminal resistance which might be indicative of pedicle twist/kink or a microcirculation issue.

If a pedicle twist or kink is found, this is immediately rectified, and resolution is obvious due to the reduced resistance during flushing. Rarely, a pedicle twist/kink might require getting the flap down and re-inset; this, however, should be counted as a 'never' event in microvascular surgery, as it is completely avoidable if all the inset steps (described in Chapters 7 and 8) have been religiously followed.

Flushing ceases once the surgeon is satisfied that there is free and uninterrupted venous return of the heparinized saline, the flushing pressure reduces, there are no leaks on the pedicle and the orientation is correct. The presence of clots and thrombi washed out the vein is a promising sign that the flap's microcirculation is still functioning.

Step 4

It is important that the recipient artery flow is evaluated. Occasionally if the flow is deemed poor to revascularize the flap another recipient vessel needs to be identified, and the free flap artery needs to be anastomosed in the new identified and prepared vessel. The reader is referred to Chapter 5 in order to evaluate, assess, and identify an alternative vessel of good flow and power to profuse the flap.

Identifying a suitable recipient vessel for a revision arterial anastomosis is a difficult task. If the facial artery has adequate length left and the vessel wall and lumen are of good quality, then this is the preferred option, due to size match. In this occasion, we prefer to tie off the external carotid artery immediately above the facial artery take off, to divert all the external carotid artery (ECA) blood pressure into the flap circulation.

Alternatively, if a higher flow is required then the external carotid artery has to be dissected, divided, and turned downwards to be used as a recipient vessel in order to successfully salvage the situation. There is always a diameter size mismatch when the ECA is utilized for head and neck (H&N) reconstruction, but this reduces at the level of the parotid, hence our preference for upwards dissection. Alternatively, the operator has to follow the steps to overcome a global size mismatch as described in Chapter 8.4.

In some instances, and only if the free flap pedicle is long enough, a new recipient vessel needs to be shown in the contralateral neck.

This step will require neck dissection in the contralateral neck, identification, and preparation of a new recipient vessel and revision of the anastomosis in the newly identified artery.

Step 5

The arterial anastomosis is done in a meticulous way as previously described (Chapter 8). The use of papaverine to flush prior to release the donor artery is of paramount importance in revision cases. A MAP of 80mmHg must be maintained once the recipient artery is released and for at least 48 hours afterwards, to ensure perfusion.

Step 6

Once the arterial anastomosis is released and the flap is running, venous outflow is checked and encouraged by using a vessel dilator at the vein side. Satisfactory venous drainage is an encouraging sign, but this must be maintained. Therefore, the vein is left in situ, covered with a heparinized saline gauze, for at least 30 minutes. The intraoral component of the flap (skin paddle) is checked; a successful arterial revision will quickly transform the skin paddle into a full, pink, well-perfused skin flap.

After 30 minutes the flap and the venous drainage is re-checked and if the flow remains satisfactory, the venous anastomosis is redone. The use of couplers or sutures is entirely up to the microvascular surgeon's preference. However, a new recipient vessel must be sought on most occasions. This will usually be the internal jugular vein, in an end to side fashion.

Step 7

The pedicle orientation is maintained with suspension sutures, the neck position is confirmed, and the wound is washed and closed. It is customary to keep the patient sedated for 24 hours, following a flap salvage revision procedure, although the evidence behind this practice is not very strong. However, cardiovascular and respiratory optimization of the patient with intensive care unit (ICU) input is crucial. Blood loses need to be replaced with transfusion and low molecular weight heparin must be administered. Whether this would be the standard prophylactic dose or treatment dose, that depends on the cause of the flap compromise and must be discussed and mutually agreed between the surgeon and the ICU team.

13.3 **Regional causes: Secondary arterial compromise**

Introduction

The most commonly encountered scenario when an artery has failed, is due to an underlying cause. In that case, the arterial anastomosis compromise is a phenomenon secondary to a cause that precipitates the first arterial spasm, in the sensitive area of the anastomosis, further resulting in a thrombus formation and occlusion of the anastomosis.

In this chapter we will discuss the most common causes of arterial spasm and the comprehensive management of addressing those in conjunction with revision (redo) of the arterial anastomosis as described in Chapter 13.2.

Infection

An infection of the neck wound can be suspected early and as soon as the problem with the anastomosis has been recognized as discussed in Chapters 11, 12, and 13.1.

In brief, evidence of a surgical site infection may be demonstrated by the patient's observations such as signs of early systemic inflammatory response or sepsis (tachycardia and/or hypotension).

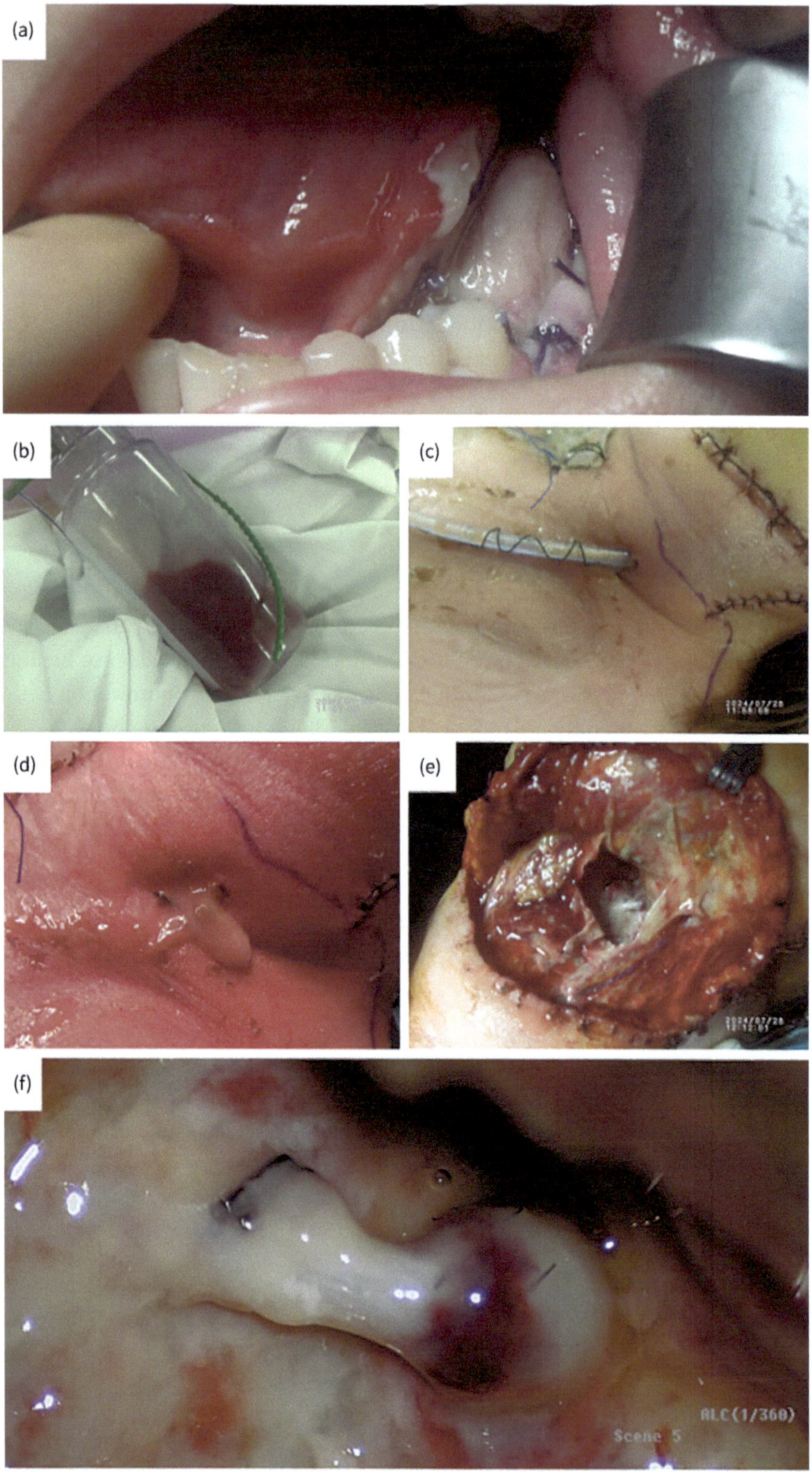
(a)
(b)
(c)
(d)
(e)
(f)
ALC(1/360)
Scene 5

Figure 13.3.1 Acute (Type A) arterial failure of a radial forearm free flap used to reconstruct the left lateral floor of mouth and ventral tongue defect. a. The clinical picture of a completely pale deflated radial forearm free flap. b. Assessment of the drain contents demonstrates turbot fluid. c. The drain is full of whiteish, turbid material. d. Assessment of the neck and removal of the drain reveals discharge of pus. e. Upon re-opening of the neck, clear evidence of infection (collection of pus, fibrin debris) is identified. f. Microscope picture showing the failed arterial anastomosis. Note the presence of a fresh thrombus on the site of the arterial anastomosis, but most importantly, the post-anastomosis narrowing (spasm) of the donor artery. Piecing the evidence together, the most likely aetiology scenario was acute infection in the neck leading to arterial spasm post anastomosis and formation of a thrombus that has completely occluded the artery. The type of anastomosis failure is under the category of regional. Unfortunately, in this case identification of the arterial failure was delayed, hence the flap was deemed unsalvageable. The flap was debrided (removed), and the defect was closed under primary intention.

In case the patient is physiologically compromised, and the infection still remains localized, the neck wound may manifest erythema and oedema. A possible swelling in the neck can be fluctuant suggestive of collection. The overlying skin is often erythematous with clinical signs of cellulitis (Figure 13.3.1).

The contents of the drain and drain exit point should be carefully assessed.

The patient should have already started on empirical broad-spectrum antimicrobials, but if not immediate administration of antibiotics is required. Supportive management to prevent further deterioration or sepsis, such as fluid administration and oxygen, are immediately given while the patient is prepared for theatre.

For cases deemed salvageable (early recognition, patient medically fit to return to theatre), a 'stat' dose of heparin 500 units intravenously to 'slow down' the thrombosis cascade is practised widely by microvascular surgeons in similar instances.

As described in the earlier subchapters upon neck wound opening a collection of pus and fibrin infection will be encountered. That will require a thorough 'washout'. Copious amounts of warm normal saline or heparinized saline are required.

The artery will then be inspected carefully and if deemed salvageable the steps as described in Chapter 13.2 will follow.

Samples are sent to the microbiology laboratory for Gram stain, cultures, and sensitivities. The patient is also provided with supportive management to prevent sepsis such as fluid administration, oxygen (if required) and postoperative admission to critical care for further monitoring and management.

Salivary collection—orocervical communication

A fluid collection in the neck that precipitates arterial spasm, and anastomotic compromise may not always be attributed to pus presence. Occasionally, technical errors such as suture gaps, or dehiscence in the free flap inset site may lead to fistulation into the neck, salivary leak, and collection.

Salivary contents may precipitate arterial spasm, as they carry digestive enzymes and oral bacteria that can trigger inflammatory response and infection.

In such a scenario asides revision of the anastomosis as described in Chapter 13.2, careful thorough evaluation of the reconstructed site is required. The flap has to be sutured in a 'watertight' fashion and closure of the fistulation is mandatory if one is to mitigate the cause that led in first instance to arterial spasm and compromise.

If re-inset proves difficult the whole flap needs to be taken down and reinserted, or a local or regional additional flap may be useful as further discussed in Chapter 13.4.

Asides orocervical communication and salivary leakage, a sialocele may be the cause of a salivary collection.

Sialoceles are best prevented at the point of the original operation:

- If the parotid duct or its orifice are included in the resection, the duct is best ligated prior to division.
- If parotid tail or parenchyma are involved in the neck dissection or resection, the gland is treated with botulinum toxin type A injections (60–80 units), best at the time of the operation, where accurate intraparenchymal injection under direct visualization can be administered.
- Postoperatively, treatment with an anticholinergic agent, transdermal hyoscine hydrobromide (1.5 mg) patches every 72 hours, can also help reduce salivary production.
- Postoperative non-infective collections such as sialoceles or seromas that have not compromised the flap can be aspirated using aseptic technique to release the tension and decompress the neck, alongside pharmaceutical treatments, as described earlier).

Chyle leak

Chyle leak is a complication of mainly left-sided neck dissections, where a tear in the thoracic duct occurs, allowing for extravasation of chylous fluid. Chyle leak can occur on the right side of the neck as well due to the presence of the right lymphatic duct. Chyle leak occurs in approximately 1–2.5% of neck dissections involving level IV, with the majority (75–92%) being on the left side. Normally the thoracic duct transports up to 4 litres of chyle per day (see Tilney et al. and de Gier et al. in 'Further reading').

Recognition

Chyle leakage can usually be recognized intraoperatively by pooling of characteristically yellow 'oily', or occasionally 'milky' fluid in the inferior medial corner of the neck dissection, and in that case it MUST be addressed immediately.

Most often, chyle leak is recognized postoperatively due to the presence of characteristic 'milky' (turbid) fluid in the drains. This is due to commencement of nutrition that contains lipid molecules that enrich the lymph.

In either case, chyle leak needs to be confirmed, and a sample of fluid must be immediately sent to the laboratory for biochemical analysis. The diagnostic criteria to confirm chyle leak are the following:

- Triglyceride levels over 1.2 mmol/L
- Fluid is composed of 4% or more of chylomicrons
- Triglyceride level over 0.5 mmol/L
- Chylomicrons confirm chyle

Chyle leak is classified into

- Low output (less than 1,000 ml/24 h) and
- High output (over 1,000 ml/24 h)

Chyle leaks can have severe complications due to the following reasons:

- Chyle is toxic for the blood vessels, leading to arterial spasm and thrombosis in the case of a free flap
- Chyle leak can lead to venous thrombosis
- Chyle leak is accompanied by a significant fluid loss and importantly electrolyte imbalance

Although there are various protocols for the management of chyle leak, in the presence of a free flap chyle leak has to be addressed decisively and proactively.

Management—intraoperative recognition of chyle leak

The best management of chyle leak is prevention.

When performing the neck dissection in level IV, we strongly advocate ligating the remaining lymphatics prior to division. Bipolar diathermy or electrocoagulation is not effective in 'sealing' lymphatic vessels because they do not contain blood cells and platelets to coagulate.

If there is an intraoperative suspicion of chyle leak, then every effort must be made in order to identify the leaking lymphatic vessels or the thoracic duct.

The patient is placed in Trendelenburg position and with raised intrathoracic pressure (Valsalva manoeuvre) the leaking lymphatics can be identified. These have to be carefully picked up in atraumatic way and sealed using multiple ligation clips.

Special absorbent and haemostatic dressings such as oxidized cellulose (Surgicel®) layered with fibrin sealants (Tisseel®) can further help 'cement' the area of the leakage.

Medical management of chyle leak

Whenever chyle leak is suspected, pharmacological management with a somatostatin or its analogue octreotide needs to commence (subcutaneous injections). The dosage is usually 100 mcg three times daily but in the literature ranges from 50 mcg twice a day to 150 mcg four times daily.

The patient must be nourished with a special regime containing medium-chain triglycerides. This is because the latter absorbs direct to the portal vein circulation bypassing the lymphatic system.

Fluid balance, electrolyte, haemoglobin, and albumin levels should be monitored carefully and replaced if required. A referral to a specialist dietician/nutritionist is advised to assist in all following parameters:

Management—postoperative recognition of chyle leak

In cases of a free flap reconstruction, upon recognition of an arterial compromise due to a chyle leak (usually low output) a sample has to be sent to biochemistry for confirmation and the patient is transported, as Category 1, to theatre for immediate neck re-exploration as discussed in Chapter 12.

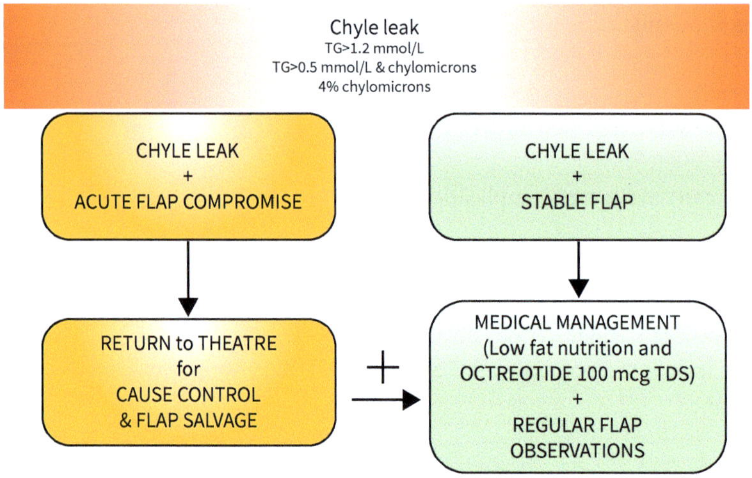

Figure 13.3.2 Algorithmic approach to the management of chyle leak. At the top of the figure, the biochemical criteria confirming the chyle leak are displayed. If a chyle leak is associated with acute flap compromise (most commonly arterial), then immediate return to theatre for flap salvage and control of chyle leak is required. The patient is placed on medical and pharmaceutical management of chyle leak (medium-chain triglycerides and low-fat nutrition, octreotide 100 mcg TDS). If there is the presence of low-volume chyle leak, however, with no sign of flap compromise, then medical management and close flap observations can be implemented. It is recommended that the patient be positioned with the head up (minimum 30 degrees) in order to avoid any chyle reaching and flooding the area of the anastomosis.

If the artery upon neck exploration is deemed salvageable then firstly the cause of compromise needs to be controlled by identifying and sealing the leaking lymphatic or thoracic duct. The arterial anastomosis is then carefully divided and the microsurgery revisited as described in the previous chapter (Chapter 13.2). The algorithm shown in Figure 13.3.2 summarizes the above.

In the postoperative management of a chyle leak, a specialist nutritionist/dietician's input is required in order to manage the electrolyte and protein deficit that may develop.

Flap failed control causes recon at later stage when chyle is ceased and the patient is physiologically and metabolically ready.

High output chyle leak will require a video-assisted thoracoscopic surgery for ligation of the thoracic duct and consideration of total parenteral nutrition (TPN) as well as critical care level support.

Thromboembolic event

Occasionally, and rather rarely, the anastomosis is compromised due to a thromboembolic event and an embolus lodged in the fresh anastomosis. This situation most commonly has an underlying cause such as arterial fibrillation or hypercoagulability.

This issue apart from revision of the anastomosis as described earlier in this subchapter will require medical management of the possible underlying cause such as cardiovascular rhythm optimization and management of atrial fibrillation or management of the underlying hypercoagulability in conjunction with haematology department.

The former and both situations need to be addressed in conjunction with the anaesthetist and the critical care unit after successful revision of the anastomosis and readmission of the patient to the intensive care unit.

In this scenario if the underlying issue is deemed difficult to address, then consideration for flap debridement and an alternative reconstructive option, such as a regional pedicle flap for closure of the defect needs to be taken.

13.4 Complex arterial compromise: Reconstructive errors and physiological causes

Introduction

Occasionally in cases of a free flap compromise with predominantly arterial component as an underlying cause of failure, the cause is far more complex than revision of the anastomosis (technical, as discussed in Chapter 13.2) or resolving a neck problem (regional, as discussed in Chapter 13.3) that has led the artery into spasm.

Complex scenarios are most often encountered in complex reconstructions such as free flaps with long pedicles, which may have been twisted, kinked, or entangled. High reconstructed sites, such as the maxilla or midface, usually require long tunnels transversing the pedicle.

Complex multisubsites, or compartmental resections, often require multiple-component free flaps that bear complex vascular branching and may include perforator segments that are subject to torsion and propagation of the thrombosis cascade.

Arterial and venous anastomosis revision required

Scenarios where the venous anastomosis needs to be divided despite the compromise is primarily attributed to arterial failure, are the following:

- When the venous drainage may have concomitantly adversely affected, or a free flap has a long pedicle that may have caused venous stasis and obliteration of the microcirculation of the flap. Flushing through the artery after division of the failed anastomosis may have increased resistance, and if there is a thrombus lodged in the venous outflow, the operator may choose to divide the venous anastomosis, in order to achieve adequate flushing of the free flap circulation.
- A different scenario when the venous anastomosis needs to be revisited is identification of a new recipient artery on a different site or in the contralateral neck. In that case, if the vein cannot be dissected and separated from the artery the best choice would be to re-site the vein on the contralateral site as well.

It is not a loss to sacrifice a venous anastomosis, the visual result of adequately flushing the failing flap circulation and the ability to confirm free drainage of heparinized saline through the divided vein can only provide the operator with further reassurance about the success of the revision surgery.

The arterial anastomosis revision steps as described in Chapter 13.2 are then followed.

Reconstructive errors—arterial venous anastomosis revision required plus flap reinsert

If the following scenarios are encountered in complex reconstructions as discussed earlier, the arterial anastomosis has failed due to either orientation issues, tunnel compression, free flap components, or has been false-orientated, which has precipitated part of the flap microcirculation to suffer.

As emphasized in Chapter 7.1, the flap inset and particularly the passage of the flap and its pedicle through the tunnel must be executed with the utmost attention!

When passing the flap through the tunnel and prior to the inset it is important that the flap is passed from the neck and through the tunnel to the defect site, as opposed to placing the flap in the defect and pulling the pedicle through the tunnel!

This manoeuvre is crucial, as pulling the pedicle through the tunnel will cause twisting or stretching with a detrimental effect on the anastomosis and the survival of the flap.

The suggested technique is to pass from the defect and through the tunnel into the neck a long pair of forceps (Spencer-Wells, or Fraser-Kelly) and grasp a point of the flap (muscle or subcutaneous fat) with its tips. Once the flap is held by the forceps it is pulled through the tunnel towards the defect with another hand gently pushing it and with extra care to avoid twisting or stretching the pedicle.

The manoeuvre must be executed slowly, gently with extreme caution and care and only after confirmation that the tunnel is of adequate width to allow the bulk of the flap to traverse through it.

Attention must be given to the dotted points on the pedicle (Figures 7.1.1 and 7.1.4). The doted surface (side) of the pedicle must remain unchanged and any for any suspicion of twisting the flap is better removed and the manoeuvre repeated, until it is established that the pedicle within the tunnel rests comfortably without pressure, twisting, stretching, or kinking.

Importantly, in complex cases when the cause is not deemed to be technical at the level of the anastomosis or secondary to a neck collection, then an inset or tunnel problem is suspected.

The venous anastomosis(es) may then need to be divided to allow pedicle alignment and re-orientation in the correct fashion.

Upon division of both the arterial and venous anastomoses, the pedicle is then traced all the way up to the intraoral component of the flap, and the tunnel patency is checked for adequacy. It is not uncommon to encounter numerous blood clots in the tunnel—these need to be carefully evacuated with warm normal saline and gentle digital dissection (finger dissection).

Simply untwisting the artery in the neck will not resolve the problem and most often a complete detachment of the flap needs to take place prior to very carefully reorientating the flap. It is prudent in those cases to try to increase space in the tunnel in order to avoid repeating the same mistake of contortion within the tunnel.

In composite oropharyngeal resections/reconstructions where a lip split approach has been utilized, this must be re-opened to ensure appropriate orientation of all the components of the pedicle. Any pedicle suspension sutures must be released. Essentially, the steps are the same as at the primary surgery, with the difference of working against the clock.

In high reconstructive sites (maxillary or mid face reconstructions), often the pedicle that goes within the long tunnel may have suffered an inadvertent twist. This leads to increased vascular resistance, turbulent flow, and eventually ischaemia and thrombosis. The thrombosis will gradually migrate down to the arterial stem at the site of the anastomosis. In those cases, early recognition and a return to theatre are of paramount importance for the salvageability of the flap.

In those cases of the flap re-inset time is of the essence. Upon adequate flushing of the flap the skin paddle is temporarily immobilized with some tacking sutures and the rest of the inset is left for after the completion of the arterial anastomosis and the flap revascularization.

Physiological causes

This comprises a completely separate category of free flap arterial failure (Type B), that manifests with a different clinical picture and natural evolution is due to slow ischaemic failure of the flap due to reduced perfusion drive.

Rarely and most often in composite free flaps, a phenomenon of progressive slow ischaemia may be encountered. The clinical signs are not consistent with *acute* arterial failure, i.e. the clinical observation of the flap does not consist of the flap being well perfused until a sudden and defined time point where signs of ischaemia (flap turns pale and empty) occur, but rather vague, slow, progressive signs of under perfusion are observed.

Those cases (type B) are most often encountered in patients with borderline physiological reserves or patients who are systemically compromised due to postoperative lower respiratory tract infections or CVS complications (Figure 13.4.1).

Careful judgement is required prior to the decision for another general anaesthetic and flap re-exploration. The microvascular surgeon needs to have clear endpoints in what is aimed to be achieved.

If the general impression or feeling is that the flap is failing due to systemic hypoperfusion and loss of cardiovascular drive, there is no point in attempting to revascularize the flap, as this will add an additional strain in the already stressed physiology of the patient. In those cases, the aim is to optimize the patient and allow the flap to slowly declare itself until a better point in time where the flap can be debrided, and an alternative reconstructive plan can be made.

With experience and a high index of suspicion, careful flap selection can prevent this challenging complication from taking place. For example, it has been discussed in Chapter 2 that, for medically compromised or frail patients, avoidance of *'high-resistance'* free flaps, i.e. reconstructions that include the bony component, may be the best choice.

Bony flaps have a complex microcirculation through the Haversian canals and require higher pressures of perfusion. If adequate perfusion pressure cannot be met due to underlying cardiovascular issues, then slowly microthrombosis in the Haversian canals occurs, which propagates a cascade of further ischaemia and failure.

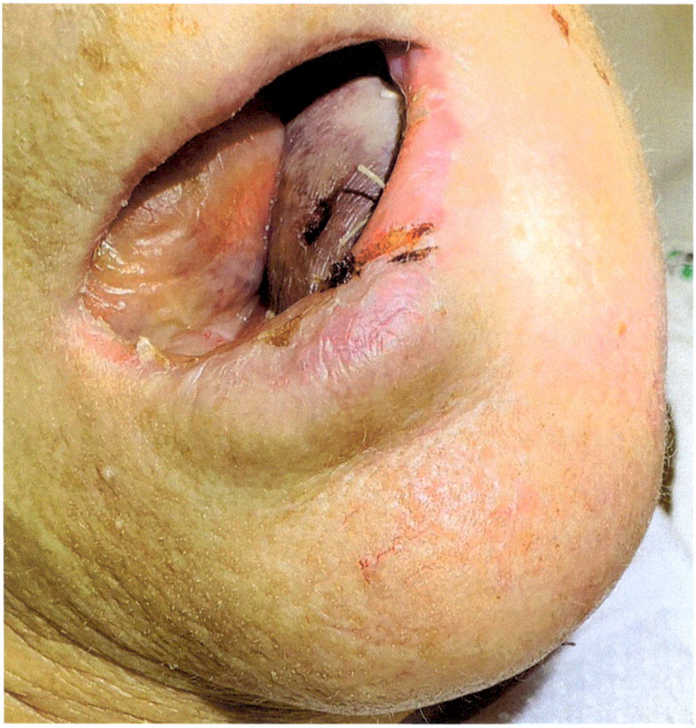

Figure 13.4.1 Slow (Type B) arterial failure of composite scapular angle flap with latissimus dorsi. The patient developed postoperative lower respiratory tract infection (LRTI), leading to hypertension and hypoperfusion of the flap, which led to slow progressive ischaemia due to reduced cardiovascular stamina. The patient was managed medically and once optimized, the flap was debrided and the defect closed primarily after removal of the plate.

A typical *'low-resistance'* system is the latissimus dorsi flap, which has widely patent microcirculation and is extremely reliable in cases that require broad surface cover, bulk, or both.

In those cases of flap reinsertion, time is of the essence. Upon adequate flushing of the flap, the skin paddle is temporarily immobilized with some tacking sutures and the rest of inset is left until after the completion of the arterial anastomosis and flap revascularization.

Further reading

Campisi CC, Boccardo F, Piazza C, Campisi C. Evolution of chylous fistula management after neck dissection. *Curr Opin Otolaryngol Head Neck Surg* 2013;21(2):150–6.

De Felice F, Musio D, Musella A, Tombolini M, Tombolini V. Chyle leak following neck dissection: could radiotherapy be considered a management option. *J Craniofac Surg* 2016;27(2):115–18.

de Gier HH, Balm AJ, Bruning PF, Gregor RT, Hilgers FJ. Systematic approach to the treatment of chylous leakage after neck dissection. *Head Neck* 1996;18(4):347–51.

Deh Carvalho Machado J, Suen VMM, Marchini JS. Is oral nutritional therapy effective for the treatment of chylothorax? A case report. *Nutrition* 2008;24:607–9.

Delaney SW, Shi H, Shokrani A, Sinha UK. Management of chyle leak after head and neck surgery: review of current treatment strategies. *Int J Otolaryngol* 2017;2017:8362874.

Lidman D, Daniel RK. Evaluation of clinical microvascular anastomoses—reasons for failure. *Ann Plast Surg* 1981;6(3):215–23.

Meyer CD, McLeod IK, Gallagher DJ. Conservative management of an intraoperative chyle leak: a case report and literature review. *Military Med* 2016;181(9):e1184.

Merki V, Pichler J, Giger R, Mantokoudis G. Chylothorax in thyroid surgery: a very rare case and systematic review of the literature. *J Otolaryngol Head Neck Surg* 2016;45(1):52.

Olsson E, Sarlomo-Rikala M, Böhling T, Asko-Seljavaara S, Lassila R. Immunohistochemical evaluation of failed vessel anastomoses in clinical microsurgery. *Br J Plast Surg* 2000;53(7):567–73.

Smoke A, DeLegge MH. Chyle leaks: consensus on management? *Nutr Clin Pract* 2008;23(5):529–32.

Sriram K, Meguid RA, Meguid MM. Nutritional support in adults with chyle leaks. *Nutrition* 2016;32:281–6.

Steven BR, Carey S. Nutritional management I patients with chyle leakage: a systematic review. *Eur J Clin Nutr* 2015;69:776–80.

Spiro JD, Spiro RH, Strong EW. The management of chyle fistula. *Laryngoscope* 1990;100(7):771–4.

Swanson MS, Hudson RL, Bhandari N, Sinha UK, Maceri DR, Kokot N. Use of octreotide for the management of chyle fistula following neck dissection. *JAMA Otolaryngol Head Neck Surg* 2015;141(8):723–7.

Talwar B, Donnelly R, Skelly R, Donaldson M. Nutritional management in head and neck cancer: United Kingdom National Multidisciplinary Guidelines. *J Laryngol Otol* 2016;130(2):32–40.

Tilney NL, Murray JE. Chronic thoracic duct fistula: operative technic and physiologic effects in man. *Ann Surg* 1968;167(1):1–8.

14
Troubleshooting and cause-directed management

Vein

Leandros Vassilios F. Vassiliou, Panayiotis Kyzas, and Nicholas Kalavrezos

14.1 Troubleshooting in venous compromise

Introduction

Venous failure is the most common cause of a return to theatre for free flap exploration and salvage. This is because venous failure has a very significantly pronounced presentation and is difficult to be missed or left unrecognized as opposed to arterial failure.

Free flap venous compromise can be crudely categorized into:

- Acute and rapidly evolving (Type A)
- Delayed and slowly progressing (Type B) (Figure 14.1.1)

Type A compromise usually manifests with a dramatic clinical presentation as described in Chapter 11. As will be described in detail in this chapter the acute and rapidly evolving scenarios of venous failure may have different underlying causes similar to the categorization of the arterial anastomosis compromise.

Causes for free flap venous compromise can be broadly divided into the following (Figure 14.1.2):

1. TECHNICAL: This refers to cases where the cause of venous failure is primarily due to technical errors in microvascular suturing.
2. REGIONAL: Venous failure is secondary to problems based on the neck such as a haematoma, or low-neck-level pedicle orientation issues.
3. COMPLEX-TECHNICAL: That refers to flap inset issues, such as tunnel compression, wrong orientation, or pedicle contortion due to errors on the free flap inset.
4. COMPLEX-PHYSIOLOGICAL: Issues that refer to underlying physiological compromise that leads to poor cardiovascular drive resulting in free flap failure.

As mentioned in Chapter 13.1, other classifications of microvascular related troubleshooting simply divide the causes in 'microvascular' related ones, implying that the issue is based on the anastomosis (technical), and 'macrovascular' ones when the root cause stems from conditions in the neck or the patient's physiology (regional and complex, based on the proposed

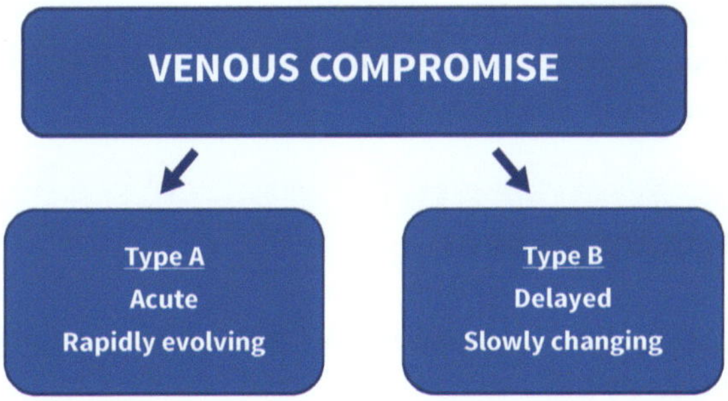

Figure 14.1.1 Broad categorization of free flap venous compromise. Type A refers to an acute and rapidly evolving clinical situation. The flap demonstrates signs of venous engorgement that quickly leads to swelling and bleeding from both the pedicle to the neck and also the free flap site. This clinical situation can be dramatic and even life-threatening. Free flap engorgement may lead to airway embarrassment (if there is no tracheostomy in place) and any airway manoeuvre can be extremely difficult due to the progressively evolving swelling. Type B refers to a slowly progressing and delayed venous compromise. This is most usually encountered due to partial venous obstruction or in free flaps with two venous systems dominance of one that has not been anastomosed. The situation is far less dramatic, and the flap may not display signs of complete venous failure. As in Type B arterial compromise, careful clinical assessment and judgement of the overall situation, including the patient's clinical condition, is required prior to decision making.

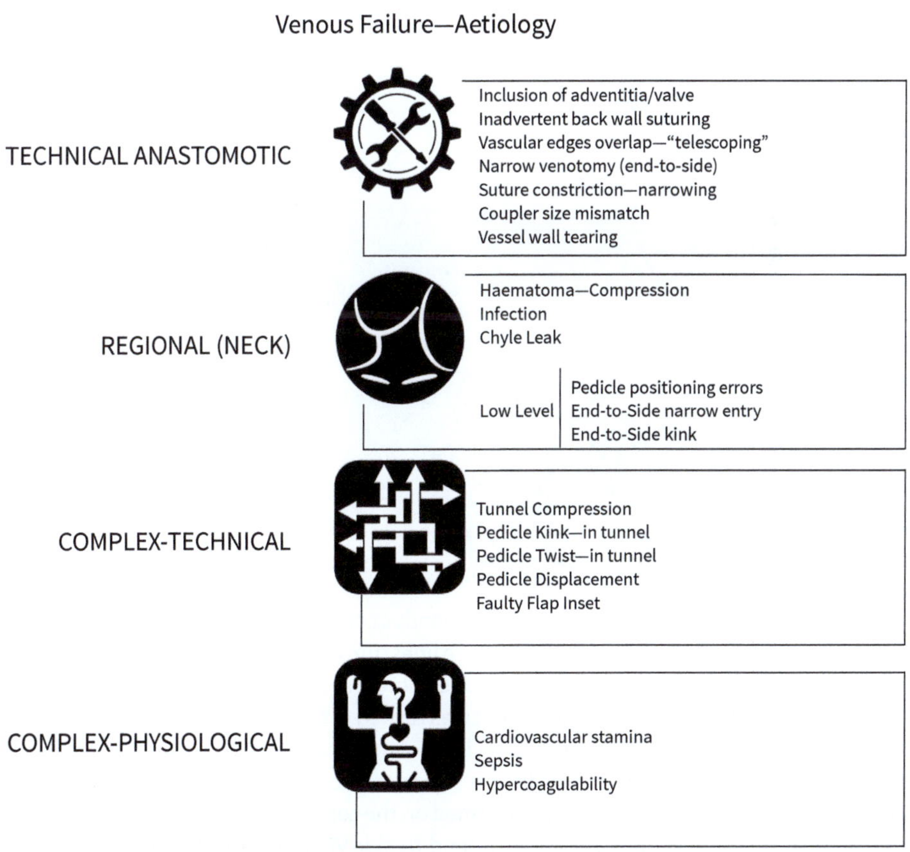

Figure 14.1.2 Summary of flap venous failure aetiology.

classification in this textbook). We prefer the categorization into technical–regional–complex as this is more analytical, helps define the cause more precisely and provides guidance towards the appropriate action plan.

Type A—Initial management

The troubleshooting starts upon recognition that there is a free flap compromise and mirrors the steps followed in Chapter 13.

The general condition of the patient including vital observations (heart rate, temperature, and blood pressure readings) in conjunction with haematological and biochemical results need to be carefully assessed.

As stated in Chapter 12, a venous compromise especially of **type A** (acute and rapidly evolving) will manifest with rapid and significant free flap purple discolouration and engorgement, neck swelling, and bleeding from both the flap sites and the neck. The airway may be quickly and severely compromised (Figure 14.1.3).

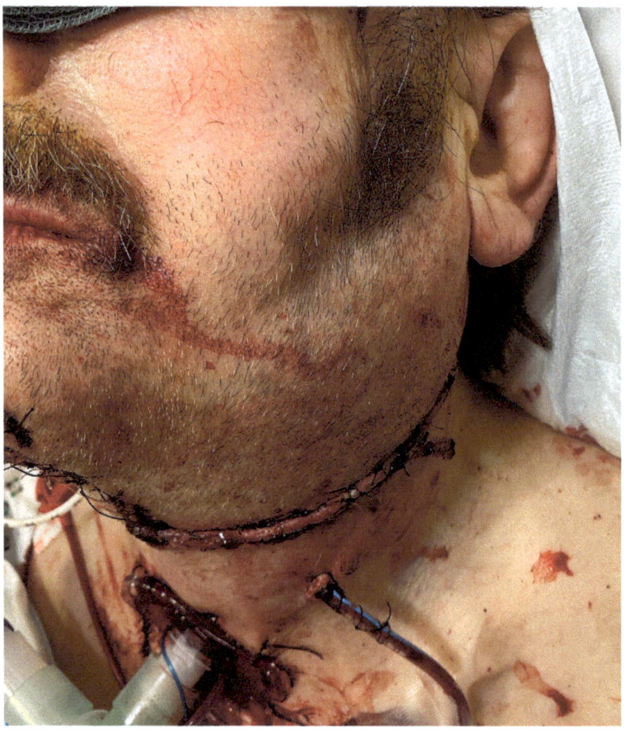

Figure 14.1.3 Typical clinical picture of Type A venous compromise manifesting with a massive neck swelling, bleeding from the suture lines, through the drain and intraoral massive engorgement of the flap, change of colour to deep blue and purple and development of bleeding from the flap insert site. The patient was rushed to the theatre as a category 1 for immediate re-exploration and immediate revision of the venous anastomosis. The free flap was successfully salvaged. The underlying cause was the dominance of the VC system. The original venous anastomosis was only performed on the cephalic vein, which was patent. Upon completion of a second venous anastomosis (end-to-side VC to IJV), the flap venous drainage was restored, and the flap was successfully salvaged.

The airway first has to be secured and the neck, if possible, can be decompressed on the bedside by quickly removing/cutting the sutures allowing drainage and decompression (see detailed management in Chapter 12.2).

The patient is supported with oxygen therapy, broad-spectrum antibiotic administration, intravenous fluids, and it is optional whether intravenous heparin to slow down the coagulation cascade can be administered.

Cross match for blood transfusion is urgently requested and the patient is returned to theatre as a Category 1.

Intraoperative steps

The real troubleshooting starts upon opening and exploration of the neck. In cases of venous compromise, the neck is likely to be full of blood clots and blood.

This raises the fundamental question of whether:

- A neck bleed has caused a haematoma leading to venous compression and obstruction,

or

- The venous anastomosis has failed. First resulting in an increased intravascular blood pressure to build up and subsequent bleeding.

Upon opening of the neck, the following may be recognized:

1. It is likely that other contents or types of fluid may be encountered such as saliva, pus (indicative of infection) or chyle which is discussed in detail in Chapters 13.3 and 14.3.
2. Once the neck is thoroughly irrigated with warm normal saline or heparinized saline and the pedicle is cleared of any blood clots or debris that obscure a detailed inspection, the microscope should be brought in and a thorough, systematic, and in-depth troubleshooting process will be commence.
3. The assessment starts from the point of the venous anastomosis and gradually tracks along the pedicle towards the flap.
4. In early venous failures thrombus may be identified at the site of the anastomosis. This could be due to technical issues with micro-suturing or the couplers.
5. Careful assessment of the pedicle position is required. As the veins are a much weaker structure than the arteries, they are easily subject to kink, torsion, or displacement resulting in turbulent flow, flow obstruction, stasis, and thrombus. The position of the pedicle needs to be assessed and in comparison, to where it was at the end of the primary operation.
6. Occasionally the pedicle may move, especially when the patient is moved from reclining to a sitting position and in cases where free flaps bear long pedicles that may lead to an acute kink. An acute angle can cause obstruction of the blood flow and hence thrombosis.
7. Any pedicle position issues close to the level of the anastomosis ('Low-Level' pedicle position problems) can be addressed as described in Chapter 14.2 alongside a primary venous anastomosis revision.

8. If no apparent cause is primarily identified by the initial inspection phase, a more complex cause needs to be suspected as will further be described in Chapter 14.4.
9. After the initial and in-depth assessment, which shouldn't take too long, the vein is then cut open (the venous anastomosis is divided) which will allow further assessment of the flap blood flow.
10. In case of a healthy and strong patent arterial anastomosis the flap congestion will slowly be relieved and with time (over a minimum of 10 minutes) warm irrigation with heparinized saline the free flap may regain a relaxed appearance and normal venous outflow. In this case, and when the cause evidently has been deemed of a technical nature then further steps as described in Chapter 14.2 concomitantly addressing the underlying cause can be followed.
11. If and despite the time allowed the venous outflow is regarded as unsatisfactory or absent the arterial anastomosis must be revised to achieve flap reperfusion (Chapter 14.3).
12. In more complex reconstructive cases or if there is a suspicion that the venous problem stems from an issue higher up in the tunnel or the flap inset itself, the whole reconstruction must be revisited to fully address the problem (Chapter 14.4).

Type B—Venous failure

In a venous failure of type B, it can be argued that a return to theatre may not be required, especially if there's an underlying medical or physiological issue with the patient. In those scenarios priority must be given to the patient's clinical optimization and the flap issue is left to be dealt with at a secondary stage when its timely more appropriate and clinically safer for the patient to undergo another procedure.

14.2 **Technical causes: Primary venous compromise**

Introduction

Technical venous anastomosis issues are not uncommon. As it has been described in Chapter 9, veins because of the very thin-walled and collapsible structure are often more challenging for the microvascular surgeon than arteries that have a stronger and more sturdy structure easier to suture.

Priority steps when recognizing venous failure in a flap is to establish whether this is a type A or type B venous failure (Figure 14.2.1) and if timely recognized, patient fit for general anaesthetic (GA) and there is merit to re-explore the anastomosis, provision is made for return to theatre.

Common causes for venous anastomosis failure could be microvascular issues, such as:

- Inclusion of adventitia or valve
- Inadvertent back wall suturing
- Vascular edges overlap—'telescoping'
- Narrow venotomy (end-to-side)
- Suture constriction—narrowing

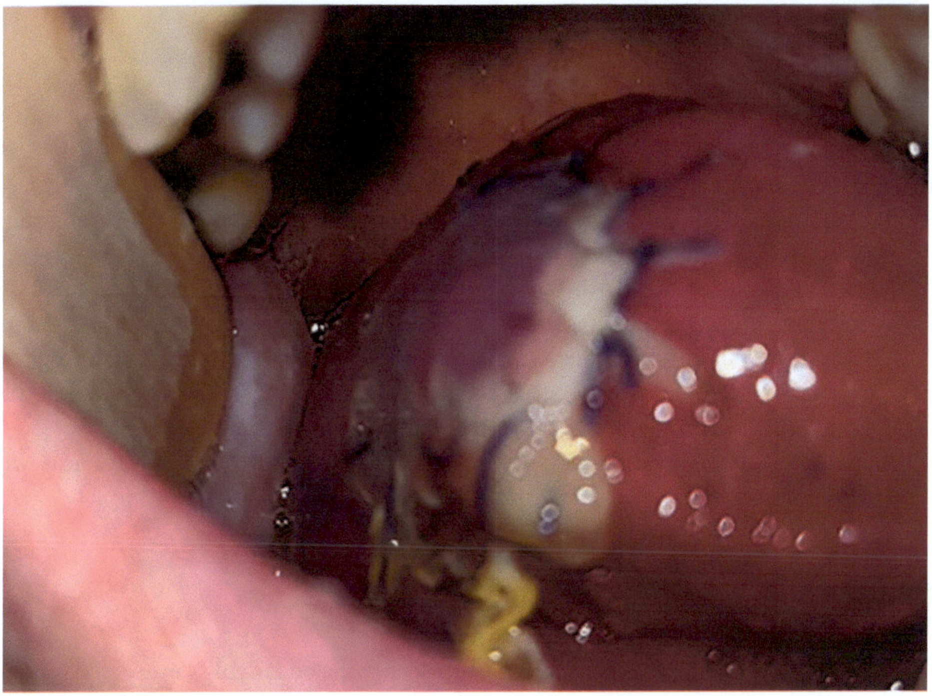

Figure 14.2.1 Clinical picture of venous failure Type B on a radial forearm free flap used for reconstruction of a partial glossectomy defect. The flap displayed slow signs of venous compromise on day 5 postoperatively. The patient was taken to the theatre for neck exploration. The cause of the venous failure was the thrombosis of the anastomosis (conjoined VC end-to-side internal jugular vein).

- Coupler size mismatch
- Vessel wall tearing

Intraoperative management

The technical steps followed for the revision of a technically failed venous anastomosis are the following:

Step 1

As described in Chapter 4, the first step is to set up the microscope as described. A 3V or an appropriately sized 'bulldog' clamp is placed on the recipient vein and the venous anastomosis is divided distally (on the donor/flap vein side):

Hand-sewn anastomoses

Upon division the anastomosis is carefully inspected under the microscope. In most cases a thrombus is present, which is gently removed, and the lumen of the anastomosis is carefully assessed. This may reveal the cause that could be:

- suturing of the back wall
- presence of suture
- adventitia inclusion in the lumen, or even
- vascular intima tear or the presence of partial valve structure.

All these are the easiest and most straightforward troubleshooting cases as in cases of early recognition and flap salvageability the next steps will only require venous anastomosis revision only.

Coupler-based anastomoses

If a coupler has been placed, careful assessment of calibre mismatch has to take place. Occasionally, and if there is a coupler size mismatch of more than two numbers, the bigger vessel, as more 'fleshy' and thick-walled may have been constricted passing through the coupler ring and that may have led to partial obstruction and then thrombosis.

Again, this can be easily addressed by replacing the coupler anastomosis with a hand-sewn suture anastomosis.

Step 2

A concise and systematic effort must be made to identify the underlying cause of the venous compromise.

Any neck haematoma, blood clots or collections must be evacuated and the whole neck has to be thoroughly irrigated with warm normal saline or heparinized normal saline. If there is a presence of a collection steps need to be taken as described Chapter 14.3.

Step 3

If no technical or local to the anastomosis cause such as pedicle mispositioning is identified, then a more complex cause must be suspected and the whole reconstruction must be revisited as described in Chapter 14.4.

Step 4

Once the problem has been identified, the vein has to be left to run and the output flow is carefully assessed. If the arterial anastomosis is healthy and strong then normal bright red blood will start flowing and the whole flap will appear relaxed after a few minutes.

It is important that the blood flow is carefully evaluated. If there any suspicion that this could be poor or unsatisfactory then provision for an arterial anastomosis revision has to be made, which is discussed further in this chapter.

Step 5

Prior to revising the venous anastomosis, ensure that the recipient vein is adequate in:

- Position
- Size
- Preparation

and the flap vein is appropriately prepared to start the microsuturing.

The venous anastomosis is redone in a thorough and meticulous fashion as described in Chapter 9.

If a second vein is available for the flap and the venous compromise is attributed to stasis due to a single-vein anastomosis, then a second vein anastomosis is carefully done after an appropriate recipient vessel or site selection is made. On certain occasions, veins accompanying the superior laryngeal artery may be of suitable calibre for end-to-end anastomosis with a VC.

Step 6

Upon revision of the venous anastomosis or performance of a second venous anastomosis, the flap perfusion is checked, and the venous outflow is thoroughly assessed as described in Chapter 10.

The empty and refill test is extremely important to validate a successful anastomosis.

Step 7

The flap is left to revascularize and the anastomosis is observed for at least 30 minutes in order to ascertain viability of the revision surgery and sustainability of the result.

Step 8

The pedicle orientation and position are carefully assessed and suspension sutures are placed in order to immobilize it in its most optimal position that promotes an unobstructed blood flow through the flap pedicle.

There is no room for failure in a case of flap re-exploration and revision of microvascular anastomosis. The operating surgeon must be 100% satisfied before closing the neck and sending the patient back to critical care.

Step 9

The patient is admitted for postoperative care to the intensive care unit (ICU) and clear instructions for cardiovascular respiratory optimization, and maintenance of MAP above 75 mmHg is given.

Narrow venotomy

A narrow or wrong-site venotomy is a common reason for venous thrombosis due to obstructed flow (Figure 14.2.2). To avoid this, the reader is reminded of the principles described in Chapter 9.3 and, in particular, that the size of the venotomy has to be 1.5× the diameter of the donor vein and the site along the line of the IJV tributaries.

Upon return to theatre and re-exploration, in cases where the venotomy is too small or on the wrong position then the anastomosis site is blocked with a Satinsky clamp or two bulldog clamps and the internal jugular vein hole is carefully closed with 5.0 round body proline sutures.

Following the above, another venotomy site is carefully selected. It is important that the new venotomy is appropriately sited (line of IJV tributaries), and sized 1.5 times the size of the donor vein, in order to maintain an unobstructed blood flow.

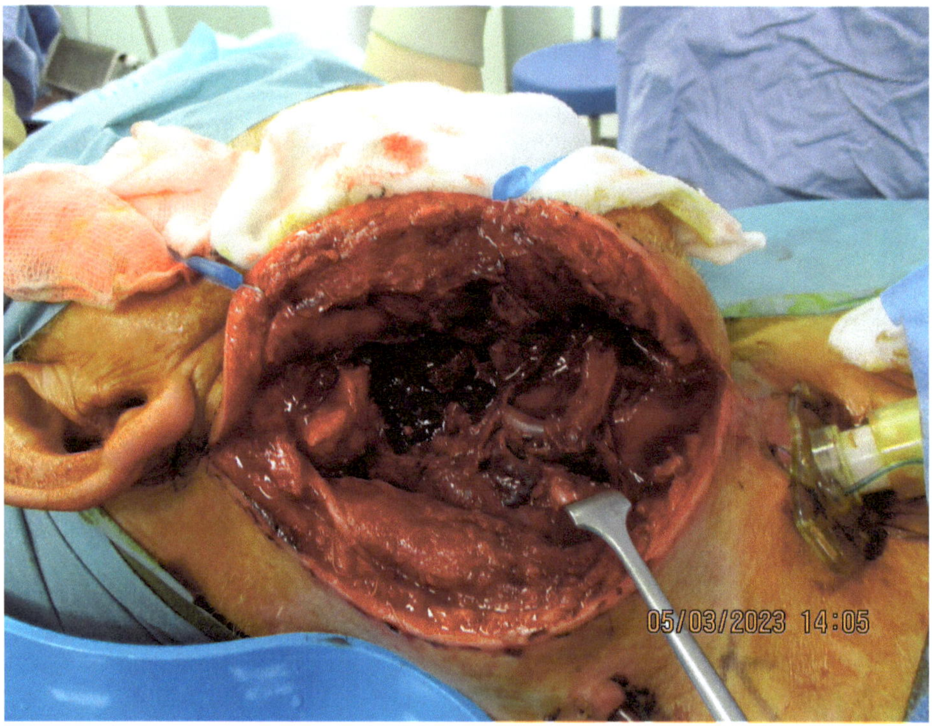

Figure 14.2.2 Neck exploration findings on late venous thrombosis of a radial forearm free flap. Thrombosed venous anastomosis at its point of junction with the internal jugular vein (end-to-side anastomosis).
Note the aggregation of blood clots, a result of flap capillary bleeding. It can be assumed that the venous failure occurred first, against a working arterial anastomosis that carried on pumping blood against a closed circuit, leading to increased pressure and bleeding.
The likely cause of the anastomosis was either kinking of the donor site or the wrong angle of entry of the donor vein into the internal jugular vein (see Chapter 6.5 and Chapter 9.3 for further explanation).

Poor blood flow rate

Occasionally the venous insufficiency is not a direct result of a technical venous anastomosis issue but precipitates from a poor blood flow rate either through the vein or due to a weak arterial drive.

Poor venous outflow rate

For the former only pre-emptive management is of value. During the free flap dissection, it is preferred to divert the blood flow into a single vein—the dominant vein. This could be the conjoined VCs in radial arm free flap or the cephalic vein. This can be assessed prior to complete flap division with the artery running and the veins divided in order to assess which stem delivers the highest blood flow.

Alternatively, and this is what we advocate further dissection in the cubital fossa will in most cases lead to a confluent single vein that concentrates the blood flow from both the deep (VCs) and the superficial (cephalic) venous systems.

Poor arterial flow

If the poor venous flow that has been the underlying cause of the venous insufficiency is not due to a venous selection or choice of anastomosis or these cannot further be corrected, then the operator should look for increasing the arterial power.

This could be addressed by the selection of a different recipient artery as described in Chapter 5. This could involve a different artery on the same side of the neck or may require, and if the pedicle length allows, contralateral neck dissection and identification of an arterial stem on the other side of the neck.

Many operators would advocate that if the facial artery was going to be used, tying off the external carotid artery higher up (more distally) in order to divert the blood flow and perfusion power to the facial artery making it effectively the terminal artery of the external carotid system.

Another solution would be to ligate the external carotid artery distally, turning it down and perform the arterial anastomosis on the external carotid artery in order to secure the highest possible blood flow rate.

Radial forearm free flap—venous failure due to VC dominance

The radial forearm free flap is drained by two distinct but interconnected venous systems. The deep venous system consists of the venae-comitantes running alongside the radial artery and the superficial system is mainly run alongside the cephalic vein. In most patients the cephalic vein is of good calibre and should be harvested with adequate fascia included with a flap. It is adequate to drain the whole forearm flap.

Many microvascular surgeons perform a single venous anastomosis of the cephalic vein into the internal jugular vein tributary (facial vein or middle thyroid vein) or the external jugular vein. The fact that the cephalic vein runs in isolation of the radial free flap and is a long good sized vessel, it gives flexibility for alignment and orientation into a different recipient vein.

There are ample articles and studies in literature describing the efficacy and sufficiency of the drainage via the cephalic system. However, there is an estimated 3-6% of radial forearms where the deep VC based system is primarily dominant. In most cases, no matter what the prime dominance is immediately post anastomosis there is a flow and drainage recalibration and adaptation and blood flow diversion through the outflow of the (patent) anastomosed vein.

If this phenomenon doesn't occur then early signs of flap congestion may become prevalent. That will manifest through mild bruising initially evident on the skin surface overlying the obstructed vein (VC) which will gradually diffuse, spread, and occupy globally the whole flap. If action is not taken then further congestion will occur leading to flap engorgement and obvious discolouration and darkening. Concomitantly the neck will swell up, the main vein system and main draining venous stem will obstruct and increasing pressures in the venous system will start precipitating bleeding and formation of a haematoma.

When the patient is immediately taken back to theatre and the neck is opened, 'tramlines' and stiff pedicle will be encountered, maybe already neck haematoma, and blood clots. The first course of action will be release of the VCs by cutting the ligatures (liga clips) that have been used to drain the veins. Within minutes the VCs will pour all the congested black blood, the pressure will decrease in the system and the pedicle will relax. Ample time should be given to the flap to recoil with constant attention to the performance of the artery. If there are any signs of arterial fatigue or dysfunction then the artery should be cut open, the whole flap should be flushed and the artery anastomosis redone.

In most cases, if the situation is recognized early before global flap skin paddle congestion and discolouration, reopening of the venae-comitantes and release of the entrapped and obstructed blood is adequate to rectify the problem. After the vascular pedicle is relaxed and normal blood flow of bright red blood is re-established a recipient vein is identified to accept the anastomosis of the VC. In most cases due to the size and small calibre of the VC a venotomy on the internal jugular vein and an end-to-side anastomosis is required.

14.3 **Regional causes: Secondary venous compromise**

Introduction

From all the collections in the neck that may cause venous compromise, a haematoma is the leading cause. Occasionally though an infection leading to a pus collection or a chyle leak may have a detrimental effect on the venous anastomosis.

Errors in the pedicle positioning close to the anastomosis ('low-level') such as lack, or loss of suspension may have altered the course of the venous outflow and may have predisposed to 'kinking' of the vein, turbulent flow, or partial obstruction that led to the compromise.

Haematoma/compression

One of the most common manifestations of venous failure is flap congestion relating to flap and neck swelling often during the exploration of the neck a haematoma is identified.

It is often a case of 'chicken and the egg' paradox to determine which was the precipitating factor.

- Was it the haematoma that led to vascular compression and venous congestion

or

- Was it the venous congestion that opened the collateral circulation due to increased pressures and led to bleeding into the neck causing a haematoma.

Intraoperative management

The neck is reopened and all the blood clots are evacuated.

The pedicle is mobilized and carefully inspected.

- If the bleeding vessel from the neck dissection caused a haematoma and venous compression then an actively bleeding vessel will be identified. In that case the vessel is ligated and the vascular pedicle carefully observed.
- If the neck bleeding led to a haematoma, which subsequently led to a venous compression and congestion, the release of the pressure and the ligation of the blood clots would allow the pedicle to relax and the blood flow will be restored. In that case careful observation and the use of a vasodilating agents will have remedied the problem.

In most occasions the neck swelling due to a haematoma is caused primarily by venous failure. In this most common scenario the neck is reopened and thoroughly irrigated with normal saline. All of the blood clots are evacuated and the pedicle is rinsed clean of any blood clots. In this scenario the veins are usually black and even a venous thrombus can be observed. The vascular pedicle is firm and stiff.

If a radial free flap or a flap with VCs (venae-comitantes) has been used then it is a usual occasion that both VCs around the artery are congested or thrombosed and gives the appearance of '*tramlines*'. That is two black lines with a pale white corridor in the middle. In that case the vein is cut open and allowed to flow. If the thrombi are established then irrigation or pooling the thrombi from a vessel dilator from inside vessel lumen can help.

In more desperate situations the artery anastomosis has to be cut open and irrigated with gentle pressure in order to flush away any blood clots from the flap vascular circuit.

Meticulous troubleshooting, as described in Chapter 14.1, has to be undertaken to identify the reasons of venous obstruction and congestion. In most cases orientation issues or a kinked/entangled vein lead to this situation.

The arterial anastomosis is redone, the vein is left to flow in order to clear up the microcirculation from the damaging radical oxygen species (ROS) and the damaged endothelial factors and then the venous anastomosis is redone with particular attention to suitable a choice of venous anastomosis in terms of site, angulation, and orientation.

Pus (infection) or chyle leak or salivary collection

In those instances, for avoidance of repetition, the reader is guided to Chapter 13.3 in order to fully address the underlying cause that has led to the venous failure.

Upon thorough irrigation of the neck and control of the underlying cause such as identification and watertight sealing of a chyle leak the venous anastomosis is revised, steps as described in Chapter 14.2 are followed.

Venous pedicle malposition close to anastomosis

Other causes of venous failure could be attributed to the changes of the pedicle positioning around the area of the anastomosis ('low-level'), excluding issues arising from higher up in the region of the tunnel or the inset of the flap.

The veins are very thin walled and delicate vessels with a soft structure that if subjected to any kind of pressure could easily lead to compression or partially obstructed or turbulent flow.

Any case of pedicle mispositioning, such as pedicle kinking as discussed in Chapter 10.3 and shown in Figure 10.3.2, or even a small amount of venous twist (torsion) described in Chapter 9 can easily lead to a compromise.

If one of these issues is identified, then the vein is redone as described in Chapter 14.2 and the pedicle observed carefully until the most optimum position that allows a fluent comfortable flow is identified. The pedicle is then suspended with 5.0 round-bodied proline sutures in a minimum of 3 points to ascertain adequate immobilization (Figure 10.3.2).

In an anastomosis where the internal jugular vein is the recipient vein often the cause is muscular compression from the overlying sternocleidomastoid muscle. If that has been the identified cause for the venous failure, then gutta or division of the sternocleidomastoid muscle above the revised new venous anastomosis must be performed in order to prevent a similar cause leading to a second failure.

14.4 Complex venous compromise: Reconstructive errors and physiological causes

Introduction

Occasionally and mostly in complex reconstructive cases a compromised flap may not be due to technical problems or neck related issues as discussed in previous subchapters (Chapter 14.2 and 14.3) but the causes may be due to pedicle orientation or compression especially in long tunnels (higher reconstructions) or even patient-related systemic factors. Occasionally and as discussed further here, a venous compromise may not necessarily require return to theatre and re-exploration especially if the patient's general condition is precarious.

The best treatment is prevention and as has been emphasized in Chapter 7.1, the flap inset and particularly the passage of the flap and its pedicle through the tunnel must be executed with the uttermost attention:

When passing the flap through the tunnel and prior to the inset it is important that the flap is passed from the neck and through the tunnel to the defect site, as opposed to placing the flap in the defect and pulling the pedicle through the tunnel!

This manoeuvre is crucial, as pulling the pedicle through the tunnel will cause twisting or stretching with detrimental effect on the anastomosis and the survival of the flap.

The suggested technique is to pass from the defect and through the tunnel into the neck a long pair of forceps (Spencer-Wells, or Fraser-Kelly) and grasp a point of the flap (muscle or subcutaneous fat) with its tips. Once the flap is held by the forceps it is pulled through the tunnel towards the defect with another hand gently pushing it and with extra care to avoid twisting or stretching the pedicle.

The manoeuvre must be executed slowly, gently with extreme caution and care and only after confirmation that the tunnel is of adequate width to allow the bulk of the flap to traverse through it.

Attention must be given to the doted points on the pedicle (Figures 7.1.1 and 7.1.4). The doted surface (side) of the pedicle must remain unchanged and any for any suspicion of twisting the flap is better removed and the manoeuvre repeated, until it is established that the pedicle withing the tunnel rests comfortably without pressure, twisting, stretching, or kinking.

Tunnel compression

Reconstruction of oral and facial defects with free tissue transfer almost always requires tunnelling for the vascular pedicle. The tunnel allows the vascular pedicle to travel from the site of the defect and reconstruction into the neck recipient vessels. In most cases the tunnels contain at least one bony wall.

Tunnels for midline defects such as glossectomy, soft palate, retromolar defects are usually created on the lingual (medial, inner) aspect of the mandible. It is important in these cases to completely strip off the posterior edge of the myeloid muscle (divide from its attachment onto mylohyoid line).

The tunnel has to be carefully and meticulously created in order to allow patency and space for the vascular pedicle without compression that will be predisposed to obstruction and thrombosis. The tunnels should be at least three, if not four fingers wide. The tunnel should be meticulously checked for haemostasis as bleeding into the tunnel will cause a haematoma and pedicle compression.

Maxillectomy defects require longer tunnels due to the distance between the defect and the neck vessels. It is even more important that tunnels created for maxillectomy defects are wide and dry of any bleeding. Cheek, lateral face, and lateral skull defects require tunnels on the lateral aspect of the mandible. The roof of the tunnel in that case is the soft tissue of the face (cheek). It is important the deep fascia is adequately released and that the tunnels are not susceptible to compression due to the soft tissue envelope/overlying cheek tissues and facial muscles oedema that will be predisposed to compression. If venous obstruction occurs at the level or in the tunnel then the characteristic appearances and flap congestion signs are the following; flap congested bruised and discoloured. The flap may be bleeding due to the internal pressures. Maxillectomy defects with congestive flaps may present with nose and mouth bleeding.

During the exploration, the neck is reopened and the veins as well as the vascular pedicle may be found completely empty and collapsed and loose. The lack of any venous congestion in the vascular pedicle within the neck points that the level of the obstruction is not at the level of the neck or the site of the anastomosis but higher indicating that the compression happened in the tunnel. This is a particularly difficult problem to solve.

In such cases the flap may have to be taken completely down, the tunnel reopened, and troubleshooting checked and the anastomosis performed again. It is extremely difficult to take the flap down and through the tunnel, especially if the flap is congested without sacrificing both anastomosis. In most cases however the tunnel congestion causes enough compression to lead the artery to fatigue and subsequent failure. Tunnel compression in most cases is detrimental to the flap. If one side of the tunnel contains skin such as a lateralized face or cheek defects then consideration should be given of an incision (full thickness/through and through) of the overlying skin in order to allow meticulous haemostasis and immediate inspection of the tunnel. This will also allow decompression of the tunnel.

For midline defects such as glossectomy or oropharyngeal reconstruction usually the native soft tissue is compliant enough to allow for some pressure build-up before congestion occurs to obstruct the pedicle. However, with a flap pedicle present which most often is already congested and bleeding surrounded by blood clots it is almost impossible to identify any bleeding vessels from the tunnel walls.

If the blood pressure is medically managed appropriately and the tunnel is thoroughly irrigated bleeding vessels may be identified and ligated. In that case which is the most favourable scenario the flap may be successfully salvaged without the need of been taken down. Lip-split and mandibulectomy defects can provide quick access however that will require a full reopening of the whole defect to allow access and reopening of the whole tunnel.

In cases of tunnel compression and compromised flap a full assessment of the patient's status should be performed in conjunction with the anaesthetist and intensivist. The troubleshooting may require several hours and even another flap in order to reconstruct the defect in case the flap is severely compromised. In that situation it may be prudent for the flap to be completely removed and a pack placed there. The patient will attend intensive care for supportive care, optimization and rescheduled for further reconstruction at a later stage.

Pedicle contortion and orientation problems

Although tunnel compression can be easily rectified by further dissection and increase in the space and patency of the tunnel, contortion issues are far more difficult to mitigate.

Pedicle contortion (twist) issues may easily affect the artery as well leading to a mixed problem, affecting both the artery and the vein. In those very difficult instances, a twisted pedicle demonstrates compromised blood flow due to intraluminal turbulence and suboptimal arterial smooth muscle propulsion. The following vicious circle will gradually lead to complete failure:

Poor perfusion → blood flow stasis → increased microcirculation resistance → further stasis arterial fatigue and thrombosis

The whole flap may need to be taken down, the arterial anastomosis redone as described in Chapter 13.4, venous anastomosis revisited, or performed in a different site.

An easier way to confirm that this is required can be done when the pathological or failed venous anastomosis is divided. If the venous flow is deemed poor or unsatisfactory it is clear proof that the arterial anastomosis is struggling, and this needs appropriate attention and revision otherwise redoing the venous anastomosis only will prove entirely futile and the flap will be effectively lost.

Type B venous failures—physiological factors

Cases where physiological factors are involved. The venous failure does not present in an acute, hyperacute, or any way dramatic fashion that calls for immediate and lifesaving return to theatre then more time consideration in rectifying systemic parameters can be given.

The venous failure could be a result of reduced cardiovascular stamina as already described in Chapter 13.4, but it could be a result of an underlying physiological compromise such as sepsis, hypercoagulability, and other circumstances such as hypothermia. In those instances the slow venous failure is due to a vicious circle similar to the one described earlier:

Poor perfusion → blood flow stasis → increased microcirculation resistance → further stasis arterial fatigue and thrombosis

If the venous compromise does not manifest with congestion or neck swelling the focus can be diverted on physiological optimization in conjunction with medical teams or readmission into the critical care unit for more comprehensive organ support.

In cases of slow and non-urgent venous congestion, classed as type B venous compromise, the free flap options could include:

- Delayed surgical intervention after physiological optimization
- Prioritization in the physiological optimization of the patient and delayed flap debridement with or without alternate flap reconstruction
- Leech therapy especially when extraoral reconstructions are concerned. Leech therapy has been described in Chapter 12.2 (Figure 14.4.1).

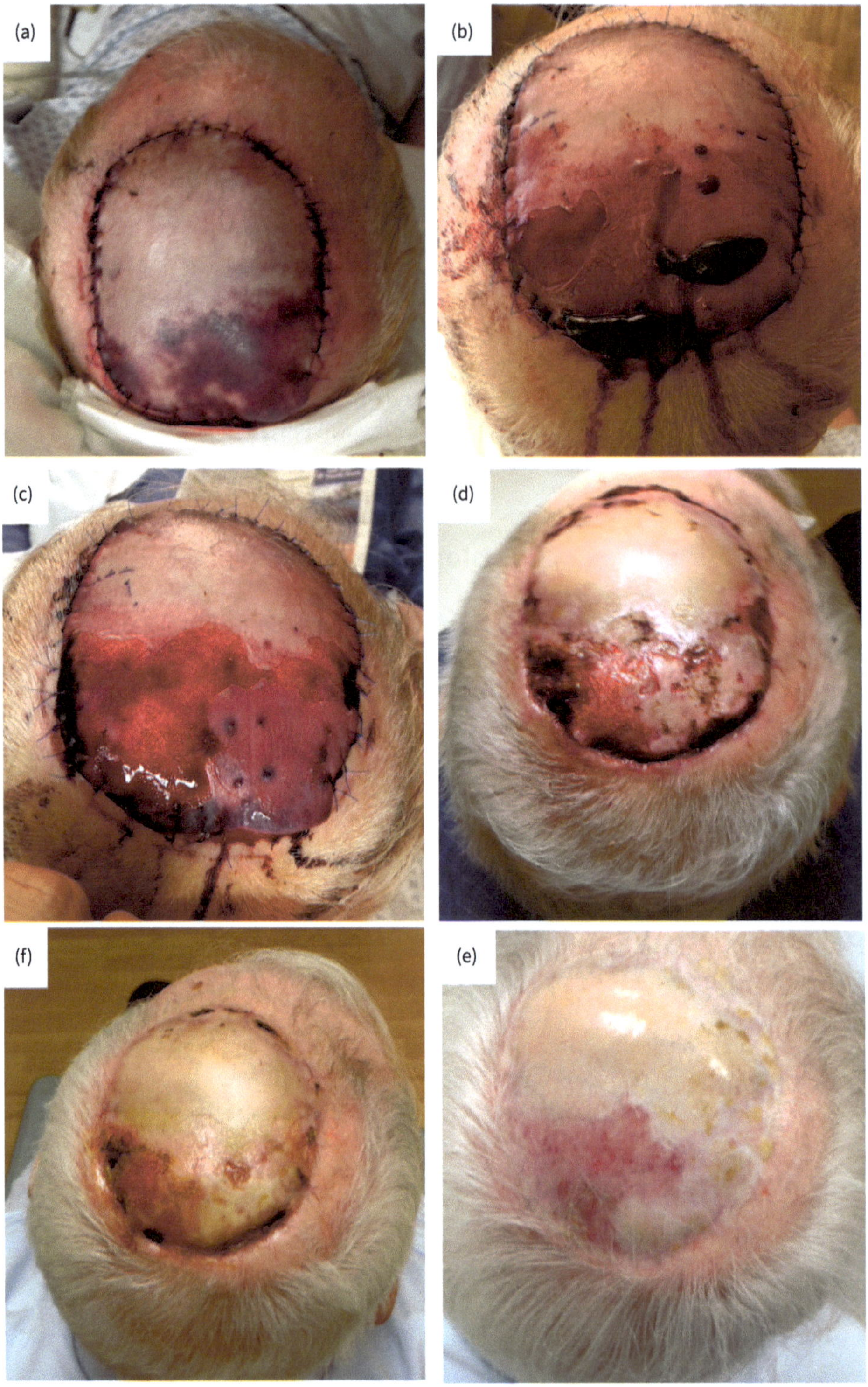

Figure 14.4.1 a. Type B congestion in a free latissimus dorsi flap used for scalp reconstruction. Note the global hyperaemia and areas of venous congestion. b. Attachment of leeches. c. Leech bites and areas of skin excoriation, consequence of leech therapy. d. Clinical photo of the flap 5 days post-leech treatment. e. Clinical photograph 1 month post-leech therapy. f. Final clinical photograph 3 months post-discharge.

Further reading

Bai S, Xu ZF, Duan WY, Liu FY, Huang DH, Sun CF. Single superficial versus dual systems venous anastomoses in radial forearm free flap: a meta-analysis. *PLoS One* 2015;10(8):e0134805.

Edmonds JL, Woodroof JM, Girod DA. Venous valves in the neck: implications for microvascular free flap reconstruction. *Arch Otolaryngol Head Neck Surg* 1999;125(10):1151–3.

Fitzgerald O'Connor E, *et al.* The microvascular anastomotic coupler for venous anastomoses in free flap breast reconstruction improves outcomes. *Gland Surg* 2016;5(2):88–92.

Fukuiwa T, Nishimoto K, Hayashi T, Kurono Y. Venous thrombosis after microvascular free-tissue transfer in head and neck cancer reconstruction. *Auris Nasus Larynx* 2008;35(3):390–6.

Galanis C, Nguyen P, Koh J, Roostaeian J, Festekjian J, Crisera C. Microvascular lifeboats: a stepwise approach to intraoperative venous congestion in DIEP flap breast reconstruction. *Plast Reconstr Surg* 2014;134(1):20–7.

Matthews JLK, Alolabi N, Farrokhyar F, Voineskos SH. One versus 2 venous anastomoses in free flap surgery: a systematic review and meta-analysis. *Plast Surg (Oakv)* 2018;26(2):91–8.

Moreno MA, Small LT, Gardner JR, Kim AH, Vural E, Sunde J. Outcomes of single anastomoses for superficial and deep-system venous drainage of radial forearm free flaps. *OTO Open* 2021;5(2):2473974X211006927.

Netscher DT, Sharma S, Alford EL, Thornby J, Leibman NS. Superficial versus deep: options in venous drainage of the radial forearm free flap. *Ann Plast Surg* 1996;36(5):536–41.

Razzano S, Esposito L, Schonauer F. The venae comitantes clipping test for the evaluation of the venous drainage of the radial forearm free flap. *Microsurgery* 2016;36(8):647–50.

Selber JC, Sanders E, Lin H, Yu P. Venous drainage of the radial forearm flap: comparison of the deep and superficial systems. *Ann Plast Surg* 2011;66(4):347–50.

Shaw RJ, Rogers SN. Venous microvascular anastomotic failure due to prothrombin gene mutation. *Plast Reconstr Surg* 2005;115(5):1451–2.

Stewart M, *et al.* Outcomes of venous end-to-side microvascular anastomoses of the head and neck. *Laryngoscope* 2021;131(6):1286–90.

Stewart M, *et al.* Anastomotic revision in head and neck free flaps. *Laryngoscope* 2021;131(5):1035–41.

Sullivan SK, Dellacroce F, Allen R. Management of significant venous discrepancy with microvascular venous coupler. *J Reconstr Microsurg* 2003;19(6):377–80.

Wittenborn J, *et al.* Numerical simulations of different configured venous anastomosis in microvascular flap transfer. *J Craniomaxillofac Surg* 2019;47(5):792–7.

15
Troubleshooting

An overview algorithm

Leandros Vassilios F. Vassiliou, Panayiotis Kyzas, and Nicholas Kalavrezos

15.1 **Summary of troubleshooting and compromised flap management algorithms**

Introduction

This chapter consolidates the information and guidance, as has been described in the troubleshooting chapters (Chapters 11, 12, 13, and 14). The summary provided here is presented in flowcharts with action steps and algorithms, in order to help the reader refresh the knowledge in the management of a compromised free flap.

Basic categories of free-flap compromise

The types that a compromised free flap is presenting as, are illustrated in Figure 15.1, which demonstrates the broad categorization of possible scenarios encountered.

A failing flap may become compromised due to predominantly arterial (A) or venous (B) failure. Any of these situations has to be viewed in relation to the acuteness of presentation and speed of evolution.

Type A flap compromise represents the majority (over 80%) of cases and refers to situations where an immediate return to theatre for exploration and salvage is required.

Type B refers to either scenarios of late flap failure recognition, insidious uncertain progression or situations where a medical emergency or life-threatening condition is not declared, and the patient happens to be unfit for a second general anaesthetic (GA), hence delayed management may be more appropriate.

Stepwise summary of actions for return to theatre

The flow chart in Figure 15.2 presents a summary of the steps required for taking the patient back to theatre for free flap salvage.

As described in Chapter 11 regarding the immediate management upon free flap compromise recognition, in type A (either arterial or venous failure) emergencies, the patient has to be deemed suitable and stable for another general anaesthetic (if not, immediate optimization and preparation is required) and the flap has to be deemed salvageable.

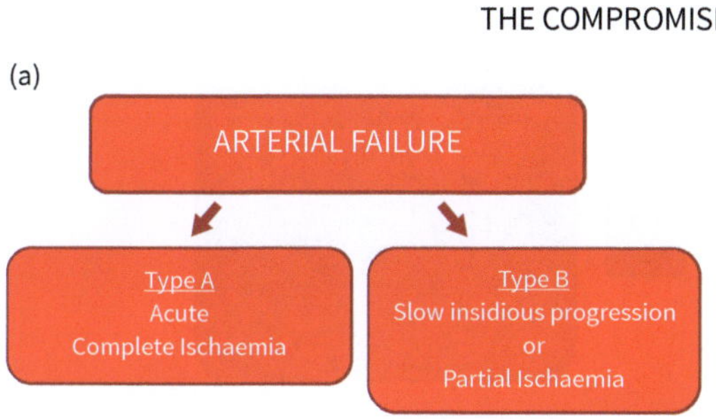

Figure 15.1 Broad categorization of free flap compromise.

When these conditions are met, ideally, involvement of two microvascular trained surgeons is required.

The underlying cause of the free flap failure (troubleshooting and root cause) must be completed and appropriate actions to remedy the underlying cause and successfully revise the anastomosis has to be taken.

Of course, in life-threatening emergencies such as airway compromise or bleeding immediate Category 1 transfer to theatre has to be undertaken.

Troubleshooting algorithms

In Figure 15.3 a general oversight and comprehensive algorithm of the actions is demonstrated depending on a thorough troubleshooting process.

The root cause of free flap compromised aetiology must be established.

As summarized in Figure 15.4 the cause of a free flap compromise could be simply technical due to anastomotic pitfalls, regional regarding to situations in the neck affecting directly the anastomosis or complex as described in Chapter 13.

The most common 'technical' anastomotic pitfalls for arterial failure are demonstrated next:

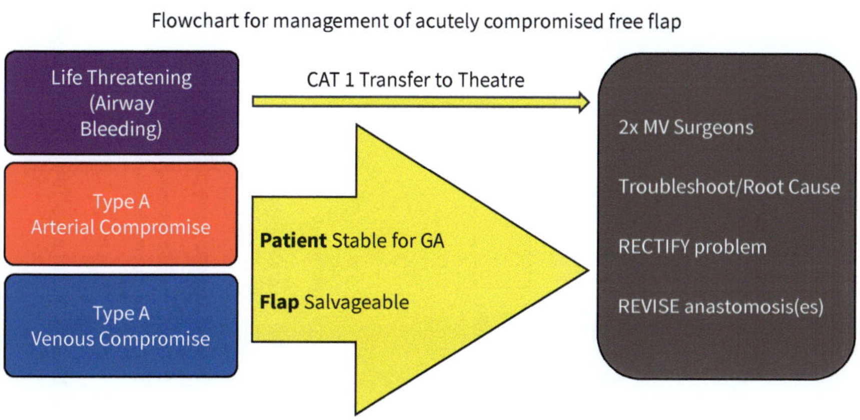

Figure 15.2 Flowchart for management of acutely compromised free flap.

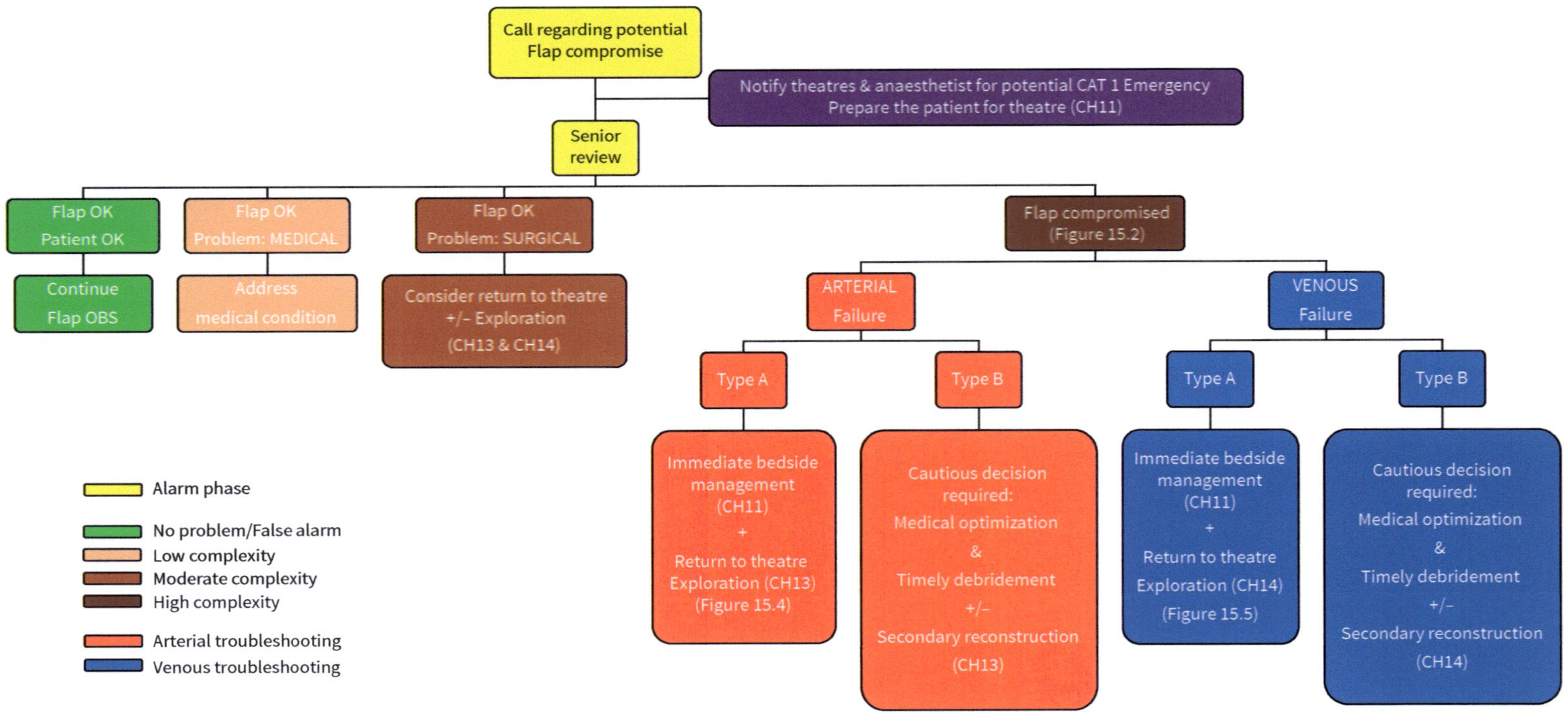

Figure 15.3 General algorithm for management of possible flap compromise.

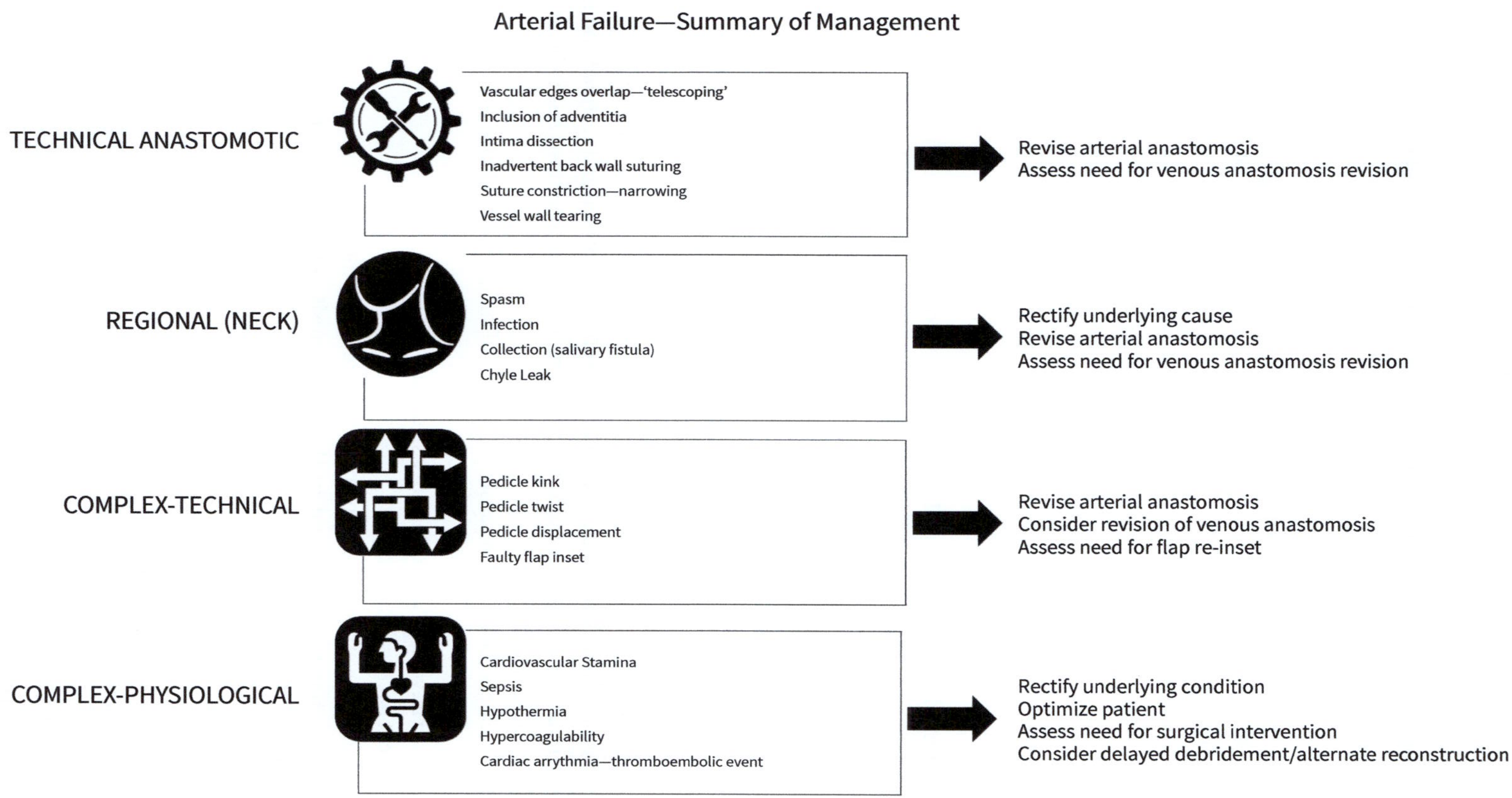

Figure 15.4 Summary of management recommendations in scenarios of free flap arterial compromise.

- Vascular edges overlap/telescoping
- Inclusion of adventitia tissue which is highly thrombotic into the anastomosis
- Intima dissection
- Inadvertent back wall suturing
- Suture constriction/narrowing due to non-equidistant placement of microvascular sutures
- Vessel wall tears

Depending on the cause and the primary vessel compromised the surgeon will have to consider revising the arterial or the venous anastomosis and even consider reinserting the flap in complex technical situations.

'Regional' causes of arterial anastomosis failure can be the following:

Arterial spasm due to:

- Infection
- Collection
- Chyle leak

'Complex technical' causes refer to pedicle displacement or free flap inset errors:

- Pedicle kink
- Pedicle twist
- Pedicle displacement
- Faulty flap insertion

Finally, 'Complex physiological' due to underlying medical conditions as described in detail in Chapter 13.4.

For venous failures again a thorough troubleshooting process must be undertaken (Figure 15.5). The cause (technical, regional, or complex) has to be identified and rectified and revision of the venous anastomosis or both the venous or arterial anastomosis has to be undertaken in order to salvage the flap.

For venous failures the common causes for 'technical' anastomotic failure are:

- Inclusion of adventitia or partial valve structure
- Inadvertent back wall suturing
- Vascular edges overlap/telescoping predisposing to turbulent flow and thrombosis
- Narrow venotomy in cases of end-to-side anastomosis causing constriction, reduced flow, congestion, and thrombosis
- Suture constriction due to non-equidistant placement of suturing and narrowing of the anastomosis
- Coupler size mismatch due to thick vessel wall edges passing through the coupler ring and occluding the anastomosis
- Vessel wall tearing

Common 'regional' causes for venous failure refer to problems in the neck leading to venous anastomosis compromise:

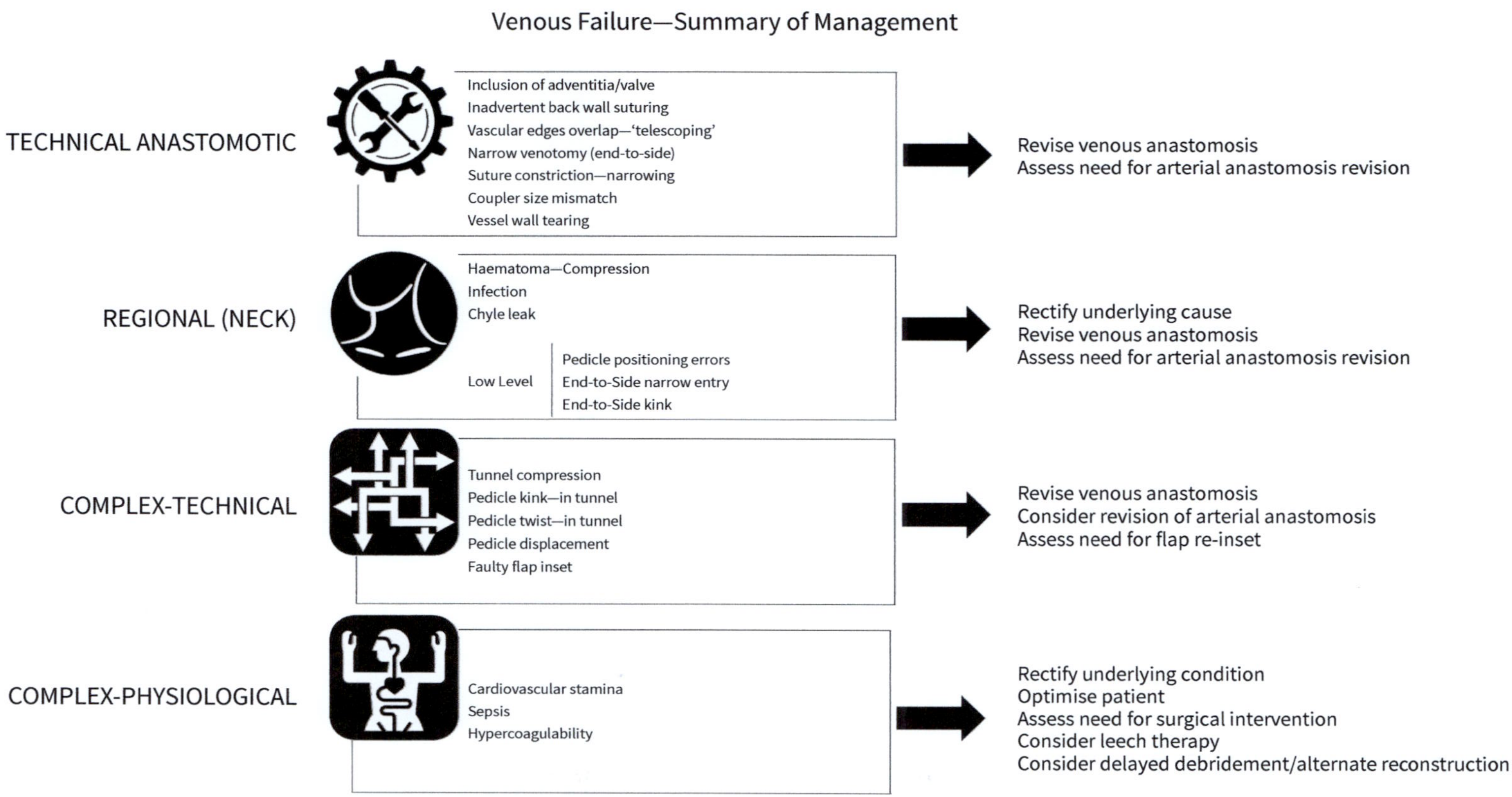

Figure 15.5 Summary of management recommendations in scenarios of free flap venous compromise.

- Haematoma compression of the thin-walled vessels (veins)
- Infection
- Chyle leak
- Low level pedicle misplacement issues

'Complex technical' issues leading to venous compromised are listed next:

- Tunnel compression
- Pedicle kink inside the tunnel
- Pedicle twist inside the tunnel
- Pedicle displacement
- Faulty flap inset causing kinking or twisting of the vessels

The 'complex physiological' causes are rarer in cases of venous anastomosis failure and are described in Chapter 14.4.

16

Vessel-depleted neck and solutions

Fu-Chan Wei, El Muiz Mustafa, Nidal Al Deek, Leandros Vassilios F. Vassiliou, Panayiotis Kyzas, and Nicholas Kalavrezos

16.1 The vessel-depleted neck

Introduction

Microsurgical reconstruction in patients who have already received free tissue transfer is not uncommon. Indications for another free flap surgery include:

- Recurrent disease
- New cancer diagnosis
- Delayed reconstruction
- Flap salvage
- Osteoradionecrosis (ORN)
- Closure of fistula
- Plate exposure
- Revision of a stenosis of the neo-pharynx or oesophagus.

The operative conditions can be challenging. 8% of patients have previously undergone a neck dissection or radiation therapy (see Kushida-Contreras et al. in 'Further reading'). At least 5–8% have osteoradionecrosis (ORN) despite improvements in the delivery of radiotherapy, such as intensity modulation and proton beam (see Frankart et al. in 'Further reading').

Large systematic reviews of flap outcomes in the referred to as vessels depleted neck (VDN) cohorts indicate that failure rates are typically higher than those in primary surgery (see Kushida-Contreras et al. and Mijiti et al. in 'Further reading'). Partial flap loss is not uncommon and returns to the operating room are reportedly as high as 18% (see Tam et al. in 'Further reading'). Peripheral dehiscence and development of cutaneous fistula is also more common in this group of patients and may require further revision surgery or additional tissue transfer (Choi et al. in 'Further reading').

The following main challenges are encountered in the previously treated neck rendering free tissue transfer far more difficult than treating a virgin neck:

Patients' general physical status

Patients needing further major head and neck (H&N) surgery are often in poor nutritional and functional status or under treatment for a systemic comorbidity which raises the risks of postoperative complications.

These patients will require thorough preassessment and optimization and careful treatment planning. Given the complexity of the operation and the higher risk of complications and return to the operating theatre, the preoperative assessment needs to consider the possibility of additional surgery and evaluate the potential physiological reserves to withstand this.

Previous operations in the neck

When recipient vessels that are routinely available for anastomosis in the neck are rendered unsuitable or absent, an even more challenging subgroup of patients emerges and often referred to as VDN patients, constituting a formidable challenge.

Previous irradiation

Surgical access is severely impeded by radiation fibrosis. The history of previous neck radiotherapy is one of the main challenges in cases of further free tissue transfer.

This chapter will focus on the VDN subgroup of patients and will discuss strategies on how to best manage free tissue transfer in this group.

Definition of vessel-depleted neck (VDN)

There are several descriptive terms in the literature such as: the difficult neck, the frozen neck or the hostile neck, previously dissected neck or 'already treated neck (ATN)'. These are open to broad interpretation. Contreras et al proposed an operative-centred definition, based on the requirement for preparation of vessels outside the external carotid or internal/external jugular vein systems, or the use of vein grafts due to radical neck dissection and radiation (see Kushida-Contreras et al. in 'Further reading').

Many series included in the authors' review report utilizing the superficial temporal vessels (when the external carotid system is intact), or the contralateral branches of the external carotid artery, and the use of vein grants. However, the threshold for using those vessels is, naturally, variable among individual surgeons. Furthermore, the requirement for a vascular graft could be related to a more distant defect location rather than availability of recipients in the anterior neck.

In the senior authors' practice, a *true*-VDN rarely exist. However, it is more appropriate to consider a *near*-VDN status in patients who require the use of uncommonly used recipient vessels because bilate ral anterior neck vessels are not available or accessible.

Uncommonly used vessels could either mean recipient vessels (see chapter 16.3) that are not a first line *per se* such as the external carotid artery itself, or not a first line for a given location as in when the superficial temporal vessels are used for a lower facial defect out of necessity not choice.

Approach to reconstruction

Principles of reconstruction broadly follow those of primary surgery. The aim of free tissue transfer is the provision of a tailored reconstruction conforming to the surgical defect thereby restoring form and re-establishing anatomic boundaries. Further benefits reported by patients with osteoradionecrosis are pain reduction, treatment of pathological fracture, closure of oro-cutaneous fistulas and improvement in quality of life (QoL) (see Baron et al. in 'Further reading'). However, functional improvement with respect to speech and swallowing is predetermined to a great extent by the previous treatment(s). Following radiotherapy, pharyngeal and masticator muscles undergo progressive radiation fibrosis. These changes are irreversible, resulting in a high prevalence of trismus, impaired peristalsis, dysphagia, reduced laryngeal elevation and silent aspiration (see Servagi-Vernat et al. in 'Further reading').

The treatment planning should take into consideration the following parameters:

- Clinical and radiographic evaluation of the location of pathology
- Anticipated extent and constitution of the resulting defect
- Previously used flaps
- Location of previous anastomoses
- Prognosis when applicable
- Prior operations findings
- Radiotherapy dose and field
- Chemotherapy protocols
- Available vessels status
- Patient's QoL
- The surgeon's expertise/experience

All these dictate the choice of flap(s).

Non-microsurgical reconstruction is an acceptable alternative in selected patients.

For vessels evaluation, magnetic resonance angiography (MRA) or dual phase CT angiography (CTA) has been advocated for vessel mapping (see Breik et al. in 'Further reading').

Demonstration of the patency of the transverse cervical artery (TCA) is beneficial, for it may be unsuitable in 8% of subjects (see Du et al. in 'Further reading').

The internal mammary artery is another back up option, but it may also be inadequate in 20% of patients (see Moran et al. in 'Further reading').

Imaging may also confirm the availability of the internal mammary veins and the patency of the proximal cephalic and the internal jugular veins.

Carotid stenosis may be assessed using duplex ultrasound scanning. This would be helpful in the assessment of the risk of cerebrovascular accidents and thus suitability for complex surgery in general.

Some of these imaging modalities are part of routine preoperative assessment and incur no additional cost but recipient selection can only be reliably achieved by direct assessment.

Flap choice and design

Flap choice involves additional considerations concerning pedicle length and position and even flow-through flaps.

The choice of flap is primarily dictated by the defect parameters (bony or soft tissue, volume, functional goals of reconstruction, and distance from recipient vessels). Donor site availability may be restricted because of previous treatment or peripheral vascular disease. Together with the limited availability of recipient vessels, the surgeon may wish to reconsider their usual choice of flap.

With respect to pedicle length, the workhorse flaps including the radial forearm (RFFF), the latissimus dorsi (LD), the anterolateral thigh (ALT), and the fibula, all provide decent pedicle length for most scenarios. These flaps were the most commonly reported in a systematic review of reconstruction in the irradiated neck (57 studies, 8,694 flaps) (see Kushida-Contreras et al. in 'Further reading'). However, with careful planning, most bone and soft tissue flaps are adaptable to provide an adequate reconstruction. Some flap choices do apply themselves more readily in particular contexts.

The radial forearm free flap (RFFF) has a long pedicle (15.0–22 cm) in the adult, with an additional two centimetres venous length conferred by the cephalic vein when available. Provision of fascial bulk is limited (e.g. with the beaver tail modification). Although harvest of skin paddles up to 30 cm long and 15 cm wide are possible, the ensuing donor site morbidity would be difficult to manage. The RFFF is thus suitable as an additional flap, a flow-through flap, or in smaller defects. The paddle and pedicle orientations with respect to each other may also limit the rotatory freedom conferred by flaps. This is always a concern in head and neck reconstruction but likely more so when few recipient vessels are available.

Perforator based flaps such as the ALT flap provide adequate pedicle length. Their advantage is versatility of soft tissue configuration possible in free flap surgery. More importantly, their reach can be greatly extended by offsetting the perforator entry point with respect to the skin paddle or oblique skin paddle orientation. They allow for multiple soft tissue components to be oriented independent of each other. This allows for additional muscle component to reduce the risk of plate exposure or salivary leak. Therefore, these flaps are a good choice for through and through defects or composite defects the involve the mandible or maxilla, or in hostile wounds as in ORN.

Reconstruction of through and through or multicompartment defects (e.g. the retromolar region that typically involves the mandible and maxillary to some extent) may be also achieved with dual flaps or single flaps such as the scapula osteo-cutaneous with dual paddle flap or perforator flaps like the ALT as described. The pedicle length in the scapula tip flap i(based on the angular artery) is usually 10–12 cm and is a good choice for reconstruction.

Reconstruction of the hypo pharynx and oesophagus is often required for post-radiotherapy salvage. The most commonly used flaps are the enteral (e.g. jejunal) flaps, fascio-cutaneous (radial forearm) or perforator flaps (ALT) (see Piazza et al. in 'Further reading'). The jejunal flap may be freely transferred or pedicled on the ileocolic vessels (oesophagus) with supercharging from the TCA to augment the blood supply in an irradiated neck. The ALT flap may be tubed or inset in a horseshoe outline sutured to the prevertebral fascia. The fascia is usually well vascularized which may be helpful in the containment of a low-grade leak. Success rates are high following chemo-radiotherapy, reported as much as 98.2% but fistula rates are encountered between 5 and 30% of cases (see Hasan et al. and Piazza et al. in 'Further reading').

16.2 **Contralateral neck anastomosis**

Introduction

In the systemic review by Contreras et al. the commonest of uncommon recipient vessels were the superficial temporal (20%) and the transverse cervical artery (TCA) followed by the contralateral branches of the external carotid artery (11%) and the ipsilateral external carotid stump (10%). Less commonly reported recipients: the internal mammary, thoraco-acromial, anastomosis to a previous flap pedicle (6%) and retrograde flow (TCA, superficial temporal, and reverse flow thoracodorsal arteries used in the scapula flap) (see Kushida-Contreras et al. and Breik et al. in 'Further reading').

In contrast to the systematic review findings, the senior authors prefer either the contralateral neck or the ipsilateral transverse cervical vessels. The decision largely depends on which of these vessels limit the need for a vein graft.

The vessels should be carefully approached and released, especially the veins. It is important to assess the lumen of the vessel before committing to them, especially in patients with vascular disease or previous radiotherapy. While vein grafts are avoided as possible, low threshold to use them is maintained, and justified to reach a wider and healthier arterial or venous stump.

Recipient veins are typically the internal jugular vein (IJV) or one of its branches or the external jugular vein (EJV). If the IJV is used, it must be adequately exposed and mobilized to the extent that it allows a comfortable end-to-side anastomosis (see Chapter 16.2).

The TCA and superficial temporal artery (STA) typically have accompanying veins of adequate calibre and can be used (see Chapter 16.3).

The overlying skin is usually tight and rigid, and the pedicle comes to lie subcutaneously in many cases. Therefore, tension-free closure is important. This can be achieved by using the flap skin paddle itself. If tunnelling is required (which it is in most cases), it must be as wide as possible.

Points of consideration in the contralateral neck anastomosis

When anastomosis is planned on the contralateral neck, a number of key points are of importance:

1. Flap pedicle length is of the essence.

It is important to maintain as much vessel length as possible, both in the flap pedicle during the harvest and also in the recipient vessels of the neck.

Flaps that offer long pedicles are the following, in descending order:

- Radial forearm free flap (Figure 16.2.1)
- Latissimus dorsi free flap
- Anterolateral thigh flap
- Fibula flap
- Scapular flap (angular artery)

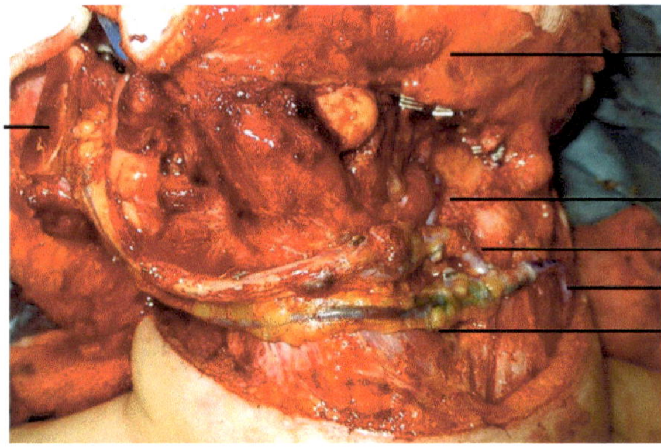

Figure 16.2.1 Contralateral neck anastomosis of a radial forearm free flap used to reconstruct an oropharyngeal defect. Note the recipient artery is the contralateral facial artery and the recipient vein the contralateral external jugular vein.

Techniques to maximize flap pedicle length are based on the following:

- o The skin paddle should be designed at the inferior-most (most distal) point possible to allow maximum pedicle length.
- o The pedicle dissection during the flap harvest should be followed to the maximum point and the flap should be divided at the highest (most proximal level possible). This for radial artery this is the bifurcation of the branchial artery into ulnar nerve radial, for latissimus dorsi flap this is at the level of the subscapular artery, for fibular flap this is at the bifurcation of the tibioperoneal trunk into peroneal and posterior tibial and for the anterolateral thigh (ALT) flap the descending branch of the lateral circumflex artery at its take off from the lateral circumflex artery.

2. Recipient vessel length.

Dissection and preparation of the recipient vessels should be meticulous. Unless the patient has risk factors for vascular disease or the field is previously irradiated when the recipient vessels flow check and lumen inspection can be omitted, the recipient vessels can remain undivided and maintain their full length until the time of the anastomosis. For example, if the anastomosis is planned to take place at the facial vessels, then the facial artery and facial vein remain intact, and dissection continues above the level of the lower border of the mandible to allow harvesting of additional length if required (Figure 16.2.2b). Similarly, the EJV remains intact, any further length is required, then dissection proceeds within the parotid gland to harvest an additional portion of the retromandibular vein for extra length.

3. Creation of the tunnel lingually.

For oral or oropharyngeal defects, the flap pedicle needs to pass through a tunnel and travel to the contralateral neck. It is natural to assume that in order to shorten the distance that the pedicle needs to travel to the recipient vessels creation of the tunnel mast take place lingually to the mandible, or else as close to the contralateral neck as possible.

4. Anterior pedicle exit.

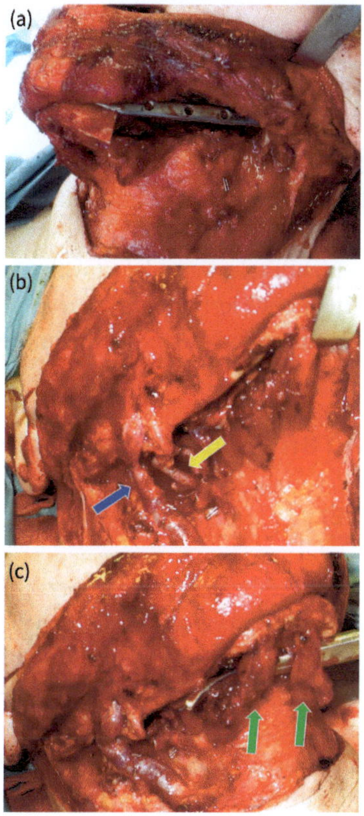

Figure 16.2.2 a. Segmental mandibulectomy defect in a previously irradiated neck requiring contralateral neck anastomosis. b. Dissection of the recipient vessels: Facial artery (yellow arrow) and facial vein (blue arrow). The vessels have been prepared further distally and above the level of the lower border of the mandible. The vessels have not been divided until the flap is inset, and the required length can be visualized. If further length is required, dissection can continue higher in order to harvest the necessary length to perform a tension-free anastomosis and avoidance of vascular grafts. c. Dissection prior to division of the anterior bellies of both digastric muscles to allow a shorter loop for the flap pedicle to reach the recipient vessels.

Care must be taken during planning and flap inset for anterior pedicle exit as a posterior exit will require substantially longer length with possible detrimental effect for the anastomosis.

5. Division of the anterior bellies of the digastric muscles.

In order to bypass the curvature of the anterior neck and shorten the arc of rotation and the required travel distance of the flap pedicle we would advocate division of the anterior bellies of both digastric muscles bilaterally (Figure 16.2.2c).

6. Inset position of the flap.

If despite all these measures, there are still issues with the pedicle reaching the recipient vessels then an alternative inset location of the flap as a final resort may make up for the distance required. Examples of this are the following:

- For a retromolar defects a more anterior location leaving the upper part of the defect to heal under secondary intention and as long as this does not predispose to fistula formation.
- For a segmental or a hemi- mandibulectomy defect with an anterior pedicle exit the bony flap can be moved further anteriorly—with some additional bone reduction in order to assist approximating the pedicle to the recipient vessels.

16.3 **Uncommon head and neck recipient vessels**

Transverse cervical artery

The transverse cervical artery (TCA) is the dominant supply of the trapezius muscle through its dorsal scapular branch. Prior to its entry point at the trapezius, it runs a long path from its origin at the thyrocervical trunk, travelling along the floor of the posterior triangle. This section allows for dissection and transposition of the vessel to the anterior neck.

Anatomical variations are not uncommon; the artery originates from the subclavian in 20% of subjects. The dorsal scapular artery (DSA) is a branch of the TCA in 30% of cases (see Rosko et al. and Moran et al. in 'Further reading'). When the DSA takes off independently from the subclavian artery, it may also be traced in the posterior triangle of the neck and utilized as a recipient. This was described previously by Rosko et al. (see 'Further reading').

The TCA is usually preserved following neck dissections as it forms the inferior boundary of level IV. Due to its position at the base of the neck, the TCA is usually outside the main radiation field.

Retrograde flow is reportedly adequate for microvascular anastomosis when the anterior segment is fibrotic (see Ciudad et al. in 'Further reading'), but we never encountered a need for retrograde flow. The TCA is usually within 10 cm of the angle of the mandible and is thus frequently accessible to a contralateral neck utilizing flaps with long vascular pedicles or a vein graft. In the study published by Tessler et al. (see 'Further reading') the TCA length ranged from 4.0 to 7.0 cm, and the mean diameter was 2.65 mm.

The vessel may be approached either by extension of the neck dissection incision, perpendicularly towards the supraclavicular fossa or through a separate incision 2 cm above and parallel to the clavicle (see Yu et al. in 'Further reading'). The dissection proceeds to the lateral border of the sternocleidomastoid and the muscle is retracted medially. The external jugular vein may be encountered. The omohyoid muscle is identified and retracted (or divided). The transverse cervical vein and artery are embedded within fatty tissue posterior to the omohyoid. Some surgeons prefer to avoid the left side of the neck due to the proximity of the thoracic duct, although this structure is occasionally at risk of injury at the level IV–V neck dissection.

Due to the position of the TCA pedicle at the root of the neck and its relatively loop-shaped appearance, it is important prior to division to mark the proximal (antegrade) side of the artery and vein in order to establish the correct orientation and avoid anastomosis in a reverse-flow manner.

The vessel can be traced distally across the posterior triangle as far as the Trapezius or the branching of the DSA (if present). The calibre of the artery is often observed to reduce along its length. It is not known to be anatomically absent, although it may lie infraclavicular in 3%.

Superficial temporal vessels

The superficial temporal vessels are the terminal branches of the external carotid. Confirmation of the artery pulsation may be achieved by palpation or Doppler ultrasonography. A vertical pre-auricular incision parallel with the vessels gives adequate exposure and allows for further extension if required. The skin and temporal fascia are dissected, and the superficial temporal vessels are isolated from a distal to proximal direction. The artery typically has an omega-shaped bend but is relatively easy to dissect. The vein has a thin wall and many branches; it is easily injured and must be handled carefully. A subcutaneous tunnel allows for the delivery of the flap pedicle for anastomosis. Aside the vessel-depleted neck, these vessels can be used for orbito-cranial reconstruction (Figure 16.3.1).

Uncommon thoracic-based recipient vessels

Subclavian vessels

For a vessel depleted neck, the use of subclavian vessels is another option (see Broderick et al. in 'Further reading'). Those vessels lie in a relatively short distance from the head and neck defect and can allow anastomosis for flaps with long pedicles.

The subclavian vessels are often outside the area of previous fibrosis (postoperative or post-radiotherapy). Dissecting and accessing the subclavian vessels requires the assistance of an experienced vascular or thoracic surgeon, as a clavicular osteotomy is necessary as well as transient clamping of the subclavian artery and vein.

There are important anatomical variations between the left and right subclavian vessels. The left subclavian artery emerges from the arch of the aorta behind the commencement of the left common carotid artery. The left subclavian vessels are in close anatomical intimacy with the thoracic duct and due to this reason are not the preferred option.

The right subclavian artery is located behind the right sternoclavicular joint, emerging from the brachiocephalic (innominate artery). Access is achieved by clavicular osteotomies at 2 cm from each side joint that allows entry into the costoclavicular space (Figure 16.3.2).

Again, an anatomical landmark of the subclavian arteries is the scalenus anterior muscle that marks the territory between the subclavian artery and vein (Figure 16.3.3). It is important to note that the course of the vessels passes intimately from the pleura of the lung apex.

Once the artery is dissected and prepared it must be temporarily clamped in order to facilitate arteriotomy. An end to side anterior anastomosis is performed, ischaemia time has to be closely monitored. Repatriation of the clavicular segment and fixation needs to avoid any compression of the underlying anastomosis.

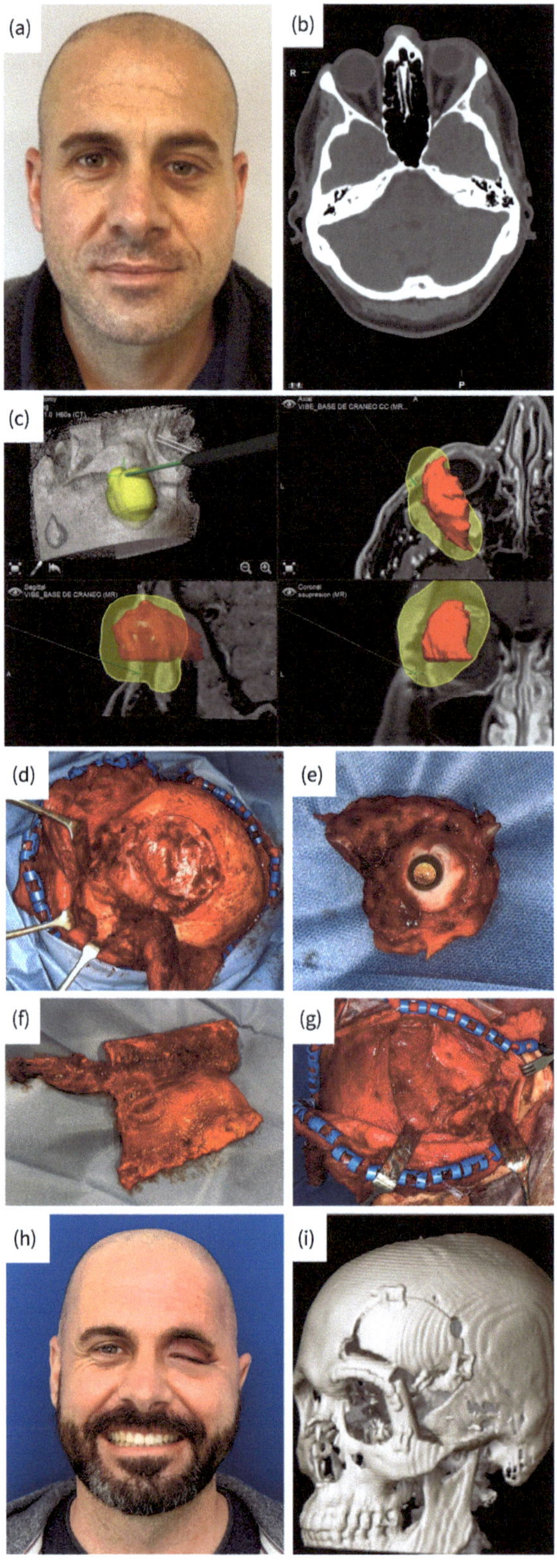
(a)
(b)
(c)
(d)
(e)
(f)
(g)
(h)
(i)

Figure 16.3.1 Complex orbito-cranial reconstruction with free flap anastomosed onto the superficial temporal vessels (courtesy of Professor Julio Acero). a. Adenoid cystic carcinoma of the lacrimal gland affecting the left orbito-cranial region. b. Axial CT. c. Virtual planning of the resection with margins in green colour. Intraoperative navigation of the resection. d. Orbito-cranial resection. e. Surgical specimen. f. Osteo-fascio-cutaneous fibula flap. g. Orbital reconstruction. Anastomosis to the temporal vessels. h. Postoperative facial aspect of the patient. i. Postoperative CT showing the orbital bone reconstruction. Courtesy of Professor Julio Acero, Madrid, Spain.

Internal mammary vessels

The internal mammary/internal thoracic vessels are a cornerstone for coronary revascularization and breast reconstruction with well-sdocumented high patency rates. Urken et al. introduced these vessels into head and neck practice in 2006 (see Urken et al. in 'Further reading'); since then over 180 cases have been reported in the literature with good outcomes (see Scaglioni et al. in 'Further reading').

The internal mammary (IMA) artery is a branch of the proximal subclavian artery in most instances. Rarely, the artery originates from the distal subclavian or the thyrocervical trunk (see Shahoud Kerndt and Burns in 'Further reading'). Moran et al. reported that in 20% of patients, the accompanying vein is unsuitable for anastomosis (see 'Further reading').

Harvesting of the IMA requires the assistance of a thoracic surgeon. The IMA runs along the inner surface of the anterior thoracic wall, 1–3 cm lateral to the sternal margin. Both artery and its accompanying internal mammary vein are accessible through an incision over the second or third rib (see Roche et al. in 'Further reading'). The muscle fibres of the pectoralis major are split parallel to their direction, revealing the intercostal muscles and rib cartilages. The muscles and perichondrium are incised, exposing the rib cartilage to enable excision of the cartilage up to the sternochondral joint. The posterior perichondrium is then incised, exposing the internal mammary vessels situated anterior to the transverses thoracic muscle.

Three to four centimetres of vessel length can be isolated after ligation of the intercostal branches. Anastomosis may be performed at this location in an antegrade flow direction.

Vein grafts may be used to bridge to flaps with shorter pedicles or positioned high in the head and neck. Pneumothorax is reported in 1.4% of cases (see Keiling et al. in 'Further reading'). It is important to note that utilizing the IMA precludes its future use as an arterial graft in cardiac surgery. Another approach is to isolate the vessel at its takeoff from the subclavian trunk.

Other vessels

There are very few reports concerning the pectoral branch of the thoraco-acromial vessels, or the occipital vessels. Not enough clinical reports are currently available to make recommendations regarding their use.

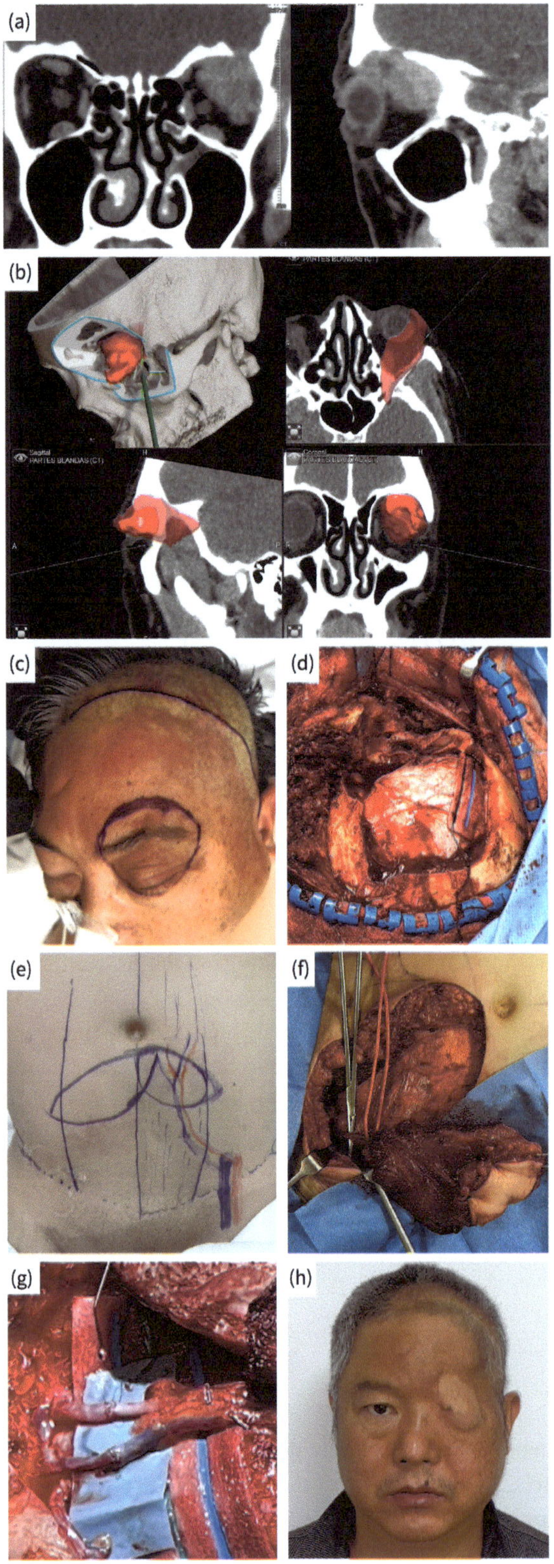

Figure 16.3.2 Complex orbito-cranial reconstruction case with rectus abdominis free flap anastomosed onto the superficial temporal vessels, adenoid cystic carcinoma of the lacrimal

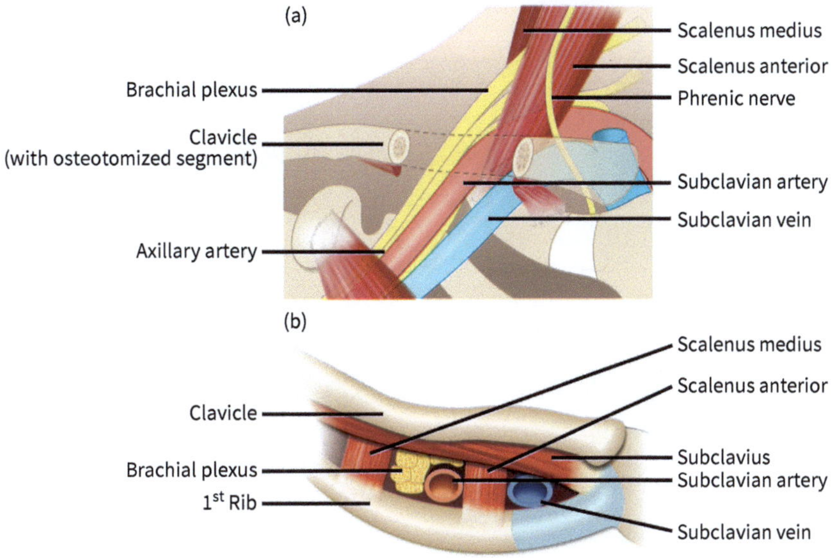

Figure 16.3.3 a. Coronal (anterior) representation of the right thoracic outlet demonstrating the subclavian vessels in relation to the scalenus anterior muscle, the phrenic nerve, and the right branchial plexus. b. Axial representation of the costoclavicular space illustrating the relationship of the subclavian vessels with the scalenus anterior muscle, subclavius muscle, and the branchial plexus.

Adapted with permission from Broderick D, Vassiliou L, Kyzas P. Use of the subclavian vessels for microvascular reconstruction in the vessel-depleted neck. Br J Oral Maxillofac Surg. 2021 Jan;59(1):114–16. doi: 10.1016/j.bjoms.2020.08.091. Epub 2020 Aug 21.

16.4 **Vascular bridges**

Several techniques are described in the head and neck literature to enable bridging the flap pedicle to a distant recipient. The options include the following:

- Autologous vein grafts (Figure 16.4.1)
- Cephalic vein techniques (transposition and Corlett loop)
- Intermediary flow-through flaps
- Re-using the vascular pedicle of a previous flap reconstruction

With the exception of vein grafts, there is a paucity of literature concerning success rates. As with venous anastomoses in general, the success of a venous bridge depends not just on microsurgical technique and the number of anastomotic joins, but also on the avoidance

Figure 16.3.2 Continued

gland. a: CT image showing orbital involvement, including the orbital roof. b. Navigation planning of the resection c. Surgical approach. d. Navigation-guided resection. e. Flap design and surface markings. f. Elevation of a rectus abdominis flap. g. Anastomosis of the flap pedicle to the temporal vessels. h. Postoperative appearance of the patient.

Reproduced courtesy of Professor Julio Acero, Ramon y Cajal University Hospital, Madrid, Spain.

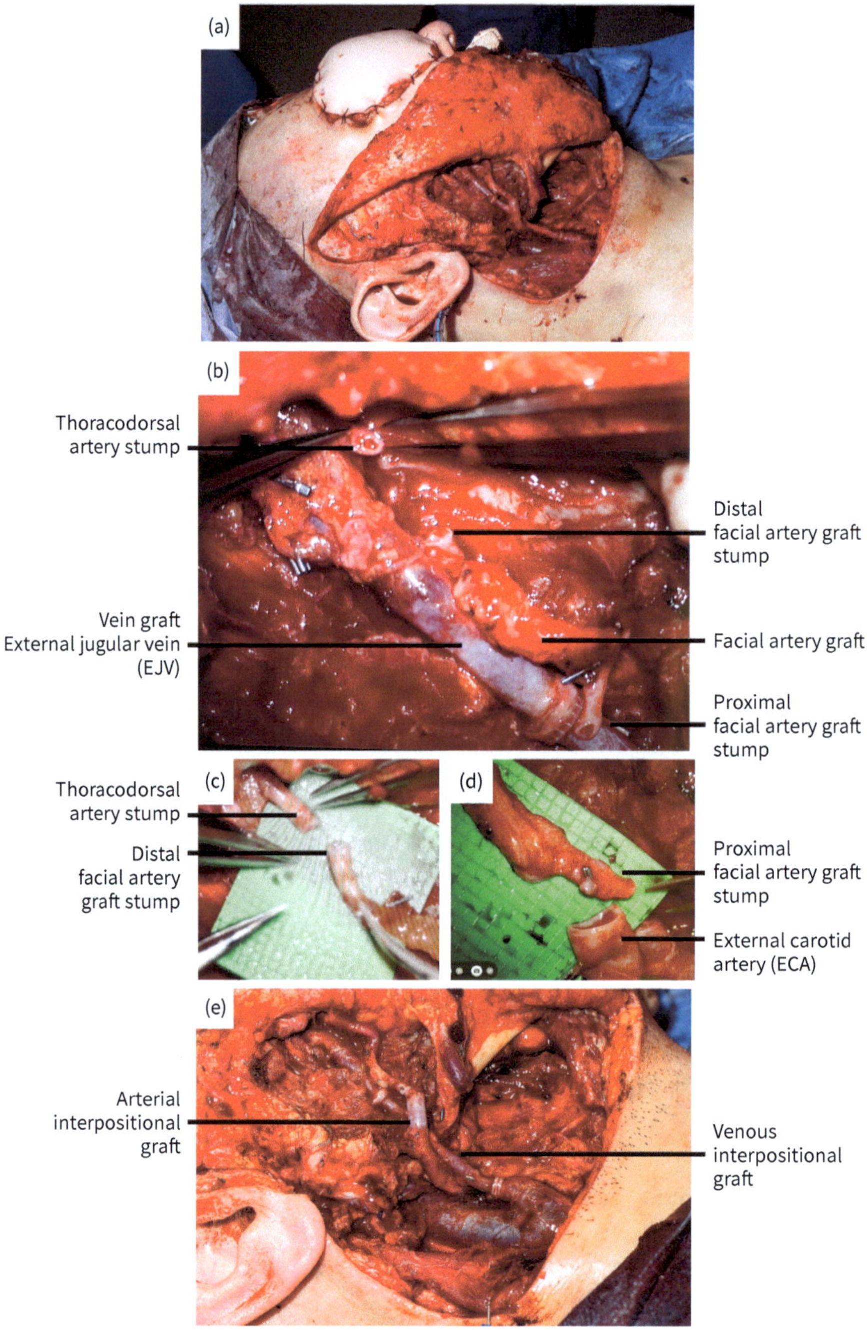

Figure 16.4.1 Vascular bridges (interpositional arterial and venous grafts). a. Macroscopic photograph showing right-sided major orbital resection and reconstruction with latissimus dorsi free flap with interpositional grafts in place and anastomoses completed. b. The upper part of the photograph shows the thoracodorsal artery stump (donor artery). The lower right quarter of the photograph displays the facial artery graft, with the upper part being the distal stump and its proximal facial artery end turned to approximate the external carotid artery (recipient artery). c. Microvascular preparation of arteries about to be anastomosed (thoracodorsal artery and distal end of facial artery graft). d. The proximal facial artery graft stump is about to be anastomosed to the external carotid artery (ECA) (recipient artery). e. Both arterial and venous anastomoses were completed. Note the arterial interpositional graft fully expanded, evidence of patent flow through the anastomoses. The venous interpositional graft has been anastomosed to the donor and recipient veins using MACD (coupler devices).

of compression, kink, twist, and the condition of the vein graft as well as the recipient vein downstream.

Studies that report venous graft outcomes also highlight the length of a vein graft and hypertension as independent predictors of flap loss in patients who have undergone previous dissection and radiotherapy (see Di Taranto et al. in 'Further reading'). Therefore, the decision to proceed with vein grafts or other vascular bridges requires an individual risk assessment based on the patient's overall condition.

Vein grafts

The use of autologous venous grafts in the head and neck has previously been linked to substantially higher rates of flap loss, but the largest series to date (309 flaps utilizing vein grafts) appears to suggest that outcomes are comparable to non-grafted flaps (3.9% success vs. 3.2%, respectively) (see Di Taranto et al. in 'Further reading'). The rate of flap compromise requiring surgical revision was 8.2%. Interestingly, it was the group of cases where the vein graft was used for both arterial and venous anastomoses that were responsible for the bulk of lost flaps. The flap failure rates for arterial only or venous only grafting were 0% and 1.4%, respectively, indicating that the procedure is inherently safe in single-stream anastomosis.

The second largest series (see Maricevich et al. in 'Further reading') on vein grafts in head and neck reconstruction (241 flaps requiring vein grafts) does report a significantly increased rate of flap loss when vein grafts were used. However, the authors stated the reasons for flap failure were reviewed in detail for each case and was clearly attributed to compression, kink, and perforator injury. They argued against anastomotic thrombosis as the aetiology for flap loss in their series.

Donor sites for vein grafts include: the greater saphenous, lesser saphenous, anterior jugular, or distal pedicle veins. The anterior jugular vein presents a convenient location for harvest of short or intermediate length grafts. In contrast with neck donor veins, graft harvest from the lower limb can proceed in tandem with vessel preparation in the neck. The long saphenous vein is a good option and can present up to 18 cm of graft length. It lies within the range of a fibula cutaneous paddle and therefore, some forward planning needs to be kept in mind. The lesser saphenous vein is easy to harvest and would be a good choice.

In the surgical protocols of the Di Tarantino study, venous graft length was found to be an important determinant of flap loss. The authors advised that an intermediary flap was indicated when the distance between the pedicle to vein graft was 10 cm or greater. Within their study, the rate of flap compromise (prompting an unplanned revision operation) was significantly lower in the vascular bridging flaps compared to venous grafts, although the number of cases was relatively low in this study.

In our practice, long venous grafts appear to carry an increased risk of complications, mainly due to possible compression or increased resistance against flow. One should shorten the length of the graft as much as possible.

Cephalic vein techniques

The cephalic vein can be exposed and controlled distally with an incision along its course in the upper arm. The proximal end may then be left intact, and the vein transposed above the clavicle to provide venous drainage in the neck.

The vessel may also be adapted to form a Corlett loop. In this technique, following the distal division of the cephalic vein the proximal end is divided, resulting in two free ends which are anastomosed to the recipient artery and vein in the neck. This forms a temporary arteriovenous fistula. Similarly, a long venous graft (typically the great saphenous vein) is harvested and arterialized by connecting to a neck recipient as described. Either immediately or, at a delayed stage, the AV fistula is divided providing two free ends that may then be attached to the flap pedicle (see Mulholland et al. in 'Further reading'). Since the original description in 1993 by Mulholland et al., there have been a number of cases reported with good success rates. A related method involves utilizing the long saphenous vein to create an AV loop between the external carotid to the jugular vein or branches thereof and then divided to connect to the flap pedicle as previously described (see Anderson et al. in 'Further reading').

16.5 Vascular bridge flaps

The concept of an arterial flow-through flap was demonstrated in a description of the radial forearm, by Soutar in 1983 (see 'Further reading'). The authors described anastomosing one end of the radial artery to the external carotid and the other to the facial artery in order to improve flap perfusion. Subsequently, these 'arterialized' flaps gained popularity in limb trauma, in particular, following the recognition that vascular patency is superior to free grafts.

Flow-through flaps used to 'piggy-back' sequential flaps can be classified based on their inflow, outflow, and the nature of the vascular conduit (see Bullocks et al. in 'Further reading').

The first description of 'chained' radial forearm flow-through flaps in the head and neck was by Chen, Tang, and Noordhoff (see 'Further reading'). This was used for total oesophageal reconstruction. In this arrangement, two free flaps are connected in series to be perfused with a single recipient artery and draining vein. The 'main' flap covers the defect. The bridging flap serves several purposes; it connects the main flap to a distant pedicle, provides additional skin for coverage or monitoring as well as reducing the need for tunnelling the pedicle. There are several descriptions of this arrangement in the head and neck literature, with the forearm flap being the commonest choice for a vascular bridge (see Di Taranto et al. in 'Further reading').

The pedicle from a previous reconstruction may also be isolated and used to perfuse a new flap (see Hanasono et al. in 'Further reading'). There is some overlap in the use of the term 'sequential flap' to describe vascular bridge flaps that are part of the same reconstruction and flaps that were connected to a pre-existing flap from a historical treatment episode. Thus, it was not possible to discern reported flap losses accurately in this group but it is likely very low.

The radial forearm flap and the anterolateral thigh flap (ALT) are most commonly reported for this purpose, perhaps not surprisingly, due to the length and reliability of the pedicle.

It is important to exclude heterotopic calcification of a previous flap pedicle on preoperative radiography. The incidence of calcified pedicle is reportedly as high as 28% depending on flap type and location (particularly in the fibula flap reconstructions of the midface) (see Knitschke et al. in 'Further reading').

For a pre-existing flap to be suitable to use as a flow-through flap, the soft/hard tissue components ought to have achieved independence from the vascular pedicle and integrated their blood supply within the vascular bed (angiogenesis, neovascularization, and collateral blood vessel supply). This is referred to as flap 'autonomation'. Several clinical and laboratory studies indicate that this is achieved in the majority of cases within weeks. There are rare instances of partial flap take years following surgical inset.

Yoon et al. (see 'Further reading') reviewed the literature concerning flap survival following pedicle compromise as an indicator of flap autonomy. They conclude that skin flaps attain vascular autonomy after a median of 10.1 days and intestinal (jejunal flaps) require substantially longer, 20.8 days to survive pedicle disruption. Experimentally, this is confirmed in several studies on animal models, which indicate that neo-vascularization within 7–10 days is enough to sustain cutaneous and myocutaneous flaps independent of the pedicle (see Gundeslioglou et al. in 'Further reading'). Other studies advise that the duration required for complete autonomy is substantially longer, in the range of 21 to 35 days (see Bradshaw et al. in 'Further reading'). It is not known whether this timeline applies when flaps are inset into an irradiated bed. Wolff et al. (2020) argued that the hypoxic gradient driving neo-vascularization is likely reversed in this situation, leading to potentially capillary ingrowth in the reverse direction, i.e. from the flap into the irradiated bed. Therefore, a pre-existing flap of recent inset is probably not recommended as a recipient.

Novel techniques

Extracorporeal perfusion

Wolff et al. in 2020 (see 'Further reading') described two extracorporeal perfusion approaches:

1. Continuous rhythmic blood infusion and
2. Connection of the flap pedicle to an extracorporeal membrane oxygenation (ECMO) circuit.

They described the use of ECMO in five patients with no suitable arterial recipients. Oxygenated blood is infused at a controlled slow rate to enable 'ischaemic conditioning' to establish a hypoxic gradient to stimulate capillary ingrowth. Venous outflow was discarded. Oral and through-and-through defects were excluded from the study and the technique restricted to thin flaps (FRFF and thinned ALT). They could not achieve full flap survival due to epithelial loss, but the resulting vascularized bed was dressed or grafted, achieving full healing in all patients.

Vessel bioengineering

Vessel bioengineering (see Fang et al. in 'Further reading') is currently and hot research topic and in the future it may prove to be a valuable asset to the microvascular surgeon alongside tissue engineering techniques.

Further reading

Anderson SR, Scott BA, Harrison LM, Wimalawansa SM, Kadakia SP. Common carotid-to-internal jugular arteriovenous loop for single-stage microsurgical reconstruction in the radiated vessel-depleted neck. *J Craniofac Surg* 2021;32(2):711–15.

Baron S, Salvan D, Cloutier L, Gharzouli I, Le Clerc N. Fibula free flap in the treatment of mandibular osteoradionecrosis. *Eur Ann Otorhinolaryngol Head Neck Dis* 2016;133(1):7–11.

Bradshaw K, Wagels M. Perfusion of muscle flaps independent of the anatomical vascular pedicle: pedicle autonomy. *J Plast Reconstr Aesthet Surg* 2017;70(11):1547–55.

Breik O, Praveen P, Parmar S. The vessel-depleted neck in head and neck microvascular reconstruction: extreme solutions for extreme situations. *Curr Opin Otolaryngol Head Neck Surg* 2020;28(2):129–35.

Bullocks J, Naik B, Lee E, Hollier L Jr. Flow-through flaps: a review of current knowledge and a novel classification system. *Microsurgery* 2006;26(6):439–49.

Chang KP, Lee HC, Lai CS, Lin SD. Use of single saphenous interposition vein graft for primary arterial circuit and secondary recipient site in head and neck reconstruction: a case report. *Head Neck* 2007;29(4):412–15.

Chen HC, Tang YB, Noordhoff MS. Reconstruction of the entire esophagus with 'chain flaps' in a patient with severe corrosive injury. *Plast Reconstr Surg* 1989;84(6):980–4.

Choi N, *et al.* Prediction of risk factors for pharyngo-cutaneous fistula after total laryngectomy using artificial intelligence. *Oral Oncol* 2021;119:105357.

Ciudad P, *et al.* The retrograde transverse cervical artery as a recipient vessel for free tissue transfer in complex head and neck reconstruction with a vessel-depleted neck. *Microsurgery* 2017;37(8):902–9.

Crowder SL, Douglas KG, Yanina Pepino M, Sarma KP, Arthur AE. Nutrition impact symptoms and associated outcomes in post-chemoradiotherapy head and neck cancer survivors: a systematic review. *J Cancer Surviv* 2018;12(4):479–94.

Di Taranto G, *et al.* Outcomes following head neck free flap reconstruction requiring interposition vein graft or vascular bridge flap. *Head Neck* 2019;41(9):2914–20.

Du E, Patel S, Huang B, Patel SN. Dual-phase CT angiography for presurgical planning in patients with vessel-depleted neck. *Head Neck* 2019;41(9):2929–36.

Fang S, Ellman DG, Andersen DC. Review: tissue engineering of small-diameter vascular grafts and their in vivo evaluation in large animals and humans. *Cells* 2021;10(3):713.

Frankart AJ, Frankart MJ, Cervenka B, Tang AL, Krishnan DG, Takiar V. Osteoradionecrosis: exposing the evidence not the bone. *Int J Radiat Oncol Biol Phys* 2021;109(5):1206–18.

Frohwitter G, Rau A, Kesting MR, Fichter A. Microvascular reconstruction in the vessel depleted neck—a systematic review. *J Craniomaxillofac Surg* 2018;46(9):1652–8.

Guelinckx PJ, Boeckx WD, Fossion E, Gruwez JA. Scanning electron microscopy of irradiated recipient blood vessels in head and neck free flaps. *Plast Reconstr Surg* 1984;74(2):217–26.

Gundeslioglu AO, Selimoglu N, Toy H, Koç O. Neo-vascularisation of musculocutaneous and muscle flaps after division of the major vascular supply: an experimental study. J *Plast Reconstr Aesthet Surg* 2013;66:978–86.

Hanasono MM, Barnea Y, Skoracki RJ. Microvascular surgery in the previously operated and irradiated neck. *Microsurgery* 2009;29(1):1–7.

Hasan Z, Dwivedi RC, Gunaratne DA, Virk SA, Palme CE, Riffat F. Systematic review and meta-analysis of the complications of salvage total laryngectomy. *Eur J Surg Oncol* 2017;43(1):42–51.

Hyodo I, Nakamura R, Okumura S, Kamei Y, Yasuda H, Suzuki H. Feasibility and safety of microvascular anastomoses within previously-dissected neck regions. *J UOEH* 2022;44(4):331–9.

Jacobson AS, Eloy JA, Park E, Roman B, Genden EM. Vessel-depleted neck: techniques for achieving microvascular reconstruction. *Head Neck* 2008;30(2):201–7.

Kelling JA, Meade A, Adkins M, Zhang AY. Risk of pneumothorax with internal mammary vessel utilization in autologous breast reconstruction. *Ann Plast Surg* 2021;86(3S Suppl 2):S184–8.

Knitschke M, Siu K, Bäcker C, Attia S, Howaldt HP, Böttger S. Heterotopic ossification of the vascular pedicle after maxillofacial reconstructive surgery using fibular free flap: introducing new classification and retrospective analysis. *J Clin Med* 2020;10(1):109.

Kushida-Contreras BH, Manrique OJ, Gaxiola-García MA. Head and neck reconstruction of the vessel-depleted neck: a systematic review of the literature. *Ann Surg Oncol* 2021;28(5):2882–95.

Mattine S, Payne KFB. The evolving role of the superficial temporal vessels as anastomotic recipients in challenging microvascular reconstruction of the upper two-thirds of the face. *J Plast Reconstr Aesthet Surg* 2022;75(9):3330–9.

Maricevich M, Lin LO, Liu J, Chang EI, Hanasono MM. Interposition vein grafting in head and neck free flap reconstruction. *Plast Reconstr Surg* 2018;142(4):1025–34.

Mijiti A, Kuerbantayi N, Zhang ZQ, Su MY, Zhang XH, Huojia M. Influence of preoperative radiotherapy on head and neck free-flap reconstruction: systematic review and meta-analysis. *Head Neck* 2020;42(8):2165–80.

Mücke T, Wolff KD, Rau A, Kehl V, Mitchell DA, Steiner T. Autonomization of free flaps in the oral cavity: a prospective clinical study. *Microsurgery* 2012;32(3):201–6.

Moran SL, Nava G, Behnam AB, Serletti JM. An outcome analysis comparing the thoracodorsal and internal mammary vessels as recipient sites for microvascular breast reconstruction: a prospective study of 100 patients. *Plast Reconstr Surg* 2003;111(6):1876–82.

Moubayed SP, Giot JP, Odobescu A, Guertin L, Harris PG, Danino MA. Arteriovenous fistulas for microvascular head and neck reconstruction. *Plast Surg (Oakv)* 2015;23(3):167–70.

Mulholland S, *et al.* Recipient vessels in head and neck microsurgery: radiation effect and vessel access. *Plast Reconstr Surg* 1993;92(4):628–32.

Piazza C, *et al.* Fascio-cutaneous-free flaps as primary reconstruction in salvage total laryngectomy. *Eur Arch Otorhinolaryngol* 2021;278(1):219–26.

Prince ADP, Broderick MT, Neal MEH, Spector ME. Head and neck reconstruction in the vessel depleted neck. *Front Oral Maxillofac Med* 2020;2:13.

Roche NA, Houtmeyers P, Vermeersch HF, Stillaert FB, Blondeel PN. The role of the internal mammary vessels as recipient vessels in secondary and tertiary head and neck reconstruction. *J Plast Reconstr Aesthet Surg* 2012;65(7):885–92.

Rosko AJ, Ryan JT, Wizauer EJ, Ibrahim M, Srinivasan A, Stucken CL, Spector ME. Dorsal scapular artery as a recipient vessel in the vessel-depleted neck during free tissue transfer in head and neck reconstruction. *Head Neck* 2017;39(7):E72–6.

Scaglioni MF, Meroni M, Fritsche E, Rajan G. Internal mammary artery perforators as recipient vessels for free tissue transfer in head and neck reconstruction: a case report and literature review. *Microsurgery* 2021;41(4):355–60.

Servagi-Vernat S, Ali D, Roubieu C, Durdux C, Laccourreye O, Giraud P. Dysphagia after radiotherapy: state of the art and prevention. *Eur Ann Otorhinolaryngol Head Neck Dis* 2015;132(1):25–9.

Shahoud JS, Kerndt CC, Burns B. Anatomy, thorax, internal mammary (internal thoracic) arteries. [Updated 26 July 2021]. In: StatPearls [Internet]. Treasure Island (FL): StatPearls Publishing; 2021 Jan. PMID: 30726022.

Soutar DS, Scheker LR, Tanner NS, McGregor IA. The radial forearm flap: a versatile method for intraoral reconstruction. *Br J Plast Surg* 1983;36(1):1–8.

Tam S, Weber RS, Liu J, Ting J, Hanson S, Lewis CM. Evaluating unplanned returns to the operating room in head and neck free flap patients. *Ann Surg Oncol* 2020;27(2):440–8.

Tessler O, *et al.* Transverse cervical artery: consistent anatomical landmarks and clinical experience with its use as a recipient artery in complex head and neck reconstruction. *Plast Reconstr Surg* 2017;139(3):745e–51e.

Urken ML, Higgins KM, Lee B, Vickery C. Internal mammary artery and vein: recipient vessels for free tissue transfer to the head and neck in the vessel-depleted neck. *Head Neck* 2006;28(9):797–801.

Wang KY, Lin YS, Chen LW, Yang KC, Huang WC, Liu WC. Risk of free flap failure in head and neck reconstruction: analysis of 21,548 cases from a nationwide database. *Ann Plast Surg* 2020;84(1S Suppl 1):S3–S6.

Wolff KD, *et al.* Free flap transplantation using an extracorporeal perfusion device: first three cases. *J Craniomaxillofac Surg* 2016;44(2):148–54.

Wolff KD, Ritschl LM, von Bomhard A, Braun C, Wolff C, Fichter AM. In vivo perfusion of free skin flaps using extracorporeal membrane oxygenation. *J Craniomaxillofac Surg* 2020;48(1):90–7.

Yoon AP, Jones NF. Critical time for neovascularization/angiogenesis to allow free flap survival after delayed postoperative anastomotic compromise without surgical intervention: a review of the literature. *Microsurgery* 2016;36(7):604–12.

Yu P. The transverse cervical vessels as recipient vessels for previously treated head and neck cancer patients. *Plast Reconstr Surg* 2005;115(5):1253–8.

List of videos

See these videos online by searching for this book's title or ISBN at https://academic.oup.com/

Chapter 3

Video 3.1.1 Virtual Laryngoscopy

Reproduced courtesy of Leandros Vassiliou, Manchester University NHS Foundation Trust, Manchester, UK

Chapter 8

Video 8.3.1 Back wall first anastomosis. Demonstration of arterial anastomosis via the back-wall-first fashion.

Reproduced courtesy of Leandros Vassiliou, Manchester University NHS Foundation Trust, Manchester, UK

Video 8.4.1 Vertical Anastomosis.

Reproduced courtesy of Leandros Vassiliou, Manchester University NHS Foundation Trust, Manchester, UK

Video 8.4.2 Management of calibre Mismatch.

Reproduced courtesy of Leandros Vassiliou, Manchester University NHS Foundation Trust, Manchester, UK

Video 8.4.3 Management of thickness Mismatch.

Reproduced courtesy of Leandros Vassiliou, Manchester University NHS Foundation Trust, Manchester, UK

Video 8.4.4 Management of global size Mismatch (calibre and thickness).

Reproduced courtesy of Leandros Vassiliou, Manchester University NHS Foundation Trust, Manchester, UK

Chapter 9

Video 9.2.1 Venous anastomosis. End-to-end with size mismatch and using hydrodistention technique

Reproduced courtesy of Leandros Vassiliou, Manchester University NHS Foundation Trust, Manchester, UK

Video 9.4.1 Sequence of venous anastomosis with a microscopic anastomotic devices (MACD).

Reproduced courtesy of Leandros Vassiliou, Manchester University NHS Foundation Trust, Manchester, UK

Video 9.4.2 Venous Coupler Closure.

Reproduced courtesy of Leandros Vassiliou, Manchester University NHS Foundation Trust, Manchester, UK

Video 9.4.3 Jammed microscopic anastomotic devices (MACD) complication.

Reproduced courtesy of Leandros Vassiliou, Manchester University NHS Foundation Trust, Manchester, UK

Chapter 10

Video 10.1.1 Vein Patency Test via the empty and refill manoeuvre.

Reproduced courtesy of Leandros Vassiliou, Manchester University NHS Foundation Trust, Manchester, UK

Video 10.1.2 Empty and Refill test for anastomosis patency. In this case an extended craniofacial resection for an adenoid cystic carcinoma of the lacrimal gland and reconstruction with a rectus abdominis flap anastomosed to the temporal vessels has been performed.

Reproduced courtesy of Professor Julio Acero, and Dr Fernando Almeida, Ramon y Cajal University Hospital, Madrid, Spain

Video 10.2.1 Suture hole leak treated with arrow.

Reproduced courtesy of Leandros Vassiliou, Manchester University NHS Foundation Trust, Manchester, UK

Video 10.2.2 Anastomotic leak due to suture gap requiring extra stitch.

Reproduced courtesy of Leandros Vassiliou, Manchester University NHS Foundation Trust, Manchester, UK

Video 10.2.3 Anastomotic leak due to suture gap requiring extra stitch in a vertical anastomosis fashion.

Reproduced courtesy of Leandros Vassiliou, Manchester University NHS Foundation Trust, Manchester, UK

Video 10.2.4 Anastomotic leak minimal misapposition treated with arrow pressure.

Reproduced courtesy of Leandros Vassiliou, Manchester University NHS Foundation Trust, Manchester, UK

Video 10.3.1 Sternocleidomastoid (SCM) gutter for Vein.

Reproduced courtesy of Leandros Vassiliou, Manchester University NHS Foundation Trust, Manchester, UK

Index

For the benefit of digital users, indexed terms that span two pages (e.g., 52–53) may, on occasion, appear on only one of those pages.

Note: Tables, figures, and boxes are indicated by an italic *t*, *f*, and *b* following the page number.